THE
TEACHING
FILES Pediatric

THE TEACHING FILES Pediatric

Sarah Sarvis Milla, MD
Assistant Professor
Department of Radiology
New York University Medical Center
New York, New York

Sarah D. Bixby, MD
Instructor
Department of Radiology
Harvard Medical School
Staff Pediatric Radiologist
Department of Radiology
Children's Hospital of Boston
Boston, Massachusetts

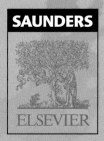

SAUNDERS

ELSEVIER

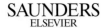

1600 John F. Kennedy Blvd.
Ste 1800
Philadelphia, PA 19103-2899

THE TEACHING FILES: PEDIATRIC

ISBN: 978-1-4160-6206-6

Library of Congress Cataloging-in-Publication Data

Milla, Sarah Sarvis.
  The teaching files. Pediatrics / Sarah Sarvis Milla, Sarah D. Bixby. -- 1st ed.
    p. ; cm.
  Other title: Pediatrics
  Includes bibliographical references and index.
  ISBN 978-1-4160-6206-6
1. Pediatrics -- Case studies. I. Bixby, Sarah D. II. Title. III. Title: Pediatrics.
  [DNLM: 1. Pediatrics--methods--Case Reports. 2. Diagnosis, Differential--Case Reports. 3. Diagnostic Imaging--methods--Case Reports. WS 141 M6435t 2010]
  RJ58.M55 2010
  618.92--dc22   2010012492

Acquisitions Editor: Rebecca Gaertner
Developmental Editor: Lora Sickora
Publishing Services Manager: Tina Rebane
Design Direction: Steve Stave

Printed in China

Last digit is the print number: 9 8 7 6 5 4 3 2 1

To my family—
My mother, Alice, an incredible woman, who gave me all the tools to succeed and showed me how to use them
  My stepfather, Cheum, for all of his support and love
James, the ultimate of big brothers and the smartest person I know, who has always guided and supported me; and
  to his wife Stacy, who is his match in mind and spirit
Robert, my "little" brother, who is charming and brilliant, and to his wife, Astrid, a budding pediatrician
  (who I hope will be able to use this book)
My stepbrothers, Richard and Steve, for their humor and love, and to their wives Dana and Melissa for their love and
  guidance in parenting
My aunt Emily, for her love and emergency babysitting
To Mimi and Joyce, who have been the sisters I never had
And my friend Allison, whose daily support has made this book possible

To my amazing friend and colleague Sarah Bixby, words will never describe how much your friendship and your
  work on this book have meant. Thanks to Children's Hospital Boston for bringing us together!

To my husband, Federico, for our past and our future. Your dedication to cardiac surgery continually inspires and
  impresses me. May we share our lives, love, careers and friendship forever.

And to the best gift I've ever received, my son Jameson. Your smile is all I need. You make me a better person and a
  better doctor. I look forward to watching you grow, learn, and experience all the joys of life.

                                                                                        Sarah Sarvis Milla

To Ava, Jack, and Kevin for being such a wonderful family, and for making each day a day to look forward to

To Sarah Milla. You continue to amaze and inspire me with your unwavering positivity and optimism. There is
  nobody else I would rather work with on this project. Thank you for keeping us focused on the goal!

                                                                                        Sarah Bixby

Preface

This book was a labor of love... and two deliveries of love. We were honored to be given the opportunity to create this collection of pediatric radiology cases for Elsevier, for which we thank Dr. Tom Slovis and Dr. Rafael Rivera. During the writing of this book we were both blessed with additions to our families, with each of us delivering a healthy and happy baby boy. Special thanks to our Elsevier editors, Colleen McGonigal and Rebecca Gaertner, for their patience and editorial guidance during these momentous life transitions. Special thanks also to our institutions, Children's Hospital of Boston and New York University Langone Medical Center.

We hope this collection of cases is useful for all in radiology and pediatric care. These cases will be a review for some and perhaps an introduction for others. As this book is not an exhaustive review or illustration, we encourage all to further investigate the entities described, as they each deserve much more attention.

Radiology is an incredible field, and it is truly fascinating to visualize the internal portions of the human body. This book presents images of both common and rare pediatric conditions. Pediatric radiology is a unique and rewarding specialty that encompasses all body parts and utilizes all the different imaging modalities including plain radiography, fluoroscopy, ultrasound (US), computed tomography (CT), and MRI. Pediatric radiologists have the additional benefit of maintaining close relationships with our pediatric colleagues and referring clinicians, as well as having hands-on interaction with our patients and their families. We hope this book may interest others in joining our small and valuable subspecialty.

Lastly, let this book serve as a reminder to us that we are surrounded by amazing children and loving parents in our communities. These cases represent our children, the children of our friends, and the children of our friends' friends. Let us treasure the health of our family and loved ones, and actively embrace each day we have with them.

Sarah Sarvis Milla
Sarah D. Bixby

Contents

THE TEACHING FILES Pediatric

Case 1

DEMOGRAPHICS/CLINICAL HISTORY

The patient is a young child with stridor.

FINDINGS

A lateral radiograph (Fig. 1) shows distention of the hypopharynx. Frontal radiograph of the neck (Fig. 2) shows the typical "steeple" appearance of the radiolucent airway.

DISCUSSION

Definition/Background

Croup is typically caused by a viral infection and typically represents inflamation of the larynx and upper trachea, characterized by a loud "barking" cough.

Characteristic Clinical Features

Patients present with a loud "barking" cough, inspiratory stridor, and respiratory distress.

Characteristic Radiologic Findings

On the frontal radiograph, the subglottic airway has a "steeple" appearance, with loss of the normal shouldering of the subglottic airway. As a result of the subglottic narrowing, the hypopharynx is often distended and air-filled.

Differential Diagnosis

■ Subglottic hemangioma

Discussion

Subglottic hemangioma tends to have a mass effect, causing narrowing. Steepling is not typically seen.

Diagnosis

Croup

Suggested Reading

Salour M: The steeple sign. Radiology 216:428-429, 2000.

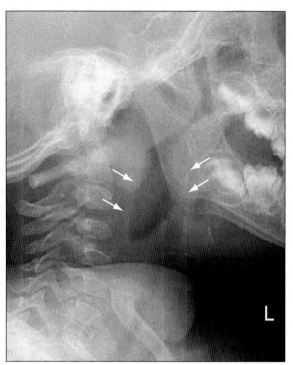

Figure 1. Lateral radiograph shows distention of the hypopharynx (*arrows*).

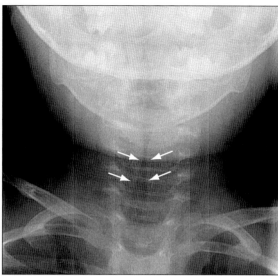

Figure 2. Frontal radiograph of neck shows typical "steeple" appearance of the radiolucent airway (*arrows*).

Case 2

DEMOGRAPHICS/CLINICAL HISTORY

The patient is a 6-month-old girl with rhinorrhea, nasal congestion, fever, and an elevated white blood cell count.

FINDINGS

Lateral view of the neck and chest (Fig. 1) shows widening of the prevertebral soft tissues and anterior displacement of the trachea. Axial contrast-enhanced computed tomography (CT) (Fig. 2) shows a rim-enhancing fluid collection in the right retropharyngeal soft tissues with surrounding inflammatory changes and a mass effect on the trachea. The right carotid artery and jugular vein are narrowed. Parasagittal reconstruction of a contrast-enhanced CT image (Fig. 3) shows the mild rim enhancement and inflammatory changes around the fluid collection. Midline sagittal reconstruction CT image (Fig. 4) shows the inflammation in the midline retropharyngeal soft tissues. Surgical drainage showed pus within the right retropharyngeal collection.

DISCUSSION

Definition/Background

Retropharyngeal abscesses typically begin as lymphadenitis, with progression to suppuration and abscess formation. The process is most common in children younger than 5 years.

Characteristic Clinical Features

Patients present with some combination of fever, an elevated white blood cell count, neck pain, and torticollis.

Characteristic Radiologic Findings

On lateral neck radiographs, increased widening of the prevertebral soft tissues can suggest a retropharyngeal abscess. Care should be taken to exclude prominence because of patient positioning. On contrast-enhanced CT, a rim-enhancing fluid collection typically represents abscess formation. Lack of rim enhancement or poor definition of a low-density area may suggest phlegmonous changes without formal abscess formation. Inflammatory changes and infected collections can extend from the retropharyngeal and danger spaces (i.e., region of the neck adjacent to the alar fascia). Patency of the carotid arteries and jugular veins should be assessed.

Less Common Radiologic Manifestations

Grisel syndrome is a rare condition of an atlantoaxial rotatory subluxation associated with a pharyngeal infection.

Differential Diagnosis

- Lymphadenitis
- Infected branchial cleft cyst (pediatric)

Discussion

Rim enhancement suggests abscess formation more than lymphadenitis. An infected branchial cleft cyst can have an appearance similar to that of suppurative lymphadenitis or a retropharyngeal abscess. The diagnosis often can be made after immediate treatment and follow-up imaging.

Diagnosis

Retropharyngeal abscess

Suggested Readings

Craig FW, Schunk JE: Retropharyngeal abscess in children: Clinical presentation, utility of imaging, and current management. Pediatrics 111(Pt 1):1394-1398, 2003.

Page NC, Bauer EM, Lieu JE: Clinical features and treatment of retropharyngeal abscess in children. Otolaryngol Head Neck Surg 138:300-306, 2008.

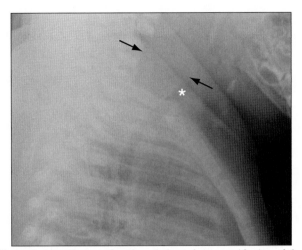

Figure 1. Lateral view of neck and chest shows a widening of the prevertebral soft tissues (*between arrows*) and anterior displacement of the trachea (*asterisk*).

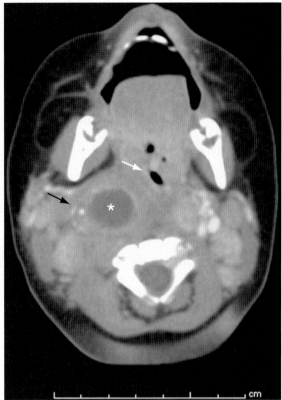

Figure 2. Axial contrast-enhanced CT image shows a rim-enhancing fluid collection (*asterisk*) in the right retropharyngeal soft tissues with surrounding inflammatory changes and mass effect on the trachea (*white arrow*). The right carotid artery and jugular vein are narrowed (*black arrow*).

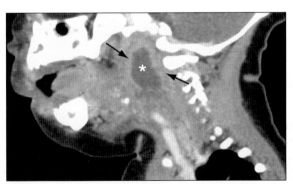

Figure 3. Parasagittal reconstruction of contrast-enhanced CT image shows mild rim enhancement and inflammatory changes (*arrows*) around the fluid collection (*asterisk*).

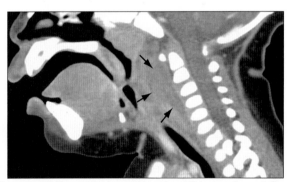

Figure 4. Midline sagittal reconstruction CT image shows inflammation in the midline retropharyngeal soft tissues (*arrows*).

Case 3

DEMOGRAPHICS/CLINICAL HISTORY

The patient is a 6-week-old girl with left-sided torticollis.

FINDINGS

Ultrasound evaluation of the neck (Figs. 1 and 2) reveals fusiform enlargement of the left sternocleidomastoid (SCM) muscle with abnormal heterogeneous echogenicity. The abnormal appearance of left SCM muscle is best appreciated when comparing it with the normal right side (Fig. 3).

DISCUSSION

Definition/Background
Fibromatosis colli often occurs in children with a history of birth trauma or difficult extraction, although this history is not present in all cases.

Characteristic Clinical Features
Infants present with torticollis, as in this case. The right side is more commonly affected, although the abnormality was on the left in the infant in this case.

Characteristic Radiologic Findings
Ultrasound is the preferred modality to evaluate an infant with a suspected neck mass. On ultrasound, the affected side exhibits an enlarged, heterogeneous SCM muscle, with no other discrete cystic or solid neck masses.

Differential Diagnosis
- Cervical lymphadenopathy
- Rhabdomyosarcoma
- Lymphoma
- Lymphatic malformation

Discussion
Cervical lymphadenopathy refers to enlarged lymph nodes in the neck, which is often secondary to viral etiologies, but also may occur in bacterial infections and neoplastic conditions, such as lymphoma. Rhabdomyosarcoma is the most common soft tissue tumor of childhood.

Diagnosis
Fibromatosis colli

Suggested Readings
Ablin DS, Jain K, Howell L, et al: Ultrasound and MR imaging of fibromatosis colli (sternomastoid tumor of infancy). Pediatr Radiol 28:230-233, 1998.

Bedi DG, John SD, Swischuk LE: Fibromatosis colli of infancy: Variability of sonographic appearance. J Clin Ultrasound 26:345-348, 1998.

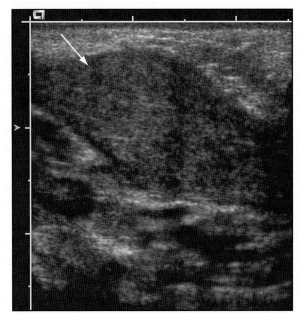

Figure 1. Longitudinal ultrasound image of the left side of the neck shows fusiform, echogenic enlargement of SCM muscle (*arrow*).

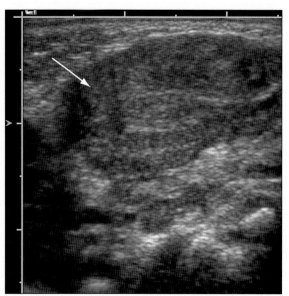

Figure 2. Transverse ultrasound image of the left side of the neck shows that SCM muscle is abnormally thickened and heterogeneous (*arrow*).

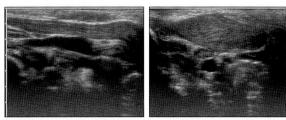

Figure 3. Dual-screen ultrasound image comparing right and left SCM muscles. Left SCM muscle appears abnormally thickened compared with normal right SCM muscle.

Case 4

DEMOGRAPHICS/CLINICAL HISTORY

The patient is a 6-week-old girl with a history of a non-mobile right neck mass.

FINDINGS

Focal masslike enlargement of the right sternocleido-mastoid (SCM) muscle is seen on longitudinal (Fig. 1) and transverse (Fig. 2) ultrasound images. The mass-like enlargement of right SCM muscle is seen best when compared with the contralateral side (Fig. 3).

DISCUSSION

Definition/Background

Fibromatosis colli is a muscular torticollis caused by shortening of SCM muscle. The condition typically manifests in infants 1 to 15 weeks old, and most patients recover completely with physical therapy.

Characteristic Clinical Features

Patients usually present with a palpable mass in the anterior neck or torticollis, with angling of the chin toward the contralateral side of the muscular abnormality.

Characteristic Radiologic Findings

Imaging shows focal hypoechoic masslike enlargement within the body of SCM muscle. Mild internal vascularity can be seen within the mass.

Less Common Radiologic Manifestations

Diffuse enlargement of SCM muscle also may be seen.

Differential Diagnosis

- Fibrosarcoma
- Rhabdomyosarcoma
- Neuroblastoma
- Infantile myofibromatosis

Discussion

Fibromatosis colli occurs within SCM muscle during the first few months of life. If imaging or clinical presentation is atypical, further investigation is recommended to exclude a sarcoma. If additional lesions are present in other muscles, infantile myofibromatosis and metastatic neuroblastoma should be considered.

Diagnosis

Fibromatosis colli

Suggested Reading

Robbin MR, Murphey MD, Temple HT, et al: Imaging of musculoskeletal fibromatosis. RadioGraphics 21:585, 2001.

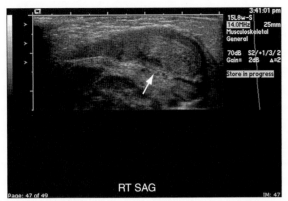

Figure 1. Longitudinal ultrasound image of right SCM muscle shows masslike focal enlargement (*arrow*).

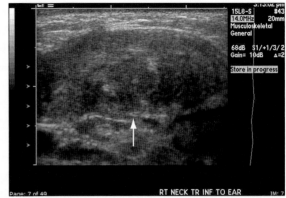

Figure 2. Transverse ultrasound image through focal enlargement within the muscle belly (*arrow*).

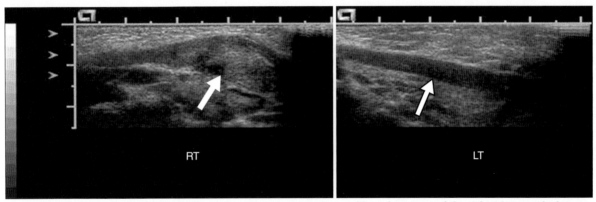

Figure 3. Longitudinal ultrasound of both SCM muscles shows asymmetric masslike enlargement of the right SCM muscle (*arrow on left image*) compared with the normal contralateral side (*arrow on right image*).

Case 5

DEMOGRAPHICS/CLINICAL HISTORY

The patient is a 9-year-old girl with enlarged thyroid and elevated thyroid-stimulating hormone.

FINDINGS

Ultrasound examination of the thyroid gland shows diffuse enlargement of the entire gland, including both lobes and the isthmus. The thyroid gland appears heterogeneously hypoechoic in Fig. 1. A longitudinal ultrasound image of the right lobe of the thyroid (Fig. 2) shows diffuse enlargement without discrete nodule. Color Doppler evaluation of the right lobe of the thyroid (Fig. 3) shows diffuse hyperemia.

DISCUSSION

Definition/Background
Hashimoto thyroiditis is the most common cause of hypothyroidism in children. It is more common in girls than in boys.

Characteristic Clinical Features
Patients may present with painless enlargement of the thyroid gland or may develop symptoms of hypothyroidism insidiously.

Characteristic Radiologic Findings
Ultrasound evaluation shows a diffusely enlarged thyroid gland that is hypoechoic and fibrotic, giving an appearance of pseudonodules without focal nodularity.

Differential Diagnosis
- Nontoxic multinodular goiter
- Thyroid lymphoma
- Graves disease

Discussion
Nontoxic multinodular goiter manifests as painless enlargement of the thyroid gland unassociated with thyroid hormone abnormality. Thyroid lymphoma most often manifests as a rapidly enlarging thyroid mass associated with neck adenopathy. Graves disease manifests with diffuse thyroid enlargement. Patients with Graves disease present with symptoms of (and laboratory tests consistent with) hyperthyroidism.

Diagnosis
Hashimoto thyroiditis

Suggested Readings
Lorini R, Gastaldi R, Traggiai C, et al: Hashimoto's thyroiditis. Pediatr Endocrinol Rev 1(Suppl 2):205-211, 2003.
Takami HE, Miyabe R, Kameyama K: Hashimoto's thyroiditis. World J Surg 32:688-692, 2008.

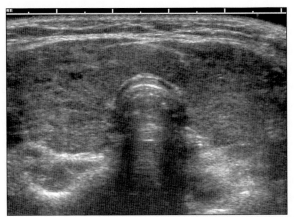

Figure 1. Ultrasound examination of the thyroid gland shows diffuse enlargement of the entire gland, including both lobes and the isthmus. The thyroid gland appears heterogeneously hypoechoic.

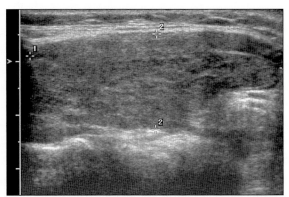

Figure 2. Longitudinal ultrasound image of the right lobe of the thyroid shows diffuse enlargement without discrete nodule.

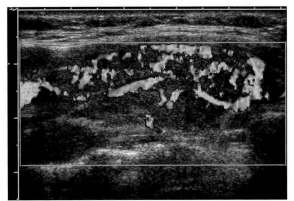

Figure 3. Color Doppler evaluation of right lobe of the thyroid shows diffuse hyperemia.

Case 6

DEMOGRAPHICS/CLINICAL HISTORY

The patient is a 12-year-old girl with enlarged thyroid and critically low thyroid-stimulating hormone.

FINDINGS

Ultrasound examination of the thyroid gland shows diffuse thyroid enlargement. The thyroid gland appears hypoechoic and coarsened in echotexture (Fig. 1). A longitudinal ultrasound image of the right lobe of the thyroid (Fig. 2) shows diffuse enlargement without a discrete nodule with pseudolobulation of the gland caused by fibrotic septations.

DISCUSSION

Definition/Background
Hashimoto thyroiditis is an autoimmune thyroiditis and is the most common cause of primary thyroiditis in North America.

Characteristic Clinical Features
Patients may present with painless enlargement of the thyroid gland or may develop symptoms of hypothyroidism insidiously. There may be an initial thyrotoxicosis, which then evolves into hypothyroidism.

Characteristic Radiologic Findings
Ultrasound evaluation shows a diffusely enlarged thyroid gland that is hypoechoic and fibrotic, giving an appearance of pseudonodules without focal nodularity.

Differential Diagnosis
- Nontoxic multinodular goiter
- Thyroid lymphoma
- Graves disease

Discussion
Nontoxic multinodular goiter manifests as painless enlargement of the thyroid gland that is not associated with thyroid hormone abnormality. Thyroid lymphoma most often manifests as a rapidly enlarging thyroid mass associated with neck adenopathy. Graves disease manifests with diffuse thyroid enlargement. Patients with Graves disease present with symptoms of (and laboratory tests consistent with) hyperthyroidism.

Diagnosis
Hashimoto thyroiditis

Suggested Readings
Lorini R, Gastaldi R, Traggiai C, et al: Hashimoto's thyroiditis. Pediatr Endocrinol Rev Suppl 2:205-211, 2003.

Takami HE, Miyabe R, Kameyama K: Hashimoto's thyroiditis. World J Surg 32:688-692, 2008.

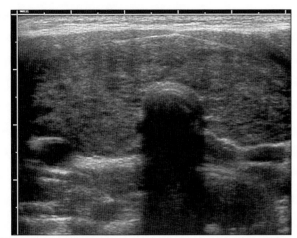

Figure 1. Transverse ultrasound image of the thyroid gland shows diffuse enlargement of the entire gland, including of both lobes and the isthmus. The thyroid gland appears heterogeneously hypoechoic.

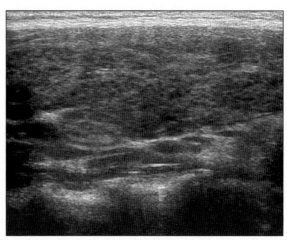

Figure 2. Longitudinal ultrasound image of right lobe of the thyroid shows diffuse enlargement with a pseudolobulated appearance to the parenchyma.

Case 7

DEMOGRAPHICS/CLINICAL HISTORY

The patient is a 16-year-old boy with acute suppurative thyroiditis.

FINDINGS

Axial contrast-enhanced computed tomography (CT) (Fig. 1) shows a complex, rim-enhancing fluid collection adjacent to a low-attenuation area within the right lobe of the thyroid gland. Barium swallow (Fig. 2) shows pooling deep to the right piriform sinus. A delayed image from the barium swallow (Fig. 3) shows barium within a sinus tract along the right side of the neck.

DISCUSSION

Definition/Background

Piriform sinus fistulas are sequelae from persistent ducts of sinuses of the third and fourth pharyngeal pouches.

Characteristic Clinical Features

Patients may present with recurrent neck swellings or infections, particularly suppurative thyroiditis.

Characteristic Radiologic Findings

Because piriform sinus fistulas are typically left-sided, imaging of acute presentations often shows an infected collection along the tract between the left piriform sinus and the left lobe of the thyroid gland. After acute infections have been treated, barium studies may show the fistulous tract. Barium studies during the acutely infected phase have a lower sensitivity, possibly because of temporary inflammatory obstruction of the tract. CT and magnetic resonance imaging (MRI) have been used to look for air and fluid within the sinus tracts. Ultrasound can be used dynamically while the patient performs a trumpet maneuver (i.e., distended cheeks while blowing) to look for the passage of air bubbles into the neck collection.

Less Common Radiologic Manifestations

Right-sided piriform sinus fistulas are less common.

Differential Diagnosis

■ Perforation from trauma

Discussion

Fistulas caused by trauma or a foreign body can simulate piriform sinus fistulas. A post-traumatic fistula is less likely to track to the thyroid gland, however, the way a piriform sinus fistula does.

Diagnosis

Piriform sinus fistula

Suggested Readings

Park SW, Han MH, Sung MH, et al: Neck infection associated with pyriform sinus fistula: Imaging findings. AJNR Am J Neuroradiol 21:817-822, 2000.

Wang HK, Tiu CM, Chou YH, Chang CY: Imaging studies of pyriform sinus fistula. Pediatr Radiol 33:328-333, 2003.

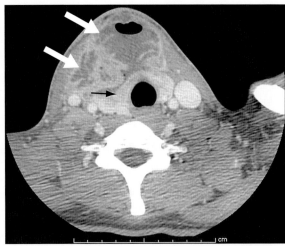

Figure 1. Axial contrast-enhanced CT scan shows complex, rim-enhancing fluid collection (*large arrows*) adjacent to a low attenuation area within the right lobe of the thyroid gland (*small arrow*).

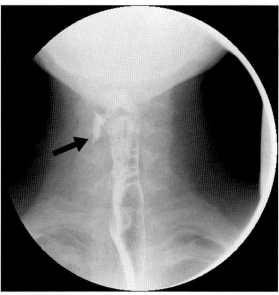

Figure 2. Barium swallow shows pooling deep to the right piriform sinus (*arrow*).

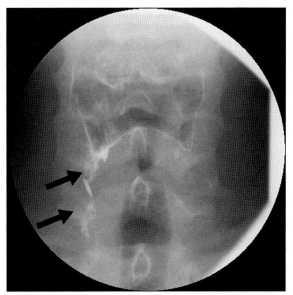

Figure 3. Delayed image from barium swallow shows barium within a sinus tract (*arrows*) along the right side of the neck.

Case 8

DEMOGRAPHICS/CLINICAL HISTORY

The patient is an 11-year-old child with a palpable left neck mass.

FINDINGS

Axial contrast-enhanced computed tomography (CT) (Fig. 1) shows a low-density mass anterior to the ster-nocleidomastoid muscle (SCM), anterior to the carotid artery and jugular vein, and extending to the lateral pharynx. Coronal reconstruction CT image (Fig. 2) shows the proximity of the cystic mass to the lateral pharynx and the SCM muscle. Axial contrast-enhanced CT scan of the temporal bone in a different patient (Fig. 3) shows a low-density mass in the external auditory canal.

DISCUSSION

Definition/Background
Branchial apparatus abnormalities include cysts, sinus tracts, and fistulas. Cysts are most common.

Characteristic Clinical Features
Branchial apparatus cysts can manifest as palpable masses, and they may be painful if they become super-infected.

Characteristic Radiologic Findings
Branchial apparatus cysts are anechoic or hypoechoic on ultrasound, hypodense on CT, and variable in signal intensity on magnetic resonance imaging (MRI), depending on the fluid and protein composition; rim enhancement and thickening of the cyst wall can be seen when cysts become superinfected. The typical locations of the cysts aid in the diagnosis. First branchial apparatus cysts are located near the external auditory canal or parotid gland. Second branchial apparatus cysts are the most common and are located anteromedial to the SCM muscle and anterior to the carotid sheath vessels. Third branchial apparatus cysts are least common and typically lie posterior to the carotid artery. Fourth branchial abnormalities usually manifest as a sinus tract.

Differential Diagnosis
- Lymphatic malformation (pediatric)
- Dermoid or epidermoid cysts
- Lymphadenitis

Discussion
Lymphatic malformations often have more than one cystic component, often contain fluid-fluid levels on MRI, and are often trans-spatial. Dermoid or epidermoid cysts are rarely in the typical locations in which branchial apparatus cysts occur and are much less common in the neck. Lymphadenitis can simulate an infected branchial apparatus cyst, and follow-up imaging can show resolution (i.e., lymphadenitis) or a residual underlying congenital cyst.

Diagnosis
Branchial apparatus cyst

Suggested Readings
Acierno SP, Waldhausen JH: Congenital cervical cysts, sinuses and fistulae. Otolaryngol Clin North Am 40:161-176, 2007.
Koch BL: Cystic malformations of the neck in children. Pediatr Radiol 35:463-477, 2005.

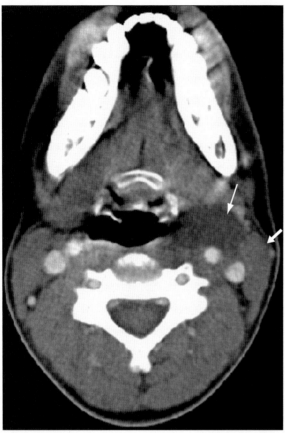

Figure 1. Axial contrast-enhanced CT scan shows low-density mass (*thin arrow*) anterior to SCM muscle (*thick arrow*), anterior to the carotid artery and jugular vein, and extending to the lateral pharynx, which was surgically confirmed to be a second branchial apparatus cyst.

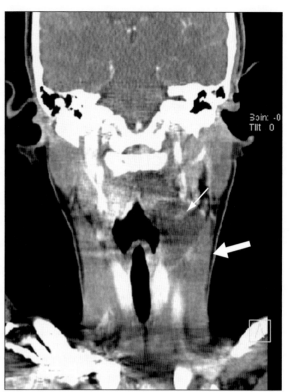

Figure 2. Coronal reconstruction shows the proximity of the cystic mass (*thin arrow*) to the lateral pharynx and the SCM muscle (*thick arrow*).

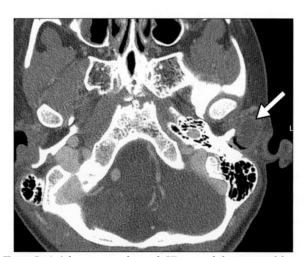

Figure 3. Axial contrast-enhanced CT scan of the temporal bone in a different patient with a first branchial apparatus cyst shows a low-density mass (*arrow*) in the external auditory canal.

Case 9

DEMOGRAPHICS/CLINICAL HISTORY

The patient is a newborn with hypothyroidism.

FINDINGS

Transverse ultrasound of the neck (Fig. 1) shows an absence of the normally positioned thyroid gland within the neck. Anterior projection of iodine 123 nuclear medicine scintigraphy (Fig. 2) shows radiotracer uptake below the nose marker, between the mouth and chin, and well above the level of the neck. In the lateral projection (Fig. 3), the radiotracer uptake is seen between the level of the mouth and chin, located posteriorly in the oropharynx in a location consistent with the base of the tongue. Transmission image (Fig. 4) shows the increased uptake with respect to the infant's outline.

DISCUSSION

Definition/Background
Ectopic thyroid tissue can occur anywhere from the foramen cecum (at the base of the tongue) to the normal pretracheal location of the thyroid, but the most common location is at the base of the tongue.

Characteristic Clinical Features
Clinical features include hypothyroidism; dysphagia; absence of normal thyroid tissue; or a midline, upper neck soft tissue mass.

Characteristic Radiologic Findings
Absence of the thyroid on an ultrasound image is typically the first radiographic suggestion of thyroid ectopia. Nuclear medicine imaging with iodine 123 radiotracer is used to locate any thyroid tissue able to take up iodine.

Less Common Radiologic Manifestations
Occasionally, patients have normal-appearing thyroid tissue in the standard pretracheal location and still have ectopic thyroid tissue.

Differential Diagnosis
- Thyroglossal duct cyst
- Lingual tonsil

Discussion
Thyroglossal duct cysts can occur in locations similar to those of ectopic thyroid tissue, but the imaging appearance has cystic characteristics instead of characteristics of solid tissue. Lingual tonsils can be prominent, particularly in obese children, but they should not take up iodine 123, and patients have a normally located thyroid gland.

Diagnosis
Ectopic thyroid

Suggested Readings
Benhammou A, Bencheikh R, Benbouzid MA, et al: Ectopic lingual thyroid. B-ENT 2:121-122, 2006.
Damiano A, Glickman AB, Rubin JS, Cohen AF: Ectopic thyroid tissue presenting as a midline neck mass. Int J Pediatr Otorhinolaryngol 34:141-148, 1996.

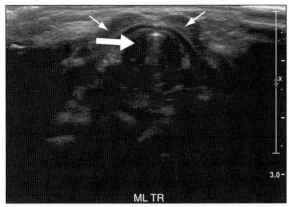

Figure 1. Transverse ultrasound of the neck shows absence of the normally positioned thyroid gland. The air-filled trachea is demonstrated (*large arrows*). within the neck (*small arrows*).

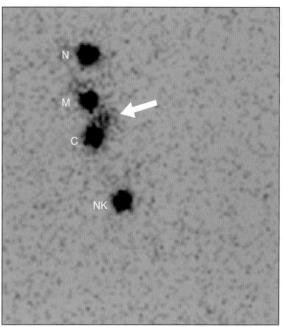

Figure 2. Anterior projection of the patient's iodine 123 nuclear medicine scintigraphy shows radiotracer uptake (*arrow*) below the nose marker (*N*), between the mouth (*M*) and chin (*C*), and well above the level of the neck (*NK*).

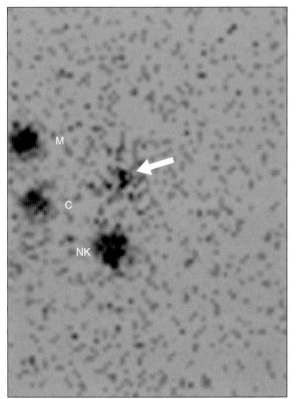

Figure 3. In the lateral projection, the radiotracer uptake (*arrow*) is seen above the level of the neck (*NK*), between the levels of the mouth (*M*) and chin (*C*), located posteriorly in the oropharynx in a location consistent with the base of the tongue.

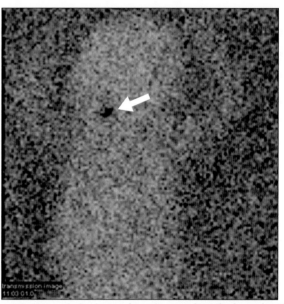

Figure 4. Transmission image shows increased uptake (*arrow*) with respect to the infant's outline.

Case 10

DEMOGRAPHICS/CLINICAL HISTORY

The patient is a 5-year-old child with painful swelling in the upper neck.

FINDINGS

Axial contrast-enhanced computed tomography (CT) (Fig. 1) shows a round, midline, hypodense mass with peripheral enhancement. Coronal CT reconstruction (Fig. 2) illustrates the relationship of the mass to the mandible and floor of the mouth. The proximity of the mass to the hyoid bone is seen on the sagittal CT reconstruction (Fig. 3).

DISCUSSION

Definition/Background

Thyroglossal duct cysts typically occur at or near midline, just inferior to the hyoid bone, but they can occur anywhere along the thyroglossal duct from the base of the tongue to the location of the thyroid gland.

Characteristic Clinical Features

A midline cystic mass in the upper neck is the typical clinical presentation. These masses are often palpated and may become clinically evident secondary to superinfection.

Characteristic Radiologic Findings

These masses can be evaluated by ultrasound, CT, or magnetic resonance imaging (MRI). On imaging, thyroglossal duct cysts are midline cystic neck masses, and they can have rim vascularity or enhancement if superinfected. Most are located at the level of or just inferior to the hyoid bone.

Less Common Radiologic Manifestations

Although typically unilocular, septations occasionally can be seen, particularly if superficial.

Differential Diagnosis

■ Dermoid

Discussion

Dermoids are midline or paramidline cystic masses, and they can be difficult to differentiate on imaging. If fat or marble-like nodules are present within the mass, dermoid cyst is the likely diagnosis.

Diagnosis

Thyroglossal duct cyst

Suggested Readings

Foley DS, Fallat ME: Thyroglossal duct and other congenital midline cervical anomalies. Semin Pediatr Surg 15:70-75, 2006.
Koch BL: Cystic malformations of the neck in children. Pediatr Radiol 35:463-477, 2005.

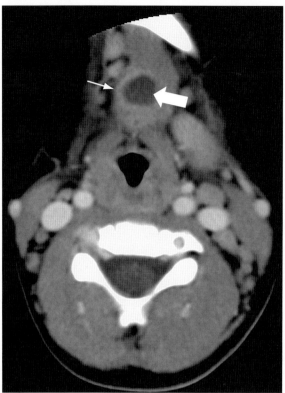

Figure 1. Axial contrast-enhanced CT image shows a round, midline, hypodense mass (*thick arrow*) with peripheral enhancement (*thin arrow*).

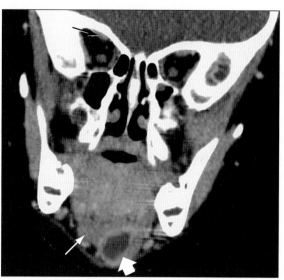

Figure 2. Coronal CT reconstruction illustrates the relationship of the mass (*thick arrow*) to the mandible and floor of the mouth. The *thin arrow* points to right digastric muscle.

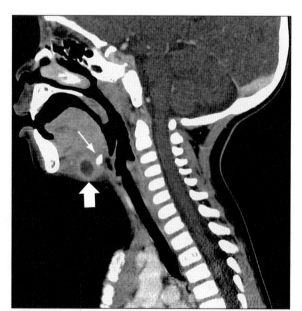

Figure 3. The proximity of the mass (*thick arrow*) to the hyoid bone (*thin arrow*) is seen on sagittal CT reconstruction.

Case 11

DEMOGRAPHICS/CLINICAL HISTORY

The patient is a 2-month-old infant with respiratory distress.

FINDINGS

A chest radiograph shows deviation of the trachea to the right (Fig. 1). Chest computed tomography (CT) shows a homogeneously enhancing paratracheal mass producing a mass effect and causing deviation of the trachea to the right (Fig. 2). The mass shows homogeneous hyperintensity on T2-weighted magnetic resonance imaging (MRI) (Fig. 3) and homogeneous enhancement after administration of contrast agent (Fig. 4). Tracheal deviation is less apparent on MRI than CT because of patient intubation.

DISCUSSION

Definition/Background
Hemangiomas are vascular tumors that manifest shortly after birth and undergo a proliferative phase that is followed by an involution phase. Patients with subglottic hemangiomas typically present with stridor in the first few months of life.

Characteristic Clinical Features
Patients with subglottic hemangiomas typically present with stridor, and 50% of these patients have cutaneous hemangiomas.

Characteristic Radiologic Findings
Radiographs of subglottic hemangiomas can show prominence of soft tissues in the posterior or lateral subglottic region. CT and MRI show homogeneous enhancement of the mass. Hemangiomas are hyperintense on T2-weighted MRI and show homogeneous enhancement. Flow voids are often seen within hemangiomas, but subglottic hemangiomas are often small when they manifest, and flow voids may be difficult to visualize on imaging.

Differential Diagnosis
- Croup
- Retropharyngeal abscess
- Vascular ring

Discussion
Stridor can have many causes. Croup has an acute presentation, and edema of the subglottic soft tissues often causes the typical tracheal "steepling" seen on radiographs. Retropharyngeal abscess manifests acutely with fever, is seen as enlargement of the prevertebral soft tissues on radiographs, and shows inflammatory changes and rim enhancement in the retropharyngeal tissues on CT. Vascular ring may have a clinical presentation similar to that of subglottic hemangiomas, but upper gastrointestinal studies may suggest a vascular ring, which can be confirmed on CT or MRI.

Diagnosis
Paratracheal hemangioma with a subglottic component

Suggested Readings
Baker LL, Dillon WP, Hieshima GB, et al: Hemangiomas and vascular malformations of the head and neck: MR characterization. AJNR Am J Neuroradiol 14:307-314, 1993.

Chetty A, Mischler E, Gregg D: Diagnosis of subglottic hemangioma by chest CT. Pediatr Pulmonol 23:464-467, 1997.

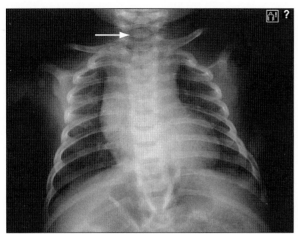

Figure 1. Chest radiograph shows deviation of the trachea (*arrow*) to the right, suggesting a left-sided mass.

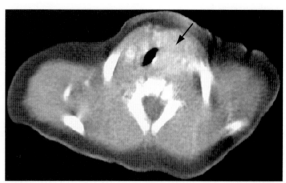

Figure 2. CT scan of the chest performed without sedation shows a homogeneously enhancing paratracheal mass (*arrow*) producing a mass effect and causing deviation of the trachea to the right.

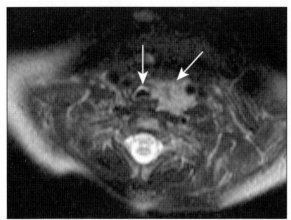

Figure 3. The mass (*black arrow*) shows fairly homogeneous hyperintensity on T2-weighted MR image. Flow voids may be seen within the mass. The mass effect on the trachea (*white arrow*) is less apparent on MRI than CT because of patient intubation.

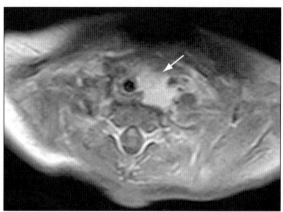

Figure 4. Postcontrast, T1-weighted, fat-saturated MR image shows homogeneous enhancement of the mass (*arrow*). Subglottic involvement and tracheal narrowing was confirmed during bronchoscopy.

Case 12

DEMOGRAPHICS/CLINICAL HISTORY

The patient is a premature infant in respiratory distress.

FINDINGS

A portable chest radiograph shows that the infant has been intubated. The lung volumes are low, and there are diffuse, bilateral granular opacities in the lungs with air bronchograms (Fig. 1).

DISCUSSION

Definition/Background

Most cases of hyaline membrane disease (HMD), also called surfactant deficiency disease and respiratory distress syndrome, occur in premature infants. HMD results from a lack of surfactant in the lungs.

Characteristic Clinical Features

Patients present with tachypnea, grunting, nasal flaring, retractions, and cyanosis.

Characteristic Radiologic Findings

Chest radiographs are valuable in the diagnosis and follow-up of patients with HMD. On radiographs, the lung volumes are low, and there is relatively symmetric parenchymal consolidation with effacement of the pulmonary vessels and air bronchograms.

Differential Diagnosis

- Transient tachypnea of the newborn
- Meconium aspiration
- Neonatal pneumonia

Discussion

Transient tachypnea of the newborn, meconium aspiration, and neonatal pneumonia tend to manifest with increased lung volumes, in contrast to HMD. Patients with transient tachypnea of the newborn have increased fetal lung fluid, which is seen on early radiographs as pulmonary edema and pleural fluid, and which resolves within 48 hours. Meconium aspiration and neonatal pneumonia may manifest with asymmetric pulmonary opacities.

Diagnosis

Hyaline membrane disease

Suggested Readings

Agrons GA, Courtney SE, Stocker JT, et al: From the archives of the AFIP: Lung disease in premature neonates: Radiologic-pathologic correlation. RadioGraphics 25:1047-1073, 2005.
Cleveland RH: A radiologic update on medical diseases of the newborn chest. Pediatr Radiol 25:631-637, 1995.

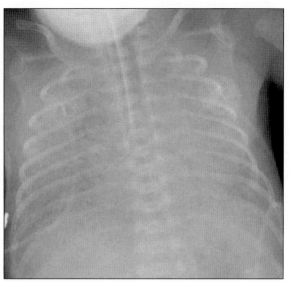

Figure 1. Portable chest radiograph shows that the infant has been intubated. The lung volumes are low, and there are diffuse, bilateral granular opacities in the lungs with air bronchograms.

Case 13

DEMOGRAPHICS/CLINICAL HISTORY

The patient is a 4-month-old infant, who was born prematurely at 25 weeks' gestation, with respiratory distress.

FINDINGS

A portable anteroposterior chest radiograph (Fig. 1) shows extensive interstitial thickening and fibrosis involving all lobes. The lungs are hyperinflated. An axial image from contrast-enhanced computed tomography (CT) of the chest (Fig. 2) also shows diffuse interstitial thickening and areas of cystic change within the right upper lobe.

DISCUSSION

Definition/Background
Bronchopulmonary dysplasia is the most common cause of chronic lung disease in neonates. It is defined clinically as oxygen dependency at 28 days old with an abnormal chest radiograph.

Characteristic Clinical Features
Patients are nearly always born prematurely and depend on supplemental oxygen for at least 1 month after birth.

Characteristic Radiologic Findings
Common CT findings include multiple areas of hyperlucency within the lungs with interspersed linear opacities.

Differential Diagnosis
- Meconium aspiration syndrome (fetal/neonatal)
- CPAM (fetal/neonatal)

Discussion
Meconium aspiration tends to occur in infants born after 40 weeks' gestation, rather than premature infants. The lung volumes are increased, and there are heterogeneous air space opacities and areas of interstitial thickening. CPAM is a congenital, hamartomatous lung lesion that may manifest as multiple cysts of varying sizes; the cysts may occupy a large portion of the lung. It is bilateral in rare cases.

Diagnosis
Bronchopulmonary dysplasia

Suggested Readings
Edwards DK, Jacob J, Gluck L: The immature lung: Radiographic appearance, course, and complications. AJR Am J Roentgenol 135:659-666, 1980.
Howling SJ, Northway WH Jr, Hansell DM, et al: Pulmonary sequelae of bronchopulmonary dysplasia survivors: High-resolution CT findings. AJR Am J Roentgenol 174:1323-1326, 2000.

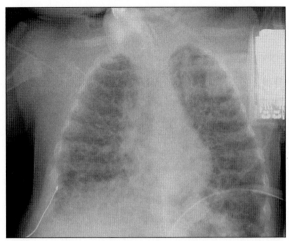

Figure 1. Portable anteroposterior chest radiograph shows a bubbly appearance of the lungs with extensive interstitial thickening and fibrosis involving all lobes. The lungs are hyperinflated. A tracheostomy tube is in place.

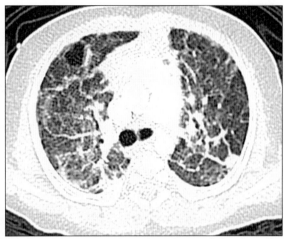

Figure 2. Axial contrast-enhanced CT image of the chest shows diffuse interstitial thickening and areas of cystic change within the right upper lobe.

Case 14

DEMOGRAPHICS/CLINICAL HISTORY

The patient is a newborn infant (born at 36 weeks' gestation) with respiratory distress, who had meconium-stained amniotic fluid at delivery and meconium seen below the vocal cords at intubation.

FINDINGS

An anteroposterior radiograph (Fig. 1) of the chest reveals increased lung volumes. The patient is intubated. There are coarsened interstitial lung markings bilaterally, with a focal opacity within the left upper lobe. Pulmonary interstitial emphysema (PIE) is noticeable in the right upper lobe.

DISCUSSION

Definition/Background

Meconium-stained amniotic fluid occurs with 10% to 15% of births, and 4% to 5% of these infants aspirate meconium. Meconium aspiration occurs most often in postmature or distressed infants.

Characteristic Clinical Features

Patients have respiratory distress and persistent pulmonary hypertension.

Characteristic Radiologic Findings

Imaging shows increased lung volumes, heterogeneous opacities bilaterally, and manifestations of air leak (e.g., PIE).

Differential Diagnosis

■ Neonatal pneumonia
■ Persistent pulmonary hypertension

Discussion

Neonatal pneumonia is most commonly caused by group B streptococcal infection, which can be acquired by passage through the birth canal. Pulmonary injuries are caused directly and indirectly by invading microorganisms or foreign material and by poorly targeted or inappropriate responses by the host defense system. Disruption of endothelial and alveolar epithelial integrity may allow surfactant to be inactivated by proteinaceous exudate, a process that may be exacerbated further by the direct effects of meconium or pathogenic microorganisms.

Persistent pulmonary hypertension (PPHN) is a failure of the circulatory transition that normally occurs after birth. During fetal life, pulmonary blood flow is low, and pulmonary vascular resistance is high. After birth, pulmonary vascular resistance decreases, and pulmonary blood flow increases as the lungs assume the function of gas exchange. When the normal decrease in pulmonary vascular tone does not occur, the result is PPHN of the newborn. PPHN can result when structurally normal pulmonary vessels constrict in response to alveolar hypoxia caused by meconium aspiration.

Diagnosis

Meconium aspiration

Suggested Readings

Cleveland RH: A radiologic update on medical diseases of the newborn chest. Pediatr Radiol 25:61-67, 1995.
Newman B: Imaging of medical disease of the newborn lung. Radiol Clin North Am 37:1049-1065, 1999.

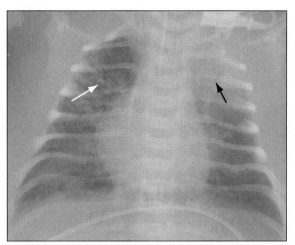

Figure 1. Anteroposterior radiograph of the chest reveals increased lung volumes, coarsened interstitial lung markings, focal left upper lobe opacity (*black arrow*), and PIE in the right upper lobe (*white arrow*).

Case 15

DEMOGRAPHICS/CLINICAL HISTORY

The patient is a 5-month-old girl transferred from an outside hospital with respiratory distress and an abnormal chest x-ray, who was treated for pneumonia 2 weeks ago.

FINDINGS

An anteroposterior radiograph of the chest reveals hyperlucency of the right upper lung with shift of the heart and mediastinum to the left (Fig. 1). Computed tomography (CT) of the chest shows hyperlucency and hyperexpansion of the right upper lobe with inferior displacement of the minor fissure (Figs. 2 and 3).

DISCUSSION

Definition/Background
Congenital lobar emphysema is more common in boys than girls, is not familial, and tends to occur in whites.

Characteristic Clinical Features
Congenital lobar emphysema most often affects the left upper lobe, followed by the right middle lobe and right upper lobe. Most patients become symptomatic in infancy, and respiratory distress is the most common symptom.

Characteristic Radiologic Findings
Radiographs and chest CT reveal hyperinflation of the affected lobe, with resultant mass effect on adjacent structures, such as the heart, mediastinum, and adjacent lung.

Differential Diagnosis
- Congenital cystic adenomatoid malformation
- Swyer-James syndrome

Discussion
Congenital cystic adenomatoid malformation, now known as *congenital pulmonary airway malformation,* is a hamartomatous lesion in which there is a proliferation of bronchial structures and cysts without alveoli. It is often detected in utero with prenatal ultrasound examination. Swyer-James syndrome is characterized by hyperlucency of the affected lung and decreased perfusion. The lung is often smaller than the opposite side. The hilum is small but present.

Diagnosis
Congenital lobar emphysema

Suggested Readings
Berrocal T, Madrid C, Novo S, et al: Congenital anomalies of the tracheobronchial tree, lung, and mediastinum: Embryology, radiology, and pathology. RadioGraphics 24:e17, 2004.
Kennedy CD, Habibi P, Matthew DJ, et al: Lobar emphysema: Long-term imaging follow-up. Radiology 180:189, 1991.

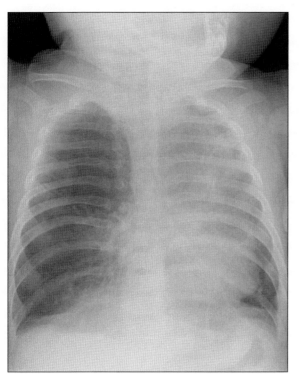

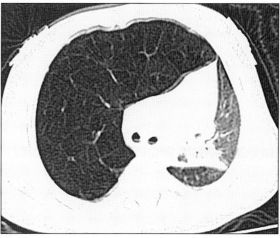

Figure 2. Axial CT scan through the level of the right upper lobe shows marked hyperinflation of the right upper lobe with extension across midline and mass effect on the mediastinum and left lung, which is compressed.

Figure 1. Anteroposterior view of the chest reveals marked hyperlucency of the right upper lobe, which extends across midline. There is compression of the right middle and lower lobes.

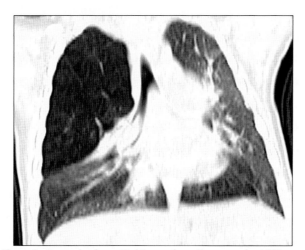

Figure 3. Coronal reformatted image from the same chest CT scan shows the hyperexpanded right upper lobe, which is causing inferior displacement of the minor fissure and the right middle lobe.

Case 16

DEMOGRAPHICS/CLINICAL HISTORY

The patient is a 3-day-old infant (born after 36 weeks' gestation) with respiratory distress after a precipitous vaginal delivery with meconium-stained amniotic fluid and now requiring ventilator support.

FINDINGS

An anteroposterior radiograph of the chest reveals bilateral, irregular, linear lucencies within the upper lobes (Fig. 1). An anteroposterior radiograph of the chest performed the next day reveals similar findings and a new right-sided pneumothorax (Fig. 2).

DISCUSSION

Definition/Background
Pulmonary interstitial emphysema (PIE) is the first imaging manifestation of barotrauma, and it occurs most often in premature, low-birth-weight infants on ventilators.

Characteristic Clinical Features
PIE can cause the lungs to be less compliant, and it further impairs gas exchange.

Characteristic Radiologic Findings
The radiographic features of PIE include multiple, linear, or bubbly lucencies within the interstitium.

Differential Diagnosis
- Congenital cystic adenomatoid malformation

Discussion
Congenital cystic adenomatoid malformation appears as a mass composed of numerous air-containing cysts scattered irregularly throughout a segment of the lung. This space-occupying mass expands the ipsilateral hemithorax and shifts the mediastinum to the contralateral side. PIE may resemble congenital cystic adenomatoid malformation when it is complicated by large air collections, but they are typically associated with linear collections and preceded by high-pressure ventilation and barotrauma. The air collections are located in the interstitial lymphatics.

Diagnosis
Pulmonary interstitial emphysema

Suggested Readings
Berk DR, Varich LJ: Localized persistent pulmonary interstitial emphysema in a preterm infant in the absence of mechanical ventilation. Pediatr Radiol 35:1243-1245, 2005.

Freysdottir D, Olutoye O, Langston C, et al: Spontaneous pulmonary interstitial emphysema in a term unventilated infant. Pediatr Pulmonol 41:374-378, 2006.

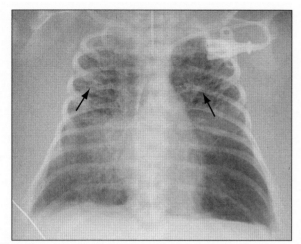

Figure 1. Anteroposterior radiograph of the chest in the intubated, ventilated infant reveals bilateral, irregular, linear, bubbly lucencies in the upper lobes (*arrows*).

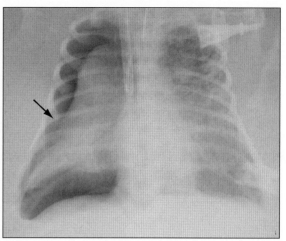

Figure 2. Anteroposterior radiograph of the chest performed 1 day later reveals a new right-sided pneumothorax (*arrow*).

Case 17

DEMOGRAPHICS/CLINICAL HISTORY

The patient is a 3-week-old boy with apnea and brady-cardia.

FINDINGS

An anteroposterior radiograph of the chest shows multiple, air-filled cystic structures occupying the left lower hemithorax (Fig. 1). A delayed radiograph of the abdomen performed approximately 16 hours after administration of oral contrast agent as part of an upper gastrointestinal examination shows contrast opacification of the colon and splenic flexure herniation into the left lower chest (Fig. 2).

DISCUSSION

Definition/Background

Congenital diaphragmatic hernia consists of a defect in the diaphragm with abdominal contents herniated into the chest cavity. It most often occurs in the left postero-lateral position.

Characteristic Clinical Features

Small hernias may be asymptomatic. Larger hernias manifest with respiratory compromise and pulmonary hypertension.

Characteristic Radiologic Findings

Chest radiographs reveal abnormal opacification of the chest, usually the left hemithorax. Lucency within the mass indicates the presence of herniated bowel loops, whereas more solid contents suggest fluid-filled bowel or solid viscera (e.g., spleen, liver).

Differential Diagnosis

- Congenital lobar emphysema
- Congenital cystic adenomatoid malformation
- Foregut duplication cyst

Diagnosis

Hernia, congenital diaphragmatic

Suggested Readings

Johnson AM, Hubbard AM: Congenital anomalies of the fetal/neonatal chest. Semin Roentgenol 39:197-214, 2004.

Sakurai M, Donnelly LF, Klosterman LA, et al: Congenital diaphragmatic hernia in neonates: Variations in umbilical catheter and enteric tube position. Radiology 216:112-116, 2000.

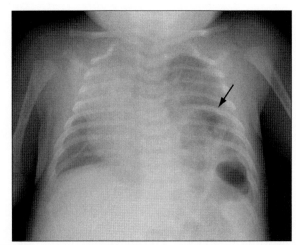

Figure 1. Anteroposterior radiograph of the chest shows multiple cystic lucencies within the left lower hemithorax that represent herniated bowel loops (*arrow*).

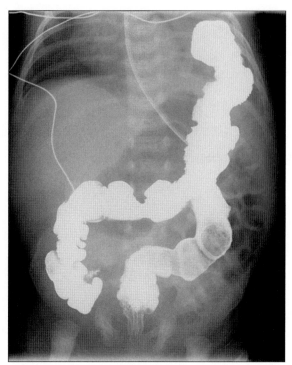

Figure 2. Anteroposterior radiograph of the abdomen obtained approximately 16 hours after administration of oral contrast agent for an upper gastrointestinal examination shows contrast material within the colon. The splenic flexure is herniated into the chest cavity; there is a nasogastric tube in the stomach.

Case 18

DEMOGRAPHICS/CLINICAL HISTORY

The patient is a 2-month-old boy with a diagnosis of cystic fibrosis.

FINDINGS

Lateral (Fig. 1) and anteroposterior (Fig. 2) radiographs of the chest show focal elevation of the right posterior hemidiaphragm. Coronal (Fig. 3) and sagittal (Fig. 4) reformatted noncontrast computed tomography (CT) images of the chest better illustrate the focal eventration of the right posterior diaphragm, with the liver riding high into the lower hemithorax just below the diaphragm.

DISCUSSION

Definition/Background

Eventration of the diaphragm consists of an intact diaphragm with a deficiency in the musculature that causes abnormal elevation of the diaphragm and paradoxical motion of the affected hemidiaphragm during breathing.

Characteristic Clinical Features

Patients may be completely asymptomatic in mild cases, whereas eventration causes respiratory compromise in more severe cases.

Characteristic Radiologic Findings

Fluoroscopic evaluation of the diaphragm during breathing shows an abnormally elevated diaphragm with paradoxical motion during inspiration and expiration.

Differential Diagnosis

- Congenital diaphragmatic hernia
- Morgagni hernia

Diagnosis

Eventration

Suggested Readings

Verhey PT, Gosselin MV, Primack SL, et al: Differentiating diaphragmatic paralysis and eventration. Acad Radiol 14:420-425, 2007.

Yazici M, Karaca I, Arikan A, et al: Congenital eventration of the diaphragm in children: 25 years' experience in three pediatric surgery centers. Eur J Pediatr Surg 13:298-301, 2003.

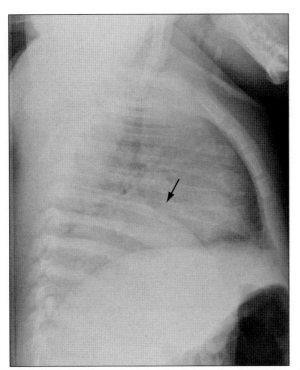

Figure 1. Lateral radiograph of the chest shows focal elevation of the posterior right hemidiaphragm (*arrow*).

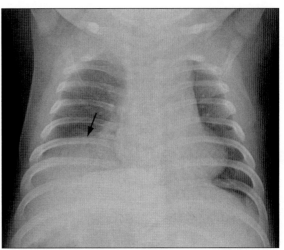

Figure 2. Anteroposterior radiograph of the chest shows elevation of the right hemidiaphragm (*arrow*).

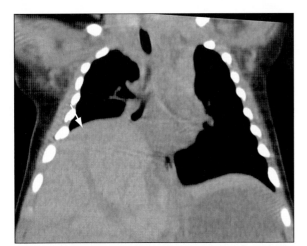

Figure 3. Coronal reformatted noncontrast CT image of the chest shows an elevated right hemidiaphragm (*arrow*). The liver is displaced into the lower hemithorax, but it is still positioned beneath the diaphragm.

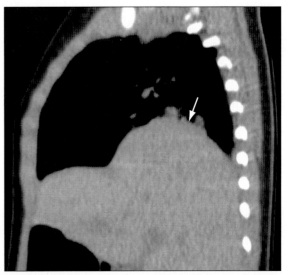

Figure 4. Sagittal reformatted noncontrast CT image of the chest shows focal elevation of the right posterior hemidiaphragm (*arrow*).

Case 19

DEMOGRAPHICS/CLINICAL HISTORY

The patient is a 1-month-old boy with increased work of breathing.

FINDINGS

Anteroposterior (Fig. 1) and lateral (Fig. 2) radiographs of the chest show midline, anterior herniation of bowel loops into the chest cavity, which is consistent with a Morgagni hernia.

DISCUSSION

Definition/Background

A Morgagni hernia is an anterior congenital diaphragmatic hernia through the foramen of Morgagni, a space usually filled with adipose tissue. The transverse colon is the most common organ to herniate through the defect.

Characteristic Clinical Features

Patients are asymptomatic or present with recurrent chest infection or gastrointestinal discomfort. Patients with Morgagni hernia have an increased risk for associated anomalies, including congenital heart disease.

Characteristic Radiologic Findings

Chest radiographs are the first-line imaging modality in the assessment of Morgagni hernia. A true lateral x-ray film is most helpful in showing the anterior location of the hernia.

Differential Diagnosis

- Eventration of the diaphragm
- Congenital diaphragmatic hernia

Diagnosis

Morgagni hernia

Suggested Readings

Al-Salem AH: Congenital hernia of Morgagni in infants and children. J Pediatr Surg 42:1539-1543, 2007.

Al-Salem AH, Nawaz A, Matta A, et al: Herniation through the foramen of Morgagni: Early diagnosis and treatment. Pediatr Surg Int 18:93-97, 2002.

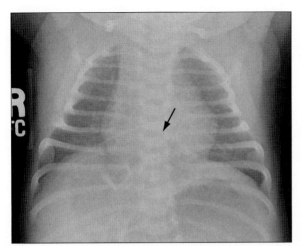

Figure 1. Anteroposterior radiograph of the chest shows a focal contour abnormality at the level of the diaphragm in the midline, with evidence of bowel loops above the level of the diaphragm (*arrow*).

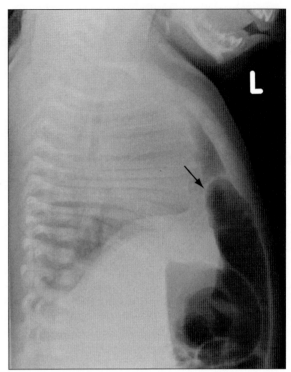

Figure 2. Lateral radiograph of the chest shows anterior location of the herniated bowel (*arrow*).

Case 20

DEMOGRAPHICS/CLINICAL HISTORY

The patient is a 1-day-old girl with a history of a chest mass identified on prenatal ultrasound examination.

FINDINGS

Contrast-enhanced computed tomography (CT) of the chest shows a well-circumscribed, subcarinal cystic lesion (Figs. 1 and 2). Barium esophagography shows mild rightward deviation of the mid-esophagus by the smoothly contoured lesion in the mediastinum, without associated esophageal narrowing (Fig. 3).

DISCUSSION

Definition/Background
Bronchogenic cysts are congenital lesions that arise from the primitive ventral foregut. Most are located within the mediastinum.

Characteristic Clinical Features
Most patients are asymptomatic, and the cyst is discovered incidentally during imaging performed for other indications.

Characteristic Radiologic Findings
Bronchogenic cysts are best evaluated with CT scan of the chest. On CT, these cysts appear as smoothly circumscribed masses of homogeneous water density without contrast enhancement.

Less Common Radiologic Manifestations
In some instances, bronchogenic cysts may become infected, which is suggested on imaging by the presence of an air-fluid level within the mass.

Differential Diagnosis
- Esophageal duplication cyst
- Neurenteric cysts

Discussion
Esophageal duplication cysts and neurenteric cysts are cysts of the primitive foregut that are related to the esophagus (esophageal duplication cysts) and spinal column (neurenteric cysts).

Diagnosis
Bronchogenic cyst

Suggested Readings

Berrocal T, Madrid C, Novo S, et al: Congenital anomalies of the tracheobronchial tree, lung, and mediastinum: Embryology, radiology, and pathology. RadioGraphics 24:e17, 2004.

Rappaport DC, Herman SJ, Weisbrod GL: Congenital bronchopulmonary disease in adults: CT findings. AJR Am J Roentgenol 162:1295-1299, 1994.

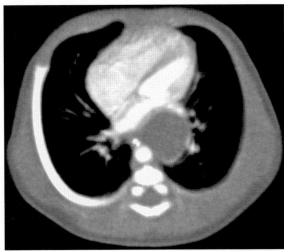

Figure 1. Axial contrast-enhanced CT image of the chest shows a smooth-walled, well-circumscribed cystic lesion in the subcarinal region.

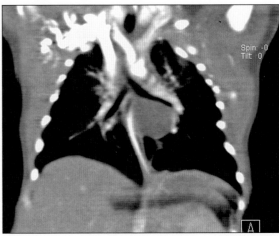

Figure 2. Coronal reformatted, contrast-enhanced CT image of the chest shows a subcarinal mass that has imaging features compatible with a simple cystic lesion.

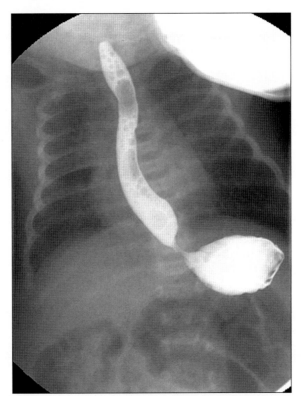

Figure 3. Fluoroscopic spot image acquired during barium esophagography shows mild rightward deviation of the esophagus by the lesion.

Case 21

DEMOGRAPHICS/CLINICAL HISTORY

The patient is a newborn with a lung mass diagnosed on prenatal ultrasound examination.

FINDINGS

An anteroposterior radiograph of the chest (Fig. 1) shows a wedge-shaped opacity in the left lower lobe. Axial contrast-enhanced computed tomography (CT) of the chest (Fig. 2) shows a focal, wedge-shaped mass within the left lower lobe, which is supplied by an arterial feeder arising directly from the aorta. Coronal reformatted, contrast-enhanced CT of the chest (Fig. 3) shows similar findings and an arterial feeder arising from the aorta.

DISCUSSION

Definition/Background

Pulmonary sequestration is a congenital bronchopulmonary malformation that often manifests as a parenchymal mass.

Characteristic Clinical Features

Early symptomatic sequestrations are associated with a large shunt or cardiovascular disease. Children who present later tend to have symptoms of infection. Many sequestrations are identified on routine screening prenatal ultrasound.

Characteristic Radiologic Findings

Radiography and chest CT show a parenchymal mass that may simulate an area of consolidation. On CT, it is usually possible to identify a feeding arterial vessel arising from the aorta.

Differential Diagnosis

- Congenital cystic airway malformation or congenital pulmonary airway malformation (CCAM/CPAM)
- Bronchogenic cyst
- Congenital diaphragmatic hernia

Discussion

CCAM/CPAM is a hamartomatous abnormality of the lung that constitutes 25% of all congenital lung lesions, and that may appear as a cystic or solid mass. Bronchogenic cysts, which are the most common cystic lesions of the mediastinum, result from anomalous development of the foregut during embryogenesis. Congenital diaphragmatic hernia is a herniation of the abdominal viscera into the chest through a defect in the diaphragm.

Diagnosis

Pulmonary sequestration

Suggested Readings

Johnson AM, Hubbard AM: Congenital anomalies of the fetal/neonatal chest. Semin Roentgenol 39:197-214, 2004.
Quinn TM, Hubbard AM, Adzick NS: Prenatal magnetic resonance imaging enhances fetal diagnosis. J Pediatr Surg 33:553-558, 1998.

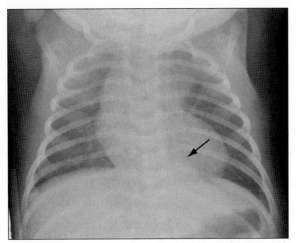

Figure 1. Anteroposterior radiograph of the chest shows a wedge-shaped opacity in the left lower lobe (*arrow*).

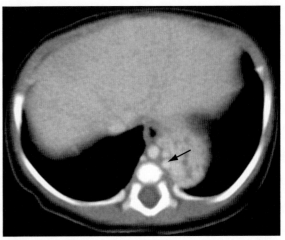

Figure 2. Axial contrast-enhanced CT image of the chest shows a focal, wedge-shaped mass within the left lower lobe that is supplied by an arterial feeder arising directly from the aorta (*arrow*).

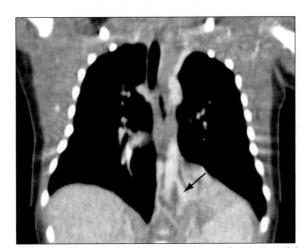

Figure 3. Coronal reformatted, contrast-enhanced CT image of the chest shows findings similar to those on other scans and an arterial feeder arising from the aorta (*arrow*).

Case 22

DEMOGRAPHICS/CLINICAL HISTORY

The patient is an infant in whom routine screening ultrasound examination revealed an abnormality in the fetal chest, and magnetic resonance imaging (MRI) was requested.

FINDINGS

Coronal (Fig. 1) and axial (Fig. 2) T2-weighted images from fetal MRI show a large, complex cystic lesion within the left lung that is displacing the heart to the right. Axial image from chest computed tomography (CT) (Fig. 3) in lung windows performed without intravenous contrast agent several days after the infant was born shows that many of these cystic spaces are now air-filled.

DISCUSSION

Definition/Background

Congenital pulmonary airway malformation (CPAM) is an abnormal mass of solid or cystic tissue that arises secondary to a defect in endodermal and mesodermal differentiation at approximately 5 to 7 weeks' gestation.

Characteristic Clinical Features

When small, CPAMs may be asymptomatic at birth. These may be incidentally discovered at routine screening. Larger lesions manifest as severe pulmonary distress in the newborn.

Characteristic Radiologic Findings

CPAMs are commonly detected on prenatal ultrasound; they appear as abnormal, hypoechoic, cystic-appearing cavities within the lung causing displacement of the heart and mediastinum to the contralateral side.

Less Common Radiologic Manifestations

At fetal MRI, CPAMs appear as lung masses (either side) with multiple T2-bright cavities of various sizes representing cystic spaces. Larger lesions may be associated with fetal hydrops.

Differential Diagnosis

- Congenital diaphragmatic hernia
- Pulmonary sequestration
- Bronchogenic cyst

Discussion

Congenital diaphragmatic hernia is a defect in the diaphragm, usually posterior, that is present at birth, and that may be associated with herniation of abdominal structures, such as bowel loops, into the chest. Pulmonary sequestration is a congenital malformation of the lung, characterized as intralobar or extralobar, in which there is an anomalous systemic arterial supply to the abnormal lung tissue. A bronchogenic cyst is a congenital, usually cystic lesion that may occur in the mediastinum or lung parenchyma.

Diagnosis

Congenital pulmonary airway malformation (fetal/neonatal)

Suggested Readings

Calvert JK, Lakhoo K: Antenatally suspected congenital cystic adenomatoid malformation of the lung: Postnatal investigation and timing of surgery. J Pediatr Surg 42:411-414, 2007.

Cass DL, Crombleholme TM, Howell LJ, et al: Cystic lung lesions with systemic arterial blood supply: A hybrid of congenital cystic adenomatoid malformation and bronchopulmonary sequestration. J Pediatr Surg 32:986-990, 1997.

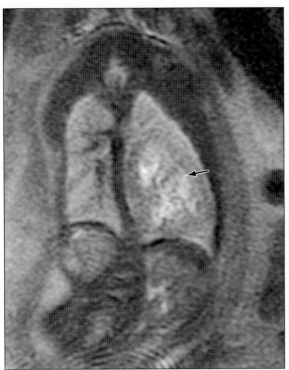

Figure 1. Coronal axial T2-weighted image from fetal MRI shows large, complex cystic lesion within the left lung (*arrow*). The diaphragm is intact.

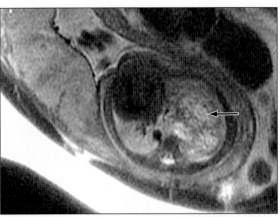

Figure 2. Axial T2-weighted image from fetal MRI shows large, complex cystic lesion within the left lung (*arrow*), which is displacing the heart to the right.

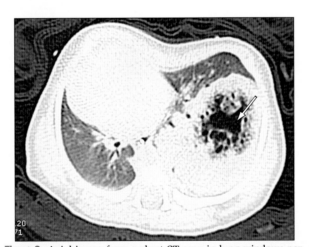

Figure 3. Axial image from a chest CT scan in lung windows performed without intravenous contrast agent several days after the infant was born shows many of these cystic spaces to be air-filled (*arrow*).

Case 23

DEMOGRAPHICS/CLINICAL HISTORY

The patient is the fetus of a 42-year-old woman with an abnormality noticed on routine ultrasound screening in her 23rd week of pregnancy.

FINDINGS

Transverse ultrasound through the fetal chest (Fig. 1) shows an abnormal cystic mass behind the heart in the left lower hemithorax. T2-weighted magnetic resonance imaging (MRI) of the fetus (Figs. 2 and 3) shows that the mass has high signal intensity, consistent with a cystic structure. The stomach, bowel, and abdominal contents appear to be appropriately positioned below the diaphragm.

DISCUSSION

Definition/Background

Congenital pulmonary airway malformation (CPAM) also called *congenital pulmonary airway malformation,* is an abnormal mass of solid or cystic tissue that is thought to result from a defect in endodermal and mesodermal differentiation at 5 to 7 weeks' gestation.

Characteristic Clinical Features

Depending on its size, CPAM may be asymptomatic at birth or manifest as severe pulmonary distress in the newborn. If detected later, symptoms are often related to a pulmonary infection that precipitates imaging investigation.

Characteristic Radiologic Findings

CPAMs are commonly detected on prenatal ultrasound and subsequently imaged with fetal MRI, which shows them as macrocystic or microcystic masses within either lung. Larger lesions may be associated with fetal hydrops.

Less Common Radiologic Manifestations

In 10% of cases, imaging may detect CPAMs in both lungs.

Differential Diagnosis
- Congenital diaphragmatic hernia (CDH)
- Pulmonary sequestration
- Bronchogenic cyst

Discussion

CDH consists of a defect in the diaphragm, with abdominal contents herniated into the chest cavity. Ultrasound examination shows that 85% of CDHs are left-sided, 13% are right-sided, and 2% are bilateral. Other findings include polyhydramnios, an absent or intrathoracic stomach bubble, and a mediastinal and cardiac shift away from the side of the hernia. A pulmonary sequestration is a portion of the lung that receives systemic, rather than pulmonary, arterial supply, and that is separated from the tracheobronchial tree. Most sequestrations that are diagnosed prenatally are extralobar. Bronchogenic cysts are congenital lesions that arise from the primitive ventral foregut, and most are located within the mediastinum. On imaging, the cysts appear as smoothly circumscribed masses of homogeneous water density. The cysts may become infected, which is suggested on imaging by the presence of an air-fluid level within the mass.

Diagnosis

Congenital pulmonary airway malformation

Suggested Readings

Calvert JK, Lakhoo K: Antenatally suspected congenital cystic adenomatoid malformation of the lung: Postnatal investigation and timing of surgery. J Pediatr Surg 42:411-414, 2007.

Cass DL, Crombleholme TM, Howell LJ, et al: Cystic lung lesions with systemic arterial blood supply: A hybrid of congenital cystic adenomatoid malformation and bronchopulmonary sequestration. J Pediatr Surg 32:986-990, 1997.

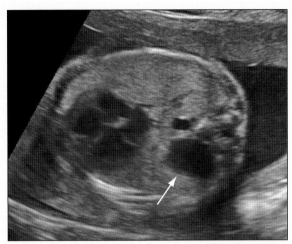

Figure 1. Transverse ultrasound through the fetal chest at the level of the heart shows a cystic mass in the left lower chest that is situated behind the heart (*arrow*).

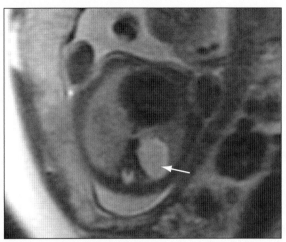

Figure 2. Axial T2-weighted MR image shows that the lesion has bright signal intensity, consistent with a cystic structure (*arrow*).

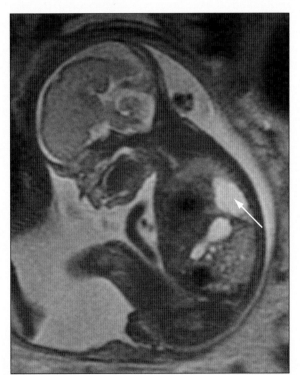

Figure 3. Sagittal T2-weighted MR image shows abnormal cystic chest lesion directly superior to the left hemidiaphragm (*arrow*). The stomach and abdominal contents appear to be appropriately positioned below the diaphragm.

Case 24

DEMOGRAPHICS/CLINICAL HISTORY

The patient is a 3-month-old boy with trouble breathing.

FINDINGS

Anteroposterior (Fig. 1) and lateral (Fig. 2) radiographs of the chest show a large, predominantly air-filled, cystic mass within the right lower lobe that occupies almost the whole right hemithorax and causes the heart and mediastinum to be shifted into the left hemithorax. Computed tomography (CT) of the chest (Fig. 3) shows that the right lower lobe is almost completely replaced by the mass, which is composed of several large, cystic structures that contain fine internal septations.

DISCUSSION

Definition/Background

Pleuropulmonary blastoma is a rare lung neoplasm occurring in children younger than 6 years. It is considered to be a dysontogenetic tumor, similar to Wilms' tumor in the kidney.

Characteristic Clinical Features

Patients present with nonspecific respiratory distress.

Characteristic Radiologic Findings

Masses are predominantly large, pleural-based, and peripherally located. Masses usually manifest with near-complete opacification of the hemithorax.

Less Common Radiologic Manifestations

Less common manifestations of pleuropulmonary blastoma include a cystic, rather than a solid, mass, such as seen in this case.

Differential Diagnosis

- Congenital diaphragmatic hernia (CDH)
- Congenital pulmonary airway malformation
- Neuroblastoma
- Ewing sarcoma
- Askin tumor
- Rhabdomyosarcoma

Discussion

Because of the large size of the mass and the cystic nature of the mass in this case, the differential diagnosis includes parenchymal diseases (i.e., congenital diaphragmatic hernia and congenital pulmonary airway malformation) and pleural or chest wall diseases.

Diagnosis

Pleuropulmonary blastoma

Suggested Readings

Naffaa LN, Donnelly LF: Imaging findings in pleuropulmonary blastoma. Pediatr Radiol 35:387-391, 2005.

Orazi C, Inserra A, Schingo PM, et al: Pleuropulmonary blastoma, a distinctive neoplasm of childhood: Report of three cases. Pediatr Radiol 37:337-344, 2007.

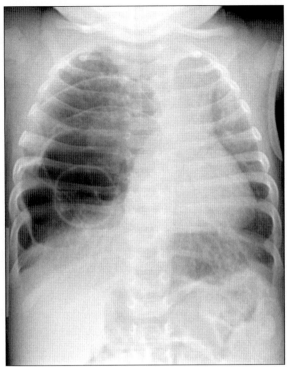

Figure 1. Anteroposterior radiograph of the chest shows a large, predominantly air-filled, cystic mass within the right lower lobe that occupies almost the whole right hemithorax, which causes the heart and mediastinum to be shifted into the left hemithorax. Because of the large size of the mass, it is difficult to discern whether it is parenchymal or pleural-based.

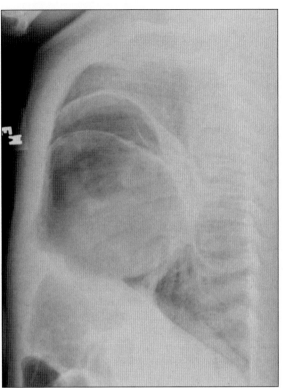

Figure 2. Lateral radiograph of the chest shows a large, predominantly air-filled, cystic mass within the right lower lobe that occupies almost the whole right hemithorax. Because of the large size of the mass, it is difficult to discern whether it is parenchymal or pleural-based.

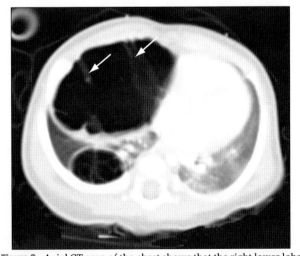

Figure 3. Axial CT scan of the chest shows that the right lower lobe is almost completely replaced by the mass, which is composed of several large, cystic structures that contain fine internal septations (*arrows*). Because of the large size of the mass, its origin is unclear, but it appears to be peripherally based, suggesting a pleural origin.

Case 25

DEMOGRAPHICS/CLINICAL HISTORY

The patient is a 1-week-old girl with a prenatal diagnosis of congenital heart disease.

FINDINGS

An anteroposterior radiograph of the chest (Fig. 1) in the intubated infant shows complete opacification of the left hemithorax, which is associated with significant volume loss. The heart and mediastinum are shifted into the left hemithorax. Contrast-enhanced computed tomography (CT) of the chest (Figs. 2 and 3) shows absence of the left lung. There is compensatory enlargement of the right lung, which crosses midline posteriorly to occupy a portion of the left hemithorax.

DISCUSSION

Definition/Background
Pulmonary agenesis is a rare congenital malformation in which the lung, including its bronchi and vascular supply, is absent. Infants often have associated congenital anomalies, including congenital heart disease and tracheoesophageal fistula.

Characteristic Clinical Features
Infants tend to present with respiratory distress, cyanosis, or feeding difficulties.

Characteristic Radiologic Findings
Chest radiographs often show an opacified hemithorax with a marked ipsilateral mediastinal shift. CT shows absence of the lung on that side, including the bronchi and vascular supply, and hyperinflation of the contralateral lung.

Differential Diagnosis
- Proximal interruption of the pulmonary artery
- Pulmonary sling
- Scimitar syndrome

Discussion
In proximal interruption of the pulmonary artery, the affected pulmonary artery terminates less than 1 cm from its origin from the main pulmonary artery. The affected lung is hypoplastic.

Diagnosis
Pulmonary agenesis

Suggested Reading
Lee EY, Boiselle PM, Cleveland RH: Multidetector CT evaluation of congenital lung anomalies. Radiology 247:632-648, 2008.

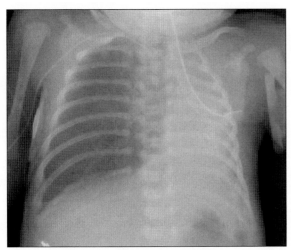

Figure 1. Anteroposterior radiograph of the chest in the intubated infant shows complete opacification of the left hemithorax, which is associated with significant volume loss. The heart and mediastinum are shifted into the left hemithorax.

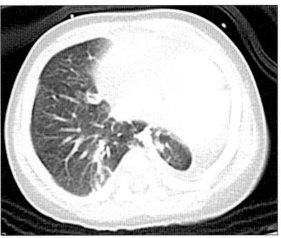

Figure 2. Axial contrast-enhanced CT image of the chest shows absence of the left lung. There is compensatory hyperinflation of the right lung, which crosses midline posteriorly to occupy a portion of the left hemithorax.

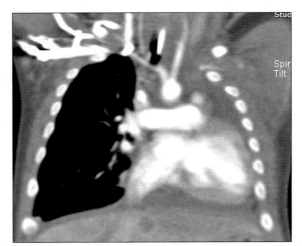

Figure 3. Coronal reformatted, contrast-enhanced CT image of the chest shows absence of the left lung. The heart and mediastinum are shifted into the left hemithorax. There is compensatory enlargement of the right lung.

Case 26

DEMOGRAPHICS/CLINICAL HISTORY

The patient is a 15-year-old girl with decreased exercise tolerance.

FINDINGS

Axial non–contrast-enhanced computed tomography (CT) scan of the chest using lung windows (Figs. 1 and 2) shows multifocal geographic areas of ground-glass attenuation in the lungs with associated interlobular septal thickening. The process is diffuse and affects all lobes, although it is more prominent in the lower lobes.

DISCUSSION

Definition/Background
Pulmonary alveolar proteinosis is most common in adults 20 to 50 years old, although it can occur in younger children and adolescents. Pulmonary alveolar proteinosis manifests as filling of the lung acini with a proteinaceous material that incites an inflammatory response in the lung.

Characteristic Clinical Features
Patients have dyspnea and cough.

Characteristic Radiologic Findings
Chest radiographs reveal bilateral, symmetric air space consolidation or ground-glass opacities. High-resolution CT shows diffuse areas of ground-glass opacities with superimposed interlobular septal thickening.

Differential Diagnosis
- *Pneumocystis jiroveci* (*carinii*) pneumonia
- Pulmonary edema
- Sarcoidosis
- Lipoid pneumonia
- Pulmonary hemorrhage (i.e., Goodpasture syndrome)

Discussion
Pneumocystis jiroveci (*carinii*) pneumonia is a pulmonary infection that most commonly occurs in patients who are severely immunocompromised. Sarcoidosis is a systemic disease characterized by noncaseating granulomas.

Diagnosis
Pulmonary alveolar proteinosis

Suggested Readings
Frazier AA, Franks TJ, Cooke EO, et al: From the archives of the AFIP: Pulmonary alveolar proteinosis. RadioGraphics 28:883-899, 2008.

Rossi SE, Erasmus JJ, Volpacchio M, et al: "Crazy-paving" pattern at thin-section CT of the lungs: Radiologic-pathologic overview. RadioGraphics 23:1509-1519, 2003.

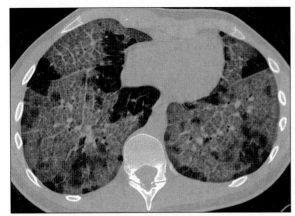

Figure 1. Axial non–contrast-enhanced CT image of the chest shows multiple geographic areas of ground-glass attenuation in the lower lobes of the lungs with associated interlobar septal thickening.

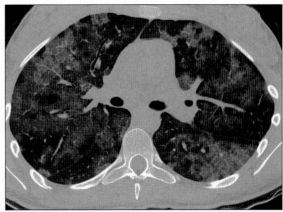

Figure 2. Axial, non–contrast-enhanced CT image of the chest slightly superior to the level in Fig. 1 shows multiple geographic areas of ground-glass attenuation in the middle, upper, and lower lobes of the lungs with associated interlobar septal thickening.

Case 27

DEMOGRAPHICS/CLINICAL HISTORY

The patient is a 17-year-old girl with a known diagnosis of cystic fibrosis.

FINDINGS

An anteroposterior radiograph of the chest (Fig. 1) reveals bronchiectasis and peribronchiolar fibrosis, predominantly involving bilateral upper lobes. An axial image from a computed tomography (CT) scan of the chest (Fig. 2) shows areas of cystic bronchiectasis within the upper lobes bilaterally. An axial CT image through the upper abdomen (Fig. 3) reveals nodularity of the liver consistent with cirrhosis and fatty replacement of the pancreas.

DISCUSSION

Definition/Background
Cystic fibrosis is a genetically transmitted disease that most commonly affects white children. It is an autosomal recessive condition that occurs in 1 in 2500 live white births.

Characteristic Clinical Features
A few cases of cystic fibrosis are diagnosed in infancy when an infant presents with meconium ileus. Most patients present later in childhood with failure to thrive, malabsorption, repeated upper respiratory tract infections, or rectal prolapse.

Characteristic Radiologic Findings
Chest radiographs and chest CT reveal hyperinflation, bronchial wall thickening, upper lobe bronchiectasis, scattered nodular opacities, and enlarged hila.

Less Common Radiologic Manifestations
A nodular cirrhotic liver with stigmata of portal hypertension and hypersplenism are less common findings on imaging.

Differential Diagnosis
- Bronchiolitis
- Primary cilia dyskinesia
- Immunodeficiency syndromes

Discussion
Bronchiolitis is a common disease in young children and is most often secondary to a virus. Chest x-ray findings include hyperinflation and peribronchiolar thickening. Primary cilia dyskinesia is an autosomal recessive condition that consists of situs inversus, sinusitis, and bronchiectasis. Immunodeficiency syndromes lead to bronchiectasis in the lungs, which is likely secondary to repeated infections.

Diagnosis
Cystic fibrosis

Suggested Readings
Moskowitz SM, Gibson RL, Effmann EL: Cystic fibrosis lung disease: Genetic influences, microbial interactions, and radiological assessment. Pediatr Radiol 35:739, 2005.

Shah RM, Sexauer W, Ostrum BJ, et al: High-resolution CT in the acute exacerbation of cystic fibrosis: Evaluation of acute findings, reversibility of those findings, and clinical correlation. AJR Am J Roentgenol 169:375, 1997.

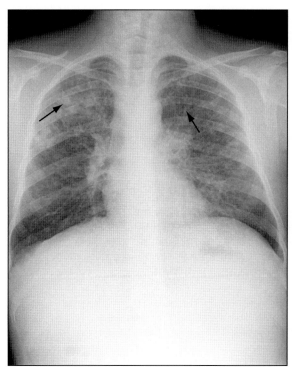

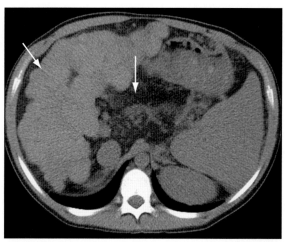

Figure 2. Axial image from non–contrast-enhanced CT through the chest reveals cystic bronchiectasis involving the upper lobes (*arrows*).

Figure 1. Anteroposterior radiograph of the chest shows hyperinflated lungs and bilateral bronchiectatic changes with bronchiolar wall thickening, primarily affecting the upper lobes (*arrows*).

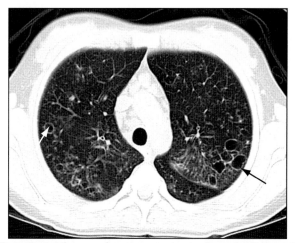

Figure 3. Axial image from non–contrast-enhanced CT through the upper abdomen shows nodular, cirrhotic liver (*black arrow*) and fatty replacement of the pancreas (*white arrow*).

Case 28

DEMOGRAPHICS/CLINICAL HISTORY

The patient is an 11-year-old boy with a known syndrome.

FINDINGS

Axial fluid attenuated inversion recovery (FLAIR) magnetic resonance imaging (MRI) (Fig. 1) shows abnormal high signal intensity in the white matter, ventriculomegaly, and dilated perivascular spaces. A lateral radiograph of the lumbar spine (Fig. 2) shows "beaking" of the L1 vertebral body, causing a focal kyphosis and scalloping of the posterior vertebral bodies. A frontal radiograph of the chest (Fig. 3) shows widened and shortened clavicles and widened "oar-shaped" ribs.

DISCUSSION

Definition/Background
Mucopolysaccharidoses (including Hurler [type I], Hunter [type II], Sanfilippo [type III], Morquio [type IV], Scheie [type V], Maroteaux-Lamy [type VI], and Sly [type VII] syndromes) are lysosomal disorders that result in the deposition and accumulation of mucopolysaccharides and their degraded products, particularly glycosaminoglycans.

Characteristic Clinical Features
Patients can present with neurologic or skeletal abnormalities, which prompt evaluation and work-up.

Characteristic Radiologic Findings
In the brain, abnormal white matter, enlarged perivascular spaces, ventriculomegaly, and atrophy are seen, particularly in Hunter and Hurler syndromes. Frontal bossing and J-shaped sella can also be present. Abnormal atlantoaxial orientation or laxity or both can be seen, particularly in Morquio syndrome. A small foramen magnum can be present. Characteristic "beaking" of the vertebral body is seen at the thoracolumbar junction. Broad "oar-shaped" ribs, short clavicles, irregularities of the acromial joints and acetabula, hypoplasia of the inferior portion of the iliac bones, and flared iliac wings are typically present.

Differential Diagnosis
- Leukodystrophy
- Achondroplasia

Discussion
Leukodystrophies can have similar white matter changes; however, the bony abnormalities and enlarged perivascular spaces are typical of mucopolysaccharidoses. Achondroplasia can have a gibbous thoracolumbar deformity, abnormal iliac bones, and hydrocephalus; however, achondroplasia also has narrowed interpediculate spaces, has a more horizontal sacrum, and does not typically have the enlarged perivascular spaces and white matter abnormalities seen in mucopolysaccharidoses.

Diagnosis
Mucopolysaccharidosis type II (Hunter)

Suggested Readings
Markowitz RI, Zackai E: A pragmatic approach to the radiologic diagnosis of pediatric syndromes and skeletal dysplasias. Radiol Clin North Am 39:791-802, 2001.

Matheus MG, Castillo M, Smith JK, et al: Brain MRI findings in patients with mucopolysaccharidosis types I and II and mild clinical presentation. Neuroradiology 46:666-672, 2004.

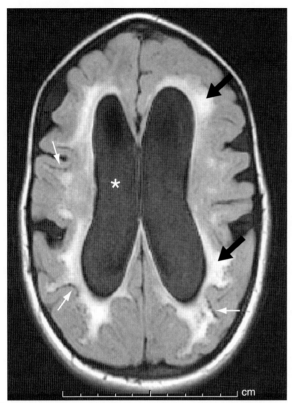

Figure 1. Axial FLAIR MR image shows abnormal high signal intensity in the white matter (*black arrows*), ventriculomegaly (*asterisk*), and dilated perivascular spaces (*white arrows*).

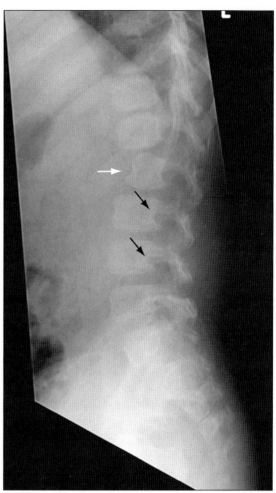

Figure 2. Lateral radiograph of lumbar spine shows "beaking" of the L1 vertebral body (*white arrow*), causing a focal kyphosis and scalloping of the posterior vertebral bodies (*black arrows*).

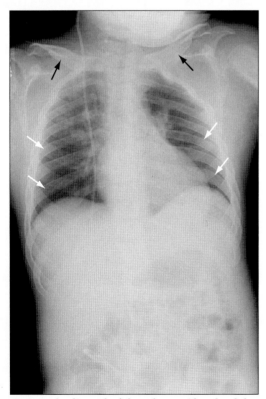

Figure 3. Frontal radiograph of chest shows widened and shortened clavicles (*black arrows*) and widened "oar-shaped" ribs (*white arrows*).

Case 29

DEMOGRAPHICS/CLINICAL HISTORY

The patient is a 17-year-old boy with hemoglobin SS disease and acute chest pain.

FINDINGS

An anteroposterior radiograph of the chest obtained on admission reveals clear lungs (Fig. 1). A radiograph performed 3 days later during hospitalization shows new, bilateral air space disease in the lower lobe (Fig. 2).

DISCUSSION

Definition/Background
Acute chest syndrome (ACS) occurs in patients with sickle cell disease (i.e., patients with homozygous inheritance of the sickle β-globin gene). In contrast to pulmonary infection, ACS tends to affect older children.

Characteristic Clinical Features
Patients may have chest pain, an elevated white blood cell count, fever, and a new pulmonary opacity seen on chest radiograph.

Characteristic Radiologic Findings
For patients with ACS, the initial chest radiograph usually is normal. Parenchymal lung opacities appear and clear rapidly, and they most often affect the lower lobes.

Differential Diagnosis
- Pneumonia
- Pulmonary hemorrhage
- Pulmonary embolus

Discussion
Pneumonia is an infection of the lung that may be caused by bacterial, viral, or fungal agents. Pulmonary hemorrhage is rare, but can occur in children with underlying lung disease. A pulmonary embolus occurs when a blood clot travels to the pulmonary artery, usually from the deep veins of the leg. Depending on the degree of parenchymal infarction, a parenchymal opacity may be seen.

Diagnosis
Sickle cell anemia and acute chest syndrome

Suggested Readings
Rucknagel DL, Kalinyak KA, Gelfand MJ: Rib infarcts and acute chest syndrome in sickle cell disease. Lancet 337:831-833, 1991.
Vichinsky EP, Neumayr LD, Earles AN, et al: Causes and outcomes of the acute chest syndrome in sickle cell disease. National Acute Chest Syndrome Study Group. N Engl J Med 342:1855-1865, 2000.

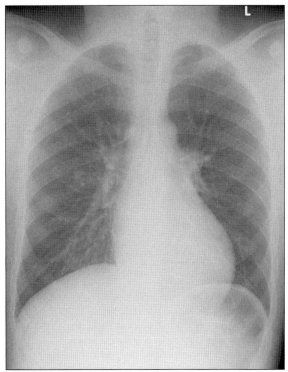

Figure 1. Anteroposterior radiograph of the chest on admission reveals clear lungs.

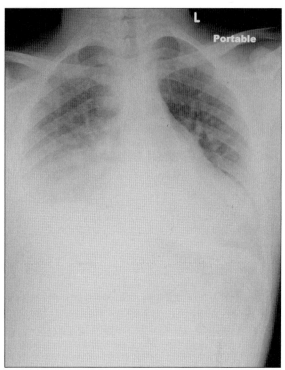

Figure 2. Anteroposterior radiograph of the chest 3 days later shows bilateral lower lobe parenchymal opacities.

Case 30

DEMOGRAPHICS/CLINICAL HISTORY

The patient is an 8-week-old girl with a cough.

FINDINGS

An anteroposterior radiograph of the chest (Fig. 1) performed on admission shows minimal increased opacity in the right lower lung adjacent to the right heart border, which likely reflects mild right middle lobe atelectasis. Two weeks later, a portable chest radiograph (Fig. 2) performed in the intensive care unit shows an endotracheal tube in place. The chest radiograph also shows a new right upper lobe opacity consistent with pneumonia.

DISCUSSION

Definition/Background

Infection caused by *Bordetella pertussis* has markedly diminished because of increased worldwide vaccination coverage, but the disease still affects infants too young to be vaccinated, adolescents, and young adults.

Characteristic Clinical Features

Patients usually present in the catarrhal stage of the illness with symptoms of upper respiratory tract infection. As the disease progresses into the paroxysmal phase, patients experience spells of coughing associated with whoop, vomiting, and sometimes apnea.

Characteristic Radiologic Findings

Radiographic findings are often nonspecific and mimic viral airways disease and pneumonia, with peribronchiolar interstitial thickening or segmental air space disease.

Differential Diagnosis

- Bacterial pneumonia
- Atelectasis
- Aspiration

Discussion

Bacterial pneumonia is caused by various organisms and is often manifested on chest radiographs as a focal segmental or lobar area of air space consolidation. Atelectasis is an area of lung collapse that may manifest as a streaky linear density in a segment of lung versus complete collapse of a lung. Aspiration pneumonia may resemble infectious causes of pneumonia and is secondary to multiple causes, including swallowing disorders, tracheoesophageal fistula, gastroesophageal reflux, and other disorders.

Diagnosis

Pertussis bronchopneumonia

Suggested Readings

Stojanov S, Liese J, Belohradsky BH: Hospitalization and complications in children under 2 years of age with Bordetella pertussis infection. Infection 28:106-110, 2000.

Tozzi AE, Celentano LP, Ciofi degli Atti ML, Salmaso S: Diagnosis and management of pertussis. CMAJ 172:509-515, 2005.

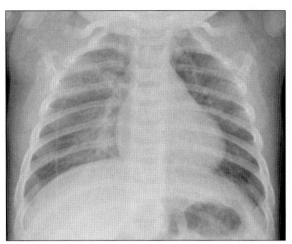

Figure 1. Anteroposterior radiograph of the chest performed on admission shows minimal increased opacity in the right lower lung adjacent to the right heart border, which likely reflects mild right middle lobe atelectasis. Mild peribronchial interstitial thickening is also noted.

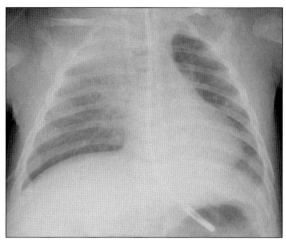

Figure 2. Anteroposterior chest radiograph performed 2 weeks later shows a new endotracheal tube in place and a new right upper lobe opacity consistent with pneumonia.

Case 31

DEMOGRAPHICS/CLINICAL HISTORY

The patient is a 19-year-old man with fever, elevated white blood cell count, and submandibular mass.

FINDINGS

Lung windows from contrast-enhanced computed tomography (CT) of the chest (Figs. 1 and 2) show multiple pulmonary nodules in a centrilobular distribution, some of which have cavitations. Axial contrast-enhanced CT image of the neck (Fig. 3) shows thrombosis of the left external jugular vein that is consistent with superficial thrombophlebitis.

DISCUSSION

Definition/Background
Septic emboli often are seen in patients with infective endocarditis, patients with indwelling central venous catheters, and patients with periodontal disease. In adolescent patients, septic emboli may be caused by thrombophlebitis resulting from infection of the oropharynx.

Characteristic Clinical Features
Patients are often very ill with fever, an elevated white blood cell count, and other signs of infection.

Characteristic Radiologic Findings
CT of the chest shows scattered parenchymal nodules, some of which may be cavitary, usually with a demonstrable feeding vessel.

Less Common Radiologic Manifestations
Imaging may show heterogeneous, subpleural, wedge-shaped densities.

Differential Diagnosis
- Bland pulmonary emboli
- Metastatic disease
- Disseminated fungal disease

Discussion
Bland pulmonary emboli are noninfected thrombi, usually from the deep veins of the lower limbs, that embolize to the pulmonary arteries.

Diagnosis
Septic pulmonary emboli

Suggested Readings
Dodd JD, Souza CA, Muller NL: High-resolution MDCT of pulmonary septic embolism: evaluation of the feeding vessel sign. AJR Am J Roentgenol 187:623-629, 2006.
Huang RM, Naidich DP, Lubat E, et al: Septic pulmonary emboli: CT-radiographic correlation. AJR Am J Roentgenol 153:41-45, 1989.

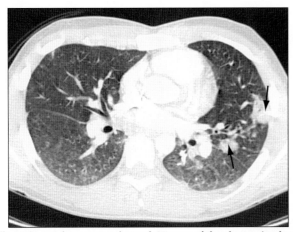

Figure 1. Axial contrast-enhanced CT scan of the chest using lung windows shows multiple pulmonary nodules in a centrilobular distribution (*arrows*).

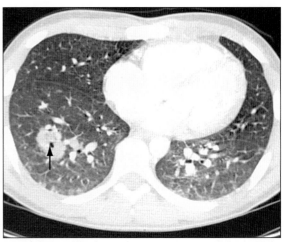

Figure 2. Axial CT scan of the chest using lung windows at a level slightly inferior to the level in Fig. 1 shows a pulmonary nodule in the right lower lobe that is beginning to cavitate centrally (*arrow*).

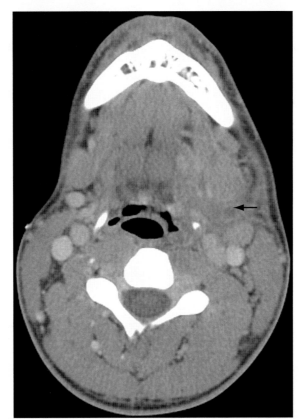

Figure 3. Axial contrast-enhanced CT scan of the neck shows thrombosis of the left external jugular vein that is consistent with superficial thrombophlebitis (*arrow*).

Case 32

DEMOGRAPHICS/CLINICAL HISTORY

The patient is a 7-year-old boy with a chronic cough.

FINDINGS

A posteroanterior radiograph of the chest (Fig. 1) shows a well-circumscribed, oblong mass projecting over the region of the right middle lung. Computed tomography (CT) of the chest (Fig. 2) shows that the soft tissue lesion is based in the parenchyma, is located in the right lower lobe of the lung, and is well circumscribed.

DISCUSSION

Definition/Background

Pulmonary inflammatory pseudotumor (i.e., plasma cell granuloma) is considered a benign entity on the spectrum of pulmonary fibrohistiocytic lesions. It is often a solitary, lobulated soft tissue mass with a predilection for the lower lobes. It is the most common primary lung mass seen in children.

Characteristic Clinical Features

Most patients have a history of lower respiratory tract infection.

Characteristic Radiologic Findings

Chest CT features of the disease are nonspecific, but pulmonary inflammatory pseudotumor usually appears as a heterogeneous mass within the lung that is sharply circumscribed. Calcification within the lesion is uncommon.

Differential Diagnosis

- Pulmonary hamartoma
- Pulmonary neoplasm
- Pulmonary chondroma

Discussion

Pulmonary hamartoma and pulmonary chondroma are benign lesions that occur in the lungs. These lesions are detected as a solitary pulmonary nodule in children who are undergoing imaging for other reasons.

Diagnosis

Plasma cell granuloma

Suggested Readings

Agrons GA, Rosada-de-Christenson ML, Kirejczyk WM, et al: Pulmonary inflammatory pseudotumor: Radiologic features. Radiology 206:511-518, 1998.

Kim TS, Han J, Kim GY, et al: Pulmonary inflammatory pseudotumor (inflammatory myofibroblastic tumor): CT features with pathologic correlation. J Comput Assist Tomogr 29:633-639, 2005.

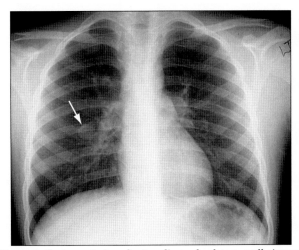

Figure 1. Posteroanterior chest radiograph shows well-circumscribed, oblong mass projecting over the region of the right middle lung (*arrow*).

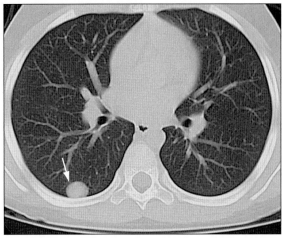

Figure 2. CT scan of the chest shows that the soft tissue lesion is based in the parenchyma, is located in the right lower lobe of the lung, and is well circumscribed (*arrow*).

Case 33

DEMOGRAPHICS/CLINICAL HISTORY

The patient is a 1-month-old boy with a prenatal diagnosis of severe Ebstein anomaly on the basis of prenatal ultrasound, presenting for routine checkup.

FINDINGS

Anteroposterior (Fig. 1) and lateral (Fig. 2) radiographs of the chest show moderate to severe cardiac enlargement, particularly the right atrium and right ventricle. Pulmonary blood flow is normal to slightly decreased.

DISCUSSION

Definition/Background
Ebstein anomaly is a rare form of congenital heart disease that accounts for less than 1% of all cases of congenital heart disease. It is frequently associated with other cardiac malformations (e.g., ventricular septal defect, tetralogy of Fallot).

Characteristic Radiologic Findings
Classic radiographic findings in Ebstein anomaly include significant enlargement of the cardiac silhouette with decreased pulmonary blood flow. In this patient, echocardiogram (images not available) revealed severe tricuspid regurgitation, poor coaptation of the tricuspid valve leaflets, and a tricuspid regurgitation jet arising low in the right ventricle.

Differential Diagnosis
■ Tricuspid regurgitation

Discussion
Tricuspid regurgitation refers to backflow of blood from the right ventricle to the right atrium, which may be caused by various conditions.

Diagnosis
Ebstein anomaly

Suggested Readings
Beerepoot JP, Woodard PK: Case 71: Ebstein anomaly. Radiology 231:747-751, 2004.
Paranon S, Acar P: Ebstein's anomaly of the tricuspid valve: From fetus to adult: Congenital heart disease. Heart 94:237-243, 2008.

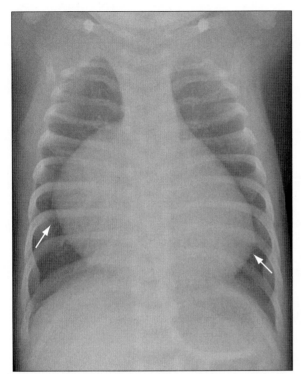

Figure 1. Anteroposterior chest radiograph reveals moderate to severe cardiac enlargement (*arrows*). The superior mediastinum appears narrow secondary to the marked cardiac enlargement.

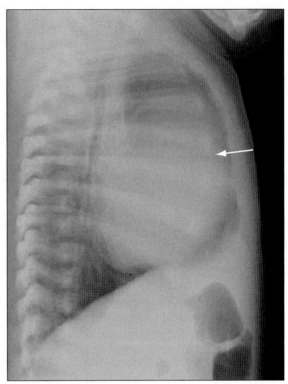

Figure 2. Lateral chest radiograph shows cardiac enlargement, which is secondary to enlargement of the right atrium and right ventricle with effacement of the retrosternal clear space (*arrow*).

Case 34

DEMOGRAPHICS/CLINICAL HISTORY

The patient is a 7-year-old girl with a history of supraventricular tachycardia in the neonatal period.

FINDINGS

Chest radiographs reveal mild increased pulmonary blood flow (Fig. 1) and mild enlargement of the right atrium and right ventricle (Fig. 2).

DISCUSSION

Definition/Background
Atrial septal defect (ASD) may be an isolated defect or associated with a larger congenital heart defect. In this patient, three secundum-type ASDs were diagnosed by echocardiography.

Characteristic Clinical Features
ASD was detected in this child on an echocardiogram performed in infancy for supraventricular tachycardia. Her ASDs have persisted; now at 7 years of age, the patient has no other cardiovascular complaints. Because her symptoms have been mild, she has required no intervention up to this point.

Characteristic Radiologic Findings
Anteroposterior and lateral radiographs of the chest reveal slight enlargement of the right-sided cardiac chambers (right atrium and right ventricle) and mild prominence of pulmonary blood flow.

Less Common Radiologic Manifestations
In many instances, the radiographic findings are very subtle.

Differential Diagnosis
- Ventricular septal defect

Discussion
Ventricular septal defect refers to a fenestration within either the muscular or the membranous portion of the interventricular septum. Chest radiographs often show increased pulmonary blood flow and left atrial prominence.

Diagnosis
Atrial septal defect (ASD)

Suggested Readings
Driscoll DJ: Left-to-right shunt lesions. Pediatr Clin North Am 46: 355-368, 1999.
Wang ZJ, Reddy GP, Gotway MB, et al: Cardiovascular shunts: MR imaging evaluation. RadioGraphics 23(Spec No):S181-S194, 2003.

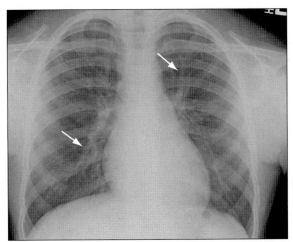

Figure 1. Posteroanterior chest radiograph reveals mild prominence of pulmonary blood flow, particularly in a perihilar distribution (*arrows*).

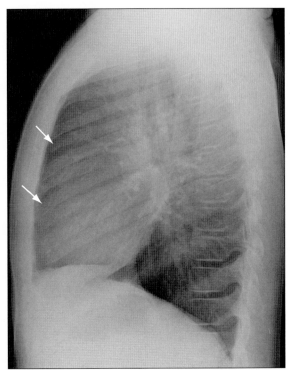

Figure 2. Lateral chest radiograph shows mild enlargement of the right atrium and right ventricle (*arrows*).

Case 35

DEMOGRAPHICS/CLINICAL HISTORY

The patient is a newborn with respiratory distress and low-set ears.

FINDINGS

Maxillofacial computed tomography (CT) scan (Fig. 1) shows bilateral choanal atresia. An enlarged heart with increased pulmonary vasculature reflects the patient's congenital heart anomaly (ventricular septal defect in this case) (Fig. 2). CT scan of the temporal bones (Fig. 3) shows decreased number of cochlear turns, dysplastic posterior and superior semicircular canals, and absence of the lateral semicircular canal.

DISCUSSION

Definition/Background

The diagnosis of CHARGE syndrome (*c*oloboma, *h*eart defect, *a*tresia choanae, *r*etarded growth and development, *g*enital hypoplasia, *e*ar anomalies) is typically made by the presence of four major criteria (ocular coloboma, choanal atresia or stenosis, cranial nerve anomalies, and characteristic ear anomalies) or three major and three minor criteria (minor criteria include cardiac malformations, genital hypoplasia, cleft lip/palate, tracheoesophageal fistula, distinctive facies, and growth and developmental delay). Mutations in the *CHD7* gene (8q12) have been found in more than 50% of patients with CHARGE syndrome in two large series.

CHARACTERISTIC CLINICAL FEATURES

Clinical findings consist of coloboma (iris or retinal), heart murmurs, genital hypoplasia, retardation, unusually shaped and low-set ears, and cranial nerve dysfunction.

Characteristic Radiologic Findings

Choanal atresia and retinal colobomas are shown on maxillofacial CT and magnetic resonance imaging (MRI). Findings of heart anomalies vary and are best shown by echocardiography and MRI. Characteristic findings on CT of the temporal bones include one or more of the following: hypoplastic incus, decreased numbers of turns to the cochlea (Mondini defect), and absent semicircular canals.

Less Common Radiologic Manifestations

Cranial nerve anomalies, renal anomalies, hand anomalies, and cleft lip/palate are less commonly shown on imaging.

Differential Diagnosis

- VACTERL association
- DiGeorge syndrome
- Velocardiofacial syndrome

Discussion

VACTERL (*v*ertebral abnormalities, *a*nal atresia, *c*ardiac abnormalities, *t*racheoesophageal fistula or *e*sophageal atresia, *r*enal agenesis and dysplasia, and *l*imb defects) association also can have cardiac, renal, and hand anomalies and tracheoesophageal fistula; however, the VACTERL association does not tend to have the other criteria necessary for CHARGE syndrome.

Diagnosis

CHARGE syndrome

Suggested Readings

Blake KD, Prasad C: CHARGE syndrome. Orphanet J Rare Dis 1:34, 2006.

Harris J, Robert E, Källén B: Epidemiology of choanal atresia with special reference to the CHARGE association. Pediatrics 99:363-367, 1997.

Morimoto AK, Wiggins RH 3rd, Hudgins PA, et al: Absent semicircular canals in CHARGE syndrome: Radiologic spectrum of findings. AJNR Am J Neuroradiol 27:1663-1671, 2006.

Tellier AL, Cormier-Daire V, Abadie V, et al: CHARGE syndrome: Report of 47 cases and review. Am J Med Genet 76:402-409, 1998.

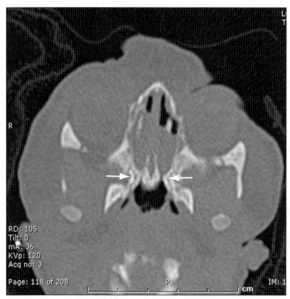

Figure 1. CT scan shows bilateral choanal atresia *(arrows)*.

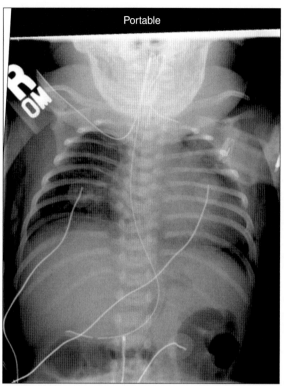

Figure 2. Radiograph shows enlarged heart with increased pulmonary vasculature, which reflects the patient's congenital heart anomaly (ventricular septal defect).

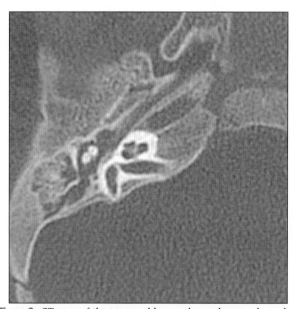

Figure 3. CT scan of the temporal bones shows decreased number of cochlear turns, dysplastic posterior and superior semicircular canals, and absence of the lateral semicircular canal.

Case 36

DEMOGRAPHICS/CLINICAL HISTORY

The patient is a 2-day-old girl diagnosed prenatally with Holt-Oram syndrome, now presenting with perioral cyanosis and trouble breastfeeding.

FINDINGS

An anteroposterior radiograph of the chest (Fig. 1) reveals an enlarged cardiac silhouette and shunt vascularity in the lungs, secondary to a large ventricular septal defect (VSD). Anteroposterior radiographs of the hands (Figs. 2 and 3) show radial ray anomalies bilaterally.

DISCUSSION

Definition/Background
This patient had a positive family history of Holt-Oram syndrome; her mother and sister had the syndrome. Holt-Oram syndrome is an autosomal dominant condition.

Characteristic Clinical Features
Cardiac anomalies are common in patients with Holt-Oram syndrome, the most common anomalies being atrial septal defect and VSD (this patient had VSD). The most common limb anomalies are radial ray anomalies.

Characteristic Radiologic Findings
An echocardiogram performed on the first day of life revealed a large VSD. This patient also has syndactyly involving the upper extremities and a triphalangeal thumb on the right side.

Differential Diagnosis
- Fanconi anemia
- VACTERL association
- Thrombocytopenia–absent radius syndrome

Discussion
Patients with Fanconi anemia have radial ray abnormalities, but they also have increased incidence of malignancy, pancytopenia, renal abnormalities, and mental retardation, among other congenital abnormalities. Thrombocytopenia–absent radius syndrome is characterized by thrombocytopenia and absent radii bilaterally. The thumb is present.

Diagnosis
Holt-Oram syndrome

Suggested Readings
Basson CT, Cowley GS, Solomon SD, et al: The clinical and genetic spectrum of the Holt-Oram syndrome (heart-hand syndrome). N Engl J Med 330:885-891, 1994.
Sletten LJ, Pierpont ME: Variation in severity of cardiac disease in Holt-Oram syndrome. Am J Med Genet 65:128-132, 1996.

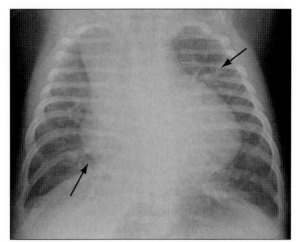

Figure 1. Anteroposterior radiograph of the chest shows enlarged cardiac silhouette (*arrow*) and enlarged pulmonary vessels indicative of shunt vascularity (*arrow*).

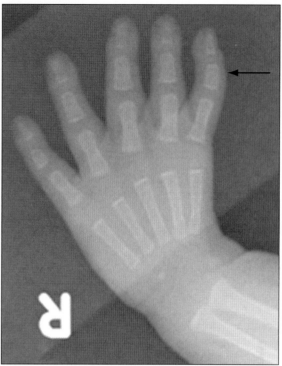

Figure 2. Anteroposterior radiograph of the right hand reveals a triphalangeal thumb (*arrow*).

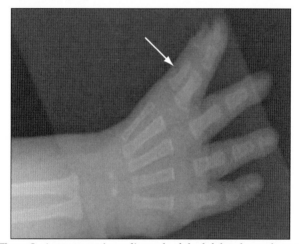

Figure 3. Anteroposterior radiograph of the left hand reveals syndactyly of the first and second digits (*arrow*).

Case 37

DEMOGRAPHICS/CLINICAL HISTORY

The patient is a newborn boy with respiratory distress.

FINDINGS

An anteroposterior radiograph of the chest (Fig. 1) reveals asymmetric lung vascularity, with increased pulmonary blood flow and pulmonary edema affecting the right lung. Contrast-enhanced computed tomography (CT) angiography (Figs. 2 and 3) shows the anomalous origin of the left pulmonary artery from the right pulmonary artery, and its anomalous course behind the trachea and anterior to the esophagus.

DISCUSSION

Definition/Background

Left pulmonary sling is a rare vascular anomaly in which the left pulmonary artery arises from the right pulmonary artery and passes posterior to the trachea and anterior to the esophagus to reach the left hilum. This anomaly produces symptoms of airway obstruction before age 1 year in most patients.

Characteristic Clinical Features

Infants present with respiratory distress. Associated tracheobronchial anomalies and heart defects are common.

Characteristic Radiologic Findings

Chest radiographs show unequal aeration of the lungs depending on the degree of tracheobronchial narrowing and diminished size of the left pulmonary artery branches. CT angiography shows the abnormal takeoff of the left pulmonary artery from the right pulmonary artery and its course between the trachea and esophagus.

Less Common Radiologic Manifestations

Barium swallow can show a smooth indentation on the anterior wall of the esophagus at the level of the carina.

Differential Diagnosis

■ Scimitar syndrome

Discussion

Scimitar syndrome is characterized by partial or total anomalous pulmonary venous return to the inferior vena cava. On chest radiography, the abnormal vein creates a curve bulging into the right chest from the mediastinum that resembles the Turkish sword called a scimitar. Patients also may have dextrocardia, hypoplasia of the right lung or pulmonary artery, malformation of the bronchi, and systemic arterial supply to the right lung. Infants usually present with congestive heart failure and severe pulmonary hypertension.

Diagnosis

Pulmonary sling

Suggested Readings

Lee KH, Yoon CS, Choe KO, et al: Use of imaging for assessing anatomical relationships of tracheobronchial anomalies associated with left pulmonary artery sling. Pediatr Radiol 31:269-278, 2001.

Newman B, Meza MP, Towbin RB, et al: Left pulmonary artery sling: Diagnosis and delineation of associated tracheobronchial anomalies with MRI. Pediatr Radiol 26:661-668, 1996.

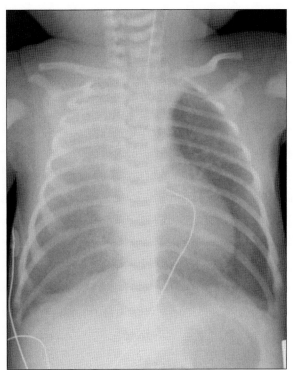

Figure 1. Anteroposterior radiograph of the infant's chest reveals asymmetric pulmonary blood flow with increased blood flow to the right lung and pulmonary edema.

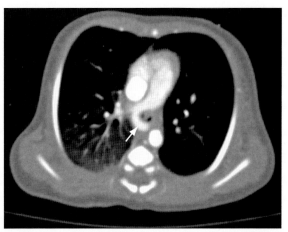

Figure 2. Axial contrast-enhanced CT angiography at the level of the main pulmonary artery shows the abnormal origin of the left pulmonary artery from the posterior aspect of the right pulmonary artery (*arrow*). The left pulmonary artery courses posterior to the trachea and anterior to the esophagus.

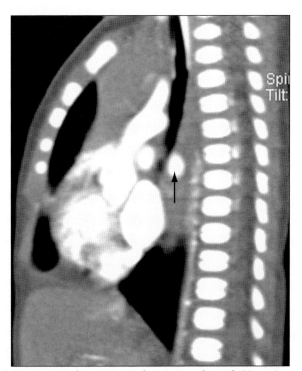

Figure 3. Sagittal reconstructed contrast-enhanced CT angiography through the chest shows the left pulmonary artery coursing posterior to the trachea (*arrow*).

Case 38

DEMOGRAPHICS/CLINICAL HISTORY

The patient is a 3-month-old boy with persistent wheezing.

FINDINGS

Fluoroscopic images acquired as part of an upper gastrointestinal (GI) examination (Figs. 1 and 2) reveal an obliquely oriented impression on the posterior esophagus. The patient has a right-sided aortic arch. Magnetic resonance imaging (MRI) of the chest (Figs. 3 and 4) shows a right-sided aortic arch and a prominent diverticulum of Kommerell arising from the proximal descending aorta.

DISCUSSION

Definition/Background
A vascular ring is a congenital condition in which the anomalous configuration of the arch and associated vessels surrounds the trachea and esophagus, forming a complete or incomplete ring around them. It constitutes 1% of all cardiovascular anomalies.

Characteristic Clinical Features
Symptoms depend on the degree of mass effect on the trachea and esophagus. Infants often present with cough, wheezing, stridor, or repeated upper respiratory tract infections.

Characteristic Radiologic Findings
A right-sided aortic arch is a component of the most common vascular rings (i.e., double aortic arch and right arch with aberrant subclavian artery). The trachea is narrowed at the level of the ring.

Differential Diagnosis
- Double aortic arch

Discussion
A double aortic arch is a complete vascular ring in which there are right and left aortic arches that encircle the trachea and esophagus. In most cases, the right arch is dominant.

Diagnosis
Vascular ring

Suggested Readings
Beekman RP, Hazekamp MG, Sobotka MA, et al: A new diagnostic approach to vascular rings and pulmonary slings: The role of MRI. Magn Reson Imaging 16:137-145, 1998.

Hernanz-Schulman M: Vascular rings: A practical approach to imaging diagnosis. Pediatr Radiol 35:961-979, 2005.

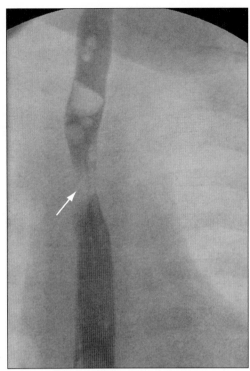

Figure 1. Anteroposterior fluoroscopic spot image of the chest obtained during upper GI study reveals obliquely oriented impression on the upper esophagus (*arrow*). The patient has a right-sided aortic arch.

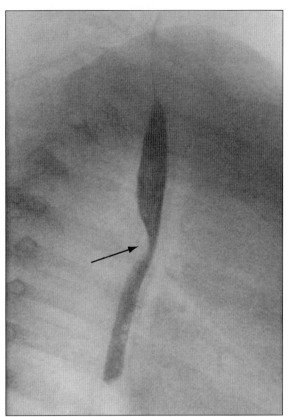

Figure 2. Lateral fluoroscopic spot image of the chest from upper GI examination reveals posterior impression on the esophagus (*arrow*).

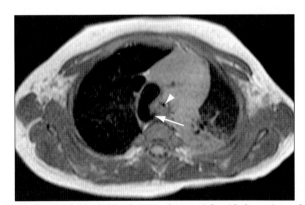

Figure 3. Axial black-blood MRI shows right-sided aortic arch with diverticulum of Kommerell projecting behind the esophagus (*arrow*). The trachea is significantly narrowed at this level (*arrowhead*).

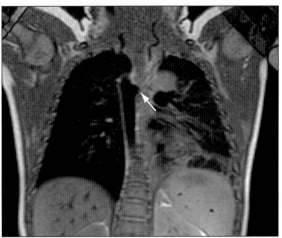

Figure 4. Coronal black-blood MRI shows right-sided aortic arch with a diverticulum of Kommerell (*arrow*).

Case 39

DEMOGRAPHICS/CLINICAL HISTORY

The patient is a newborn boy (born at 33 weeks' gestation) with dysmorphic features, cyanosis, and a heart murmur.

FINDINGS

An anteroposterior chest radiograph (Fig. 1) shows enlargement of the cardiac silhouette and increased pulmonary blood flow. The superior mediastinal contour is relatively narrow.

DISCUSSION

Definition/Background
Truncus arteriosus consists of a single vessel arising from the right and left ventricles and a ventricular septal defect.

Characteristic Clinical Features
The left-to-right shunting of blood that occurs in truncus arteriosus causes heart failure in infancy, which can manifest as tachycardia, tachypnea, cyanosis, and failure to thrive.

Characteristic Radiologic Findings
Plain radiographs show increased pulmonary vascular markings related to pulmonary overcirculation and interstitial edema. The heart is enlarged. Echocardiography is the modality of choice for more definitive evaluation.

Less Common Radiologic Manifestations
Right aortic arch is present in 30% of patients. Thymic atrophy may also be present; it causes the superior mediastinal contour to appear narrow.

Differential Diagnosis
- Transposition of the great vessels
- Total anomalous pulmonary venous return
- Hypoplastic left heart
- Single ventricle

Discussion
Total anomalous pulmonary venous connection (TAPVC) is a cyanotic congenital heart defect in which the pulmonary veins do not drain directly into the left atrium of the heart. Single-ventricle cardiac lesions consist of various disorders in which there is only a single functional ventricle. Hypoplastic left heart syndrome is a type of single-ventricle disorder.

Diagnosis
Truncus arteriosus

Suggested Readings
Kelley MJ, Jaffe CC, Shoum SM, et al: A radiographic and echocardiographic approach to cyanotic congenital heart disease. Radiol Clin North Am 18:411-440, 1980.

Waldman JD, Wernly JA: Cyanotic congenital heart disease with decreased pulmonary blood flow in children. Pediatr Clin North Am 46:385-404, 1999.

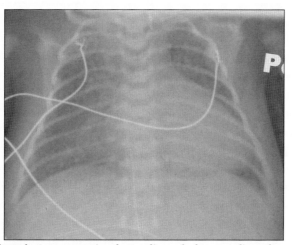

Figure 1. Anteroposterior chest radiograph shows cardiac enlargement, increased pulmonary blood flow, and a relatively narrow superior mediastinal contour.

Case 40

DEMOGRAPHICS/CLINICAL HISTORY

The patient is a 1-year-old girl with a family history of hereditary hemorrhagic telangiectasia.

FINDINGS

Fluoroscopic spot images were obtained as part of a pulmonary angiogram after a catheter was placed in the right descending pulmonary artery branches and contrast agent was injected. An image acquired during injection (Fig. 1) reveals many enlarged feeding arterial branches in the right lower lobe. An image acquired several seconds later (Fig. 2) shows contrast agent within a pulmonary vein entering the left atrium. The findings are consistent with an arteriovenous malformation in the right lower lobe.

DISCUSSION

Definition/Background

Hereditary hemorrhagic telangiectasia, also known as Osler-Weber-Rendu syndrome, consists of arteriovenous malformations (AVMs) of the skin, mucous membranes, and viscera.

Characteristic Clinical Features

Although AVMs are present since birth, patients without a known family history may present later in adult life. In some instances, patients may present with history of embolic stroke.

Characteristic Radiologic Findings

Most pulmonary AVMs occur in the lower lobes. They appear on chest radiographs as soft tissue nodules of various sizes.

Less Common Radiologic Manifestations

Computed tomography (CT) angiography, or dedicated angiography, shows enlarged feeding arteries and an early draining vein.

Differential Diagnosis

- Pulmonary artery aneurysm
- Pulmonary varix

Discussion

Pulmonary artery aneurysm is a focal dilation of a pulmonary artery branch, and it occurs rarely in children. Pulmonary varix usually occurs on the right side, and it consists of dilation of a pulmonary vein, often at the level of the hilum.

Diagnosis

Hemorrhagic telangiectasia, hereditary

Suggested Readings

Jaskolka J, Wu L, Chan RP, et al: Imaging of hereditary hemorrhagic telangiectasia. AJR Am J Roentgenol 183:307-314, 2004.

Manson D, Traubici J, Mei-Zahav M, et al: Pulmonary nodular opacities in children with hereditary hemorrhagic telangiectasia. Pediatr Radiol 37:264-268, 2007.

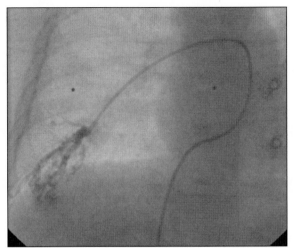

Figure 1. Fluoroscopic spot image obtained during pulmonary artery angiography shows a catheter with its tip in the right descending pulmonary artery and contrast agent opacifying several enlarged feeding arterial branches in the right lower lobe.

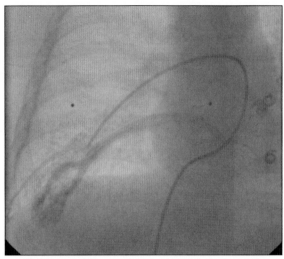

Figure 2. Fluoroscopic spot image obtained during pulmonary artery angiography several seconds later shows contrast agent quickly opacifying a pulmonary vein that drains into the left atrium.

Case 41

DEMOGRAPHICS/CLINICAL HISTORY

The patient is a newborn boy with a prenatal diagnosis of hypoplastic left heart syndrome (HLHS).

FINDINGS

Chest radiograph (Fig. 1) performed on the first day of life shows a relatively normal heart size and normal pulmonary vasculature. An anteroposterior chest radiograph performed after a Norwood procedure shows persistent cardiomegaly and mild worsening of pulmonary edema (Fig. 2).

DISCUSSION

Definition/Background

HLHS accounts for 2% of all congenital heart disease, and two thirds of these patients are male. HLHS encompasses a spectrum of diseases characterized by a hypoplastic left ventricle associated with obstruction of inflow and outflow to and from the ventricle.

Characteristic Clinical Features

HLHS consists of a hypoplastic ascending aorta, aortic valve, left ventricle, left atrium, mitral atresia or stenosis, and patent ductus arteriosus. Coarctation of the aorta coexists in 80% of patients. Most patients present within the first 2 weeks of life with cyanosis and tachypnea.

Characteristic Radiologic Findings

Findings on chest radiography may be normal. Pulmonary vascularity is normal in the first few days, but progressively increases with development of pulmonary venous congestion. Echocardiography is required for the diagnosis.

Less Common Radiologic Manifestations

In severe cases of HLHS, there is cardiomegaly with globular cardiac silhouette.

Differential Diagnosis

- Total anomalous pulmonary venous connection with obstruction
- Pulmonic atresia
- Cor triatriatum
- Mitral atresia
- Aortic stenosis (critical)
- Aortic coarctation (severe)
- Cardiomyopathy

Discussion

Cor triatriatum refers to an anomaly of pulmonary venous development in which the pulmonary veins connect to an accessory chamber of the left atrium with a small opening into the true left atrium.

Diagnosis

Hypoplastic left heart syndrome

Suggested Reading

Bardo DM, Frankel DG, Applegate KE, et al: Hypoplastic left heart syndrome. RadioGraphics 21:705-717, 2001.

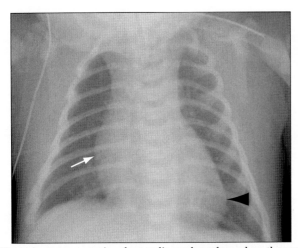

Figure 1. Anteroposterior chest radiograph performed on the second day of life reveals a mildly increased heart size with prominence of the right atrium (*arrow*) and right ventricle, which forms the left heart border (*arrowhead*). The patient has mild pulmonary edema and has been intubated.

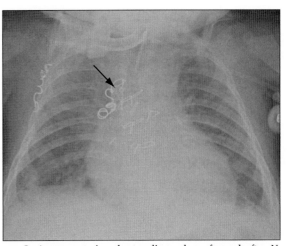

Figure 2. Anteroposterior chest radiograph performed after Norwood procedure shows persistent cardiomegaly and mild worsening of pulmonary edema. This patient has a stent projecting over the superior vena cava (*arrow*) and several vascular embolization coils.

Case 42

DEMOGRAPHICS/CLINICAL HISTORY

The patient is a 3-month-old girl with cyanosis.

FINDINGS

An anteroposterior portable chest radiograph (Fig. 1) shows an enlarged cardiac silhouette. The normal contour of the aortic arch along the left superior mediastinum is not appreciated on chest radiograph. Axial images from a contrast-enhanced computed tomography (CT) scan of the chest shows a significant narrowing in the caliber of the aorta at the level of the isthmus (Fig. 2) with normal caliber distal to this level (Fig. 3). A sagittal reformatted image (Fig. 4) shows the level of the coarctation better.

DISCUSSION

Definition/Background
Coarctations are most often juxtaductal in location, just distal to the origin of the left subclavian artery.

Characteristic Clinical Features
Anomalies that are commonly associated with aortic coarctation include bicuspid aortic valve, ventricular septal defect, patent ductus arteriosus, and hypoplastic left heart syndrome.

Characteristic Radiologic Findings
Chest radiographs show cardiomegaly and pulmonary edema. A "figure-3" sign is often seen along the left upper mediastinal border, which is secondary to prominence of the aortic knob above the level of the coarctation.

Less Common Radiologic Manifestations
Contrast-enhanced chest CT is the modality of choice to show the aortic arch anatomy. A focal or segmental narrowing of the arch at the level of the ductus arteriosus is best appreciated on oblique sagittal reformatted images.

Differential Diagnosis
- Pseudocoarctation of the aorta
- Aortic stenosis (congenital)
- Hypoplastic left heart syndrome

Discussion
Pseudocoarctation of the aorta refers to kinking of the aorta at the level of the ligamentum arteriosum without hemodynamically significant narrowing. Aortic stenosis (congenital) may be caused by a unicuspid or bicuspid aortic valve (valvular stenosis), a thin fibromuscular diaphragm encircling the left ventricular outflow tract (subvalvular stenosis), or a narrowing of the ascending aorta above the sinuses of Valsalva (supravalvular stenosis). Hypoplastic left heart syndrome is a spectrum of disease that is characterized by hypoplasia of the left ventricle and by various degrees of obstruction of the inflow in and outflow from the left ventricle.

Diagnosis
Coarctation, aortic

Suggested Readings

Abbruzzese PA, Aidala E: Aortic coarctation: An overview. J Cardiovasc Med 8:123-128, 2007.

Van Son JA, Falk V, Schneider P, et al: Repair of coarctation of the aorta in neonates and young infants. J Card Surg 12:139-146, 1997.

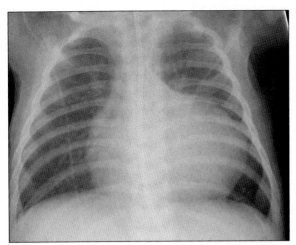

Figure 1. Anteroposterior portable chest radiograph shows enlarged cardiac silhouette. Normal contour of the aortic arch along the left superior mediastinum is not appreciated.

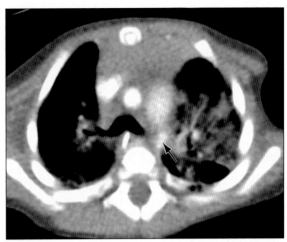

Figure 2. Axial image from contrast-enhanced CT scan of the chest shows significant narrowing in the caliber of the aorta at the level of the isthmus (*arrow*).

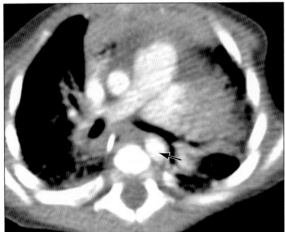

Figure 3. Axial image from contrast-enhanced CT scan of the chest shows normal caliber of the aorta distal to the level of coarctation (*arrow*).

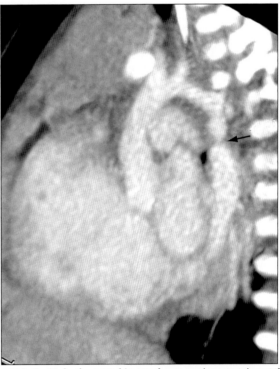

Figure 4. Sagittal reformatted image shows aortic narrowing at the level of coarctation better (*arrow*).

Case 43

DEMOGRAPHICS/CLINICAL HISTORY

The patient is a newborn boy with prenatally diagnosed tetralogy of Fallot (TOF).

FINDINGS

An anteroposterior radiograph of the chest (Fig. 1) reveals cardiac enlargement with an upturned cardiac apex. The aortic arch is right-sided, and there is an abnormal concavity at the pulmonary artery. The pulmonary vascularity appears normal in this patient.

DISCUSSION

Definition/Background
TOF is a common form of congenital heart disease that accounts for 4% to 8% of all congenital cardiac lesions.

Characteristic Clinical Features
Patients present with cyanosis, usually by age 3 months.

Characteristic Radiologic Findings
TOF consists of ventricular septal defect, anterior displacement of the aortic valve, right ventricular outflow tract obstruction, and right ventricular hypertrophy. Radiographs show a slightly enlarged cardiac silhouette with an upturned apex and a concave pulmonary artery segment.

Less Common Radiologic Manifestations
Right-sided aortic arch is present in approximately 25% of cases.

Differential Diagnosis
- Truncus arteriosus
- Pulmonic stenosis

Discussion
Truncus arteriosus is a congenital heart disease characterized by a single great artery that leaves the base of the heart and gives rise to the coronary, pulmonary, and systemic arteries. Affected infants appear physically underdeveloped and cyanotic. Chest radiography usually shows increased pulmonary arterial blood flow manifesting as increased pulmonary vascular markings. A right-sided aortic arch, cardiomegaly, and increased pulmonary vascularity strongly suggest truncus arteriosus. Pulmonic stenosis refers to abnormal stenosis of the pulmonic valve, a feature that may be present in TOF.

Diagnosis
Tetralogy of Fallot

Suggested Readings

Boechat MI, Ratib O, Williams PL, et al: Cardiac MR imaging and MR angiography for assessment of complex tetralogy of Fallot and pulmonary atresia. RadioGraphics 25:1535-1546, 2005.

Fellows KE, Weinberg PM, Baffa JM, et al: Evaluation of congenital heart disease with MR imaging: Current and coming attractions. AJR Am J Roentgenol 159:925-931, 1992.

Norton KI, Tong C, Glass RB, et al: Cardiac MR imaging assessment following tetralogy of Fallot repair. RadioGraphics 26:197-211, 2006.

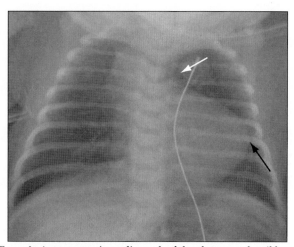

Figure 1. Anteroposterior radiograph of the chest reveals mild cardiomegaly with an upturned cardiac apex (*black arrow*), a concave pulmonary artery segment (*white arrow*), and a right-sided aortic arch. Pulmonary blood flow is normal.

Case 44

DEMOGRAPHICS/CLINICAL HISTORY

The patient is a 2-week-old boy with respiratory distress and cardiac abnormalities noticed on prenatal ultrasound.

FINDINGS

An anteroposterior chest radiograph (Fig. 1) shows a markedly enlarged cardiac silhouette and signs of pulmonary edema. A four-chamber view from a cardiac magnetic resonance imaging (MRI) examination (Fig. 2) shows marked thickening of the interventricular septum and the free wall of the left ventricle.

DISCUSSION

Definition/Background

Cardiomyopathy refers to chronic myocardial dysfunction. There are four major types: dilated, hypertrophic, restrictive, and arrhythmogenic.

Characteristic Clinical Features

This patient had severe hypertrophic cardiomyopathy, and he required cardiac transplantation for severe cardiac failure when he was 2 weeks old. As with most cases, the cause was unknown.

Characteristic Radiologic Findings

Cardiac MRI examination in patients with hypertrophic cardiomyopathy shows thickening of the wall of the left ventricle, including the interventricular septum.

Differential Diagnosis

- Complex heart disease
- Glycogen storage disease
- Pericardial effusion
- Aortic coarctation (prenatal/neonatal)

Discussion

Glycogen storage diseases result from an enzyme defect that leads to abnormal glycogen deposition in the heart, which can lead to cardiac failure. A large pericardial effusion leading to cardiac tamponade can result in enlargement of the cardiac silhouette on the chest radiograph and signs of heart failure.

Diagnosis

Cardiomyopathy

Suggested Readings

Braunwald E, Seidman CE, Sigwart U: Contemporary evaluation and management of hypertrophic cardiomyopathy. Circulation 106:1312-1316, 2002.

Nishimura RA, Holmes DR Jr: Clinical practice: Hypertrophic obstructive cardiomyopathy. N Engl J Med 350:1320-1327, 2004.

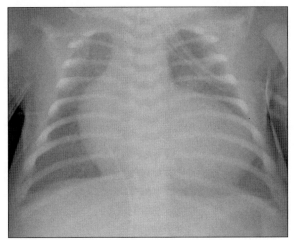

Figure 1. Anteroposterior chest radiograph shows marked enlargement of the cardiac silhouette and signs of pulmonary edema.

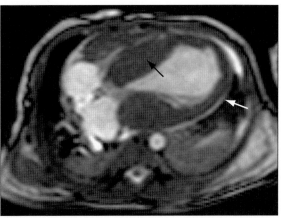

Figure 2. Four-chamber cine MRI view at end diastole from cardiac MRI examination shows severe asymmetric hypertrophy of the left ventricle, leading to severe left ventricular outflow tract obstruction and severe left ventricle dysfunction. The ventricular septum is abnormally thickened (*black arrow*). The patient also has a membranous ventricular septal defect and a trace pericardial effusion (*white arrow*).

Case 45

DEMOGRAPHICS/CLINICAL HISTORY

The patient is a 1-day-old girl with marked cyanosis.

FINDINGS

A portable chest radiograph (Fig. 1) shows a normal-sized cardiac silhouette and signs of pulmonary edema. Magnetic resonance angiography (MRA) examination of the pulmonary veins (Fig. 2) shows a common vein draining the right and left pulmonary veins, which drains into the infradiaphragmatic inferior vena cava.

DISCUSSION

Definition/Background

Total anomalous pulmonary venous return (TAPVR) is a congenital anomaly of the pulmonary veins, which connect to the systemic circulation rather than connecting normally with the left atrium. There are three types: supracardiac (type 1), cardiac (type 2), and infradiaphragmatic (type 3).

Characteristic Clinical Features

Most patients with infradiaphragmatic TAPVR (type 3) present with obstruction to pulmonary venous flow, which manifests as cyanosis, feeding difficulties, and respiratory distress.

Characteristic Radiologic Findings

Chest radiographs of infants with obstructive-type TAPVR often show evidence of pulmonary venous congestion and a normal heart size.

Less Common Radiologic Manifestations

Patients with type 1 TAPVR often present with the classic "snowman heart" configuration, which results from pulmonary venous drainage into the superior mediastinum.

Differential Diagnosis

- Hypoplastic left heart syndrome
- Truncus arteriosus
- Transposition of the great vessels

Discussion

Hypoplastic left heart syndrome is a cardiac abnormality in which the left-sided cardiac structures, including the left ventricle and aorta, are underdeveloped. Truncus arteriosus is a congenital heart condition in which the aorta and pulmonary artery arise from a common trunk. Transposition of the great arteries refers to several conditions in which the aorta and pulmonary artery are reversed (i.e., the aorta arises from the morphologic right ventricle, and the pulmonary artery arises from the morphologic left ventricle).

Diagnosis

Total anomalous pulmonary venous return

Suggested Readings

Ferguson EC, Krishnamurthy R, Oldham SA: Classic imaging signs of congenital cardiovascular abnormalities. RadioGraphics 27:1323-1334, 2007.

Valsangiacomo ER, Levasseur S, McCrindle BW, et al: Contrast-enhanced MR angiography of pulmonary venous abnormalities in children. Pediatr Radiol 22:92-98, 2003.

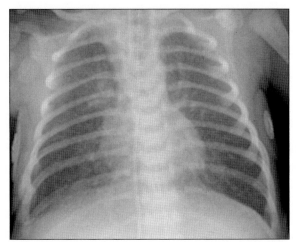

Figure 1. Portable chest radiograph shows that the infant has been intubated. Heart size is normal, and there is evidence of pulmonary venous congestion as shown by enlarged and indistinct pulmonary vascular markings extending to the periphery of the lungs bilaterally.

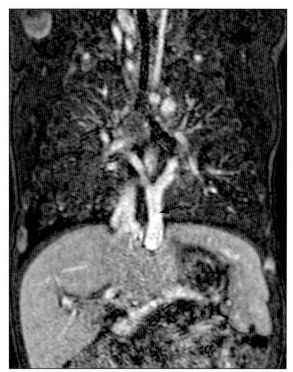

Figure 2. Coronal MRA of the chest shows common draining pulmonary vein connecting the common right and left pulmonary veins in a Y-shaped fashion (*arrow*). This draining vein crosses below the diaphragm and joins the inferior vena cava through a ductus venosus–hepatic vein connection.

Case 46

DEMOGRAPHICS/CLINICAL HISTORY

The patient is a 1-week-old infant with cyanosis.

FINDINGS

Anteroposterior and lateral chest radiographs (Figs. 1 and 2) show increased pulmonary blood flow to the lungs bilaterally. The cardiac silhouette is mildly enlarged, and the superior mediastinum is narrow, giving the heart an "egg-on-a-string" configuration.

DISCUSSION

Definition/Background

With transposition of the great arteries, there is a situation of ventriculoarterial discordance in which the aorta is anterior to the main pulmonary artery (i.e., opposite to the normal configuration). Blood from the right ventricle flows into the aorta, and blood from the left ventricle flows into the pulmonary artery.

Characteristic Clinical Features

Infants often present with various degrees of cyanosis within the first weeks of life, depending on the presence of a ventricular septal defect or pulmonary stenosis.

Characteristic Radiologic Findings

Chest radiographs vary, but they often reveal increased pulmonary vascularity. The heart has an "egg-on-a-string" appearance, with an ovoid, enlarged heart and a narrowed superior mediastinum, which appears narrow because of thymic atrophy and the arrangement of the great vessels.

Less Common Radiologic Manifestations

Other radiographic findings include cardiomegaly, lung hyperinflation, and depression of the diaphragms.

Differential Diagnosis

- Truncus arteriosus
- Total anomalous pulmonary venous return
- Hypoplastic left heart syndrome

Discussion

Truncus arteriosus is a congenital heart condition in which the aorta and pulmonary artery arise from a common trunk. In total anomalous pulmonary venous return, the pulmonary venous drainage does not return to the left atrium, but rather connects to a systemic supracardiac, cardiac, or infracardiac venous structure (i.e., inferior vena cava), which returns the blood to the right atrium. Hypoplastic left heart syndrome is a congenital lung disease characterized by hypoplasia of left-sided cardiac structures, including the left ventricle and aorta.

Diagnosis

Transposition of the great arteries

Suggested Readings

Ferguson EC, Krishnamurthy R, Oldham SA: Classic imaging signs of congenital cardiovascular abnormalities. RadioGraphics 27: 1323-1334, 2007.

Warnes CA: Transposition of the great arteries. Circulation 114: 2699-2709, 2006.

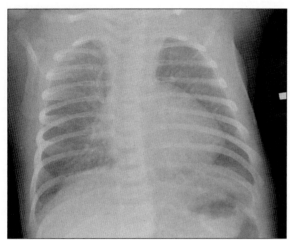

Figure 1. Anteroposterior chest radiograph shows mild cardiomegaly. Superior mediastinum is narrow, giving the heart an "egg-on-a-string" appearance. Pulmonary blood flow is increased.

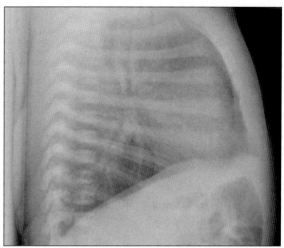

Figure 2. Lateral chest radiograph reveals hyperinflation of lungs with flattening of hemidiaphragms.

Case 47

DEMOGRAPHICS/CLINICAL HISTORY

The patient is a newborn girl born at 39 weeks' gestation with tachypnea and duskiness.

FINDINGS

A portable anteroposterior chest radiograph (Fig. 1) shows right lung hypoplasia, dextroposition of the heart, and a faint outline of a scimitar vein in the right lower lobe. Axial (Fig. 2) and coronal reformatted (Fig. 3) images from a contrast-enhanced computed tomography (CT) scan of the chest also shows right lung hypoplasia and dextroposition. The scimitar vein can be appreciated in the right lower lobe.

DISCUSSION

Definition/Background

Scimitar syndrome consists of hypoplasia of the right lung and right pulmonary artery, dextroposition of the heart, anomalous drainage of the right lung to the inferior vena cava, and pulmonary hypertension.

Characteristic Clinical Features

Patients usually present with respiratory distress. In some cases, the condition may go undetected for many years until patients present with symptoms of dyspnea.

Characteristic Radiologic Findings

Chest radiograph reveals a scimitar-shaped shadow in the right lower lung. The right lung may appear hypoplastic, as may the right hilum, with heart and mediastinal shift to the right.

Less Common Radiologic Manifestations

Multidetector CT with three-dimensional reconstructions is an effective means of showing the anatomy of the pulmonary venous drainage and clearly shows the anomalous right scimitar vein draining aberrantly into the inferior vena cava.

Differential Diagnosis

- Pulmonary hypoplasia
- Swyer-James-Macleod syndrome (pediatric lungs)
- Dextrocardia

Discussion

Pulmonary hypoplasia is a malformation characterized by incomplete development of lung tissue. It may represent a primary abnormality, although in many cases the pulmonary hypoplasia is secondary to another process, such as a congenital diaphragmatic hernia or a large abdominal mass. Chest radiographs show a small hemithorax on the ipsilateral side with shift of heart and mediastinal structures. Swyer-James-Macleod syndrome is a cause of a hyperlucent lung, which is believed to result from a prior childhood infection that leads to an obliterative bronchiolitis. Radiographs show a small, hyperlucent lung with diminished pulmonary vasculature and small hilum on the affected side. In dextrocardia, the heart is positioned on the right side of the body.

Diagnosis

Scimitar syndrome

Suggested Readings

Hornero F, Canovas S, Estornell J, et al: Scimitar syndrome: Multislice computer tomography with three dimensional reconstruction. Interact Cardiovasc Thorac Surg 2:341-344, 2003.

Wang CC, Wu ET, Chen SJ, et al: Scimitar syndrome: Incidence, treatment, and prognosis. Eur J Pediatr 167:155-160, 2008.

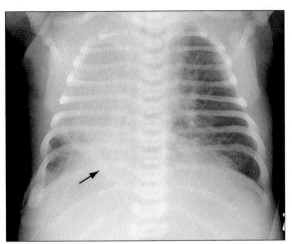

Figure 1. Portable anteroposterior chest radiograph shows right lung hypoplasia, dextroposition of the heart, and faint outline of a scimitar vein in the right lower lobe (*arrow*).

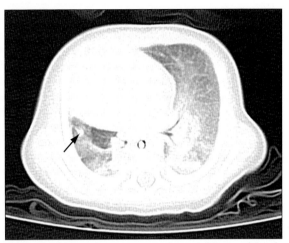

Figure 2. Axial image from contrast-enhanced CT scan of the chest in lung windows shows right lung hypoplasia and dextroposition. The scimitar vein can be appreciated in the right lower lobe (*arrow*).

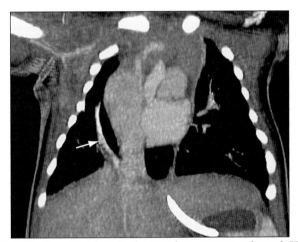

Figure 3. Coronal reformatted image from contrast-enhanced CT scan of the chest better illustrates the course of the scimitar vein (*arrow*).

Case 48

DEMOGRAPHICS/CLINICAL HISTORY

The patient is a 6-week-old girl with projectile vomiting.

FINDINGS

Anteroposterior radiograph of the abdomen (Fig. 1) shows a markedly distended stomach. Ultrasound of the pyloric region of the stomach (Fig. 2) shows thickening and elongation of the pyloric channel. No fluid passed through the pylorus during the entire scanning time.

DISCUSSION

Definition/Background
Pyloric stenosis occurs in approximately 2 to 5 neonates per 1000 births (in most white populations), and it is more common in boys.

Characteristic Clinical Features
Infants are normal at birth and then develop forceful, nonbilious vomiting when they are 3 to 6 weeks old.

Characteristic Radiologic Findings
Ultrasound reveals an abnormally thickened and elongated pylorus that is more than 3 mm thick and more than 14 mm long.

Less Common Radiologic Manifestations
On an upper gastrointestinal examination, the thickened, narrowed, elongated pyloric channel produces a "string" sign—a thin trickle of contrast material that resembles a frayed cotton string.

Differential Diagnosis
- Pylorospasm

Discussion
Pylorospasm is a transient spasm of the pylorus that may simulate pyloric stenosis, but the findings are not fixed, and the wall thickness is typically less than 3 mm.

Diagnosis
Pyloric stenosis

Suggested Readings
Hernanz-Schulman M: Infantile hypertrophic pyloric stenosis. Radiology 227:319-331, 2003.
Teele RL, Smith EH: Ultrasound in the diagnosis of idiopathic hypertrophic pyloric stenosis. N Eng J Med 296:1149-1150, 1977.

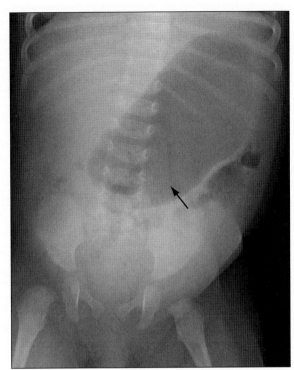

Figure 1. Anteroposterior abdominal radiograph shows markedly gas-distended stomach (*arrow*). Remainder of the bowel is decompressed.

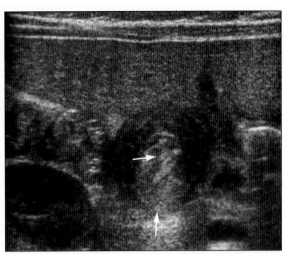

Figure 2. Transverse ultrasound image through pylorus reveals thickening of pylorus muscle (*arrow*) and redundancy of the mucosa, which has a pseudorosette appearance (*arrow*).

Case 49

DEMOGRAPHICS/CLINICAL HISTORY

The patient is a 2-year-old child with fever and abdominal pain.

FINDINGS

Longitudinal ultrasound scan of the right lower quadrant (Fig. 1) shows a tubular structure with internal echoes containing a large echogenic focus. A transverse view (Fig. 2) shows the tubular structure in cross section. A coronal reconstructed image (Fig. 3) from a computed tomography (CT) scan confirms the tubular structure as the significantly dilated inflamed appendix with surrounding inflammatory changes. Another coronal image (Fig. 4) shows a large density representing an appendicolith, corresponding to the echogenic structure seen on ultrasound.

DISCUSSION

Definition/Background

Appendicitis is a common cause of abdominal pain in children.

Characteristic Clinical Features

Classic clinical features include a history of periumbilical pain that migrated to the right lower quadrant, loss of appetite, fever, and increased white blood cell count.

Characteristic Radiologic Findings

The inflamed appendix is dilated and measures greater than 6 mm, and may contain internal debris or echogenic or dense foci representing appendicoliths. Doppler may show increased vascularity in the bowel wall. Surrounding inflammatory changes can be seen on ultrasound as increased periappendiceal echogenicity or increased attenuation in the fat surrounding the appendix. Free fluid can be seen, particularly in the right lower quadrant. Signs that indicate perforation include foci of free air and separate enhancing/fluid collections. Magnetic resonance imaging (MRI) is being used in older pediatric patients to reduce radiation exposure, with similar findings.

Differential Diagnosis

- Crohn disease (pediatric)
- Henoch-Schönlein purpura
- Cystic fibrosis (pediatric lungs)

Discussion

Crohn disease often causes inflammation in the terminal ileum and adjacent soft tissues and can mimic appendicitis. Henoch-Schönlein purpura can cause bowel wall thickening, making an ultrasound diagnosis more difficult, but clinical history can help. The appendix in patients with cystic fibrosis can be mildly enlarged as the result of inspissated mucus and can mimic appendicitis.

Diagnosis

Appendicitis

Suggested Readings

Darge K, Anupindi SA, Jaramillo D: MR imaging of the bowel: Pediatric applications. Magn Reson Imaging Clin N Am 16:467-478, 2008.

Doria AS, Moineddin R, Kellenberger CJ, et al: US or CT for diagnosis of appendicitis in children and adults? A meta-analysis. Radiology 241:83-94, 2006.

Peletti AB, Baldisserotto M: Optimizing US examination to detect the normal and abnormal appendix in children. Pediatr Radiol 36:1171-1176, 2006.

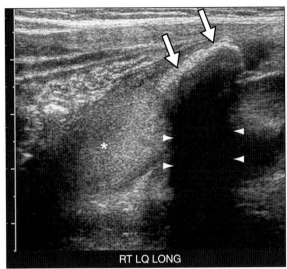

Figure 1. Longitudinal ultrasound of right lower quadrant shows a tubular structure with internal echoes (*asterisk*) containing an echogenic focus (*arrows*), with shadows (*arrowheads*), representing an appendicolith.

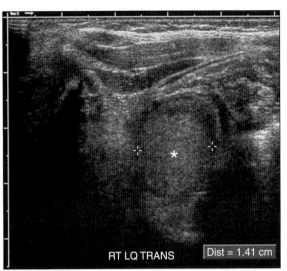

Figure 2. Transverse view shows tubular structure in cross section, with internal echoes (*asterisk*) and a diameter of 1.4 cm. Additional images showed the structure to be blind-ending (not shown).

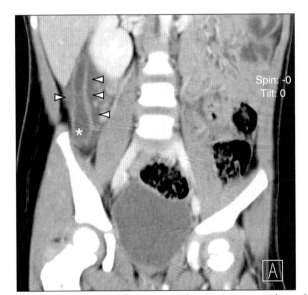

Figure 3. Coronal reconstructed image from a CT scan performed on the same patient confirms the tubular structure as the significantly dilated inflamed appendix (*asterisk*) with surrounding inflammatory changes (*arrowheads*).

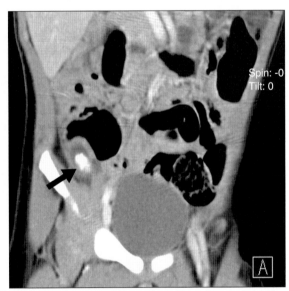

Figure 4. Another coronal image shows large density (*arrow*) representing an appendicolith, corresponding to the echogenic structure seen on ultrasound.

Case 50

DEMOGRAPHICS/CLINICAL HISTORY

The patient is a 10-day-old, premature infant with abdominal distention.

FINDINGS

An anteroposterior radiograph of the abdomen (Fig. 1) shows several mildly dilated loops of bowel in the mid-abdomen, mottled lucencies in the lower abdomen representing pneumatosis, and portal venous gas.

DISCUSSION

Definition/Background

Necrotizing enterocolitis (NEC) occurs mainly in premature infants, and it typically develops in the first 2 weeks of life.

Characteristic Clinical Features

Patients with NEC may have increased abdominal distention and bilious aspirates. They also may have guaiac-positive stools.

Characteristic Radiologic Findings

The hallmark of NEC on radiographs is dilated loops of bowel with mottled, cystic lucencies overlying the bowel wall, representing pneumatosis. Portal venous gas usually develops later in the disease process, as does pneumoperitoneum.

Less Common Radiologic Manifestations

Ultrasound shows echogenic gas within the bowel wall in infants with NEC. Ultrasound also can detect echogenic free intraperitoneal air in some cases.

Differential Diagnosis

■ Bowel ischemia

Discussion

Bowel ischemia may have many causes (e.g., severe cardiac disease) and may result in pneumatosis, portal venous gas, and bowel rupture.

Diagnosis

Necrotizing enterocolitis

Suggested Readings

Daneman A, Woodward S, de Silva M: The radiology of neonatal necrotizing enterocolitis (NEC): A review of 47 cases and the literature. Pediatr Radiol 7:70-77, 1978.

Epelman M, Daneman A, Navarro OM, et al: Necrotizing enterocolitis: Review of state-of-the-art imaging findings with pathologic correlation. RadioGraphics 27:285-305, 2007.

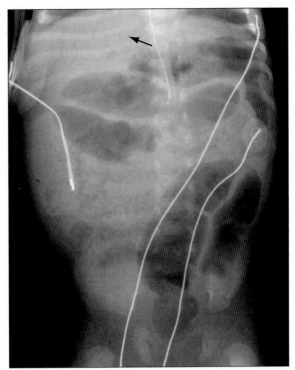

Figure 1. Anteroposterior abdominal radiograph shows diffuse mottled lucencies overlying multiple loops of bowel consistent with pneumatosis. Branching lucencies over the liver are consistent with portal venous gas (*arrow*).

Case 51

DEMOGRAPHICS/CLINICAL HISTORY

The patient is a 3-month-old infant presenting to the emergency department with bloody stool and lethargy.

FINDINGS

Anteroposterior radiographs of the abdomen (Figs. 1 and 2) reveal mildly dilated loops of small bowel with air-fluid levels and a paucity of gas in the right lower quadrant. Ultrasound scans of the abdomen (Figs. 3 and 4) reveal a heterogeneous mass within the right lower quadrant with alternating hypoechoic and hyperechoic layers, consistent with intussusception.

DISCUSSION

Definition/Background

Intussusception is prolapse of one part of the intestine into the lumen of an adjoining part, causing a bowel obstruction. It is most common in children 5 months to 3 years old.

Characteristic Clinical Features

Patients may present with abdominal pain, vomiting, lethargy, a palpable abdominal mass, or bloody, "currant jelly" stool.

Characteristic Radiologic Findings

Radiographic features of intussusception include a lack of air within the cecum and evidence of a soft tissue mass projecting within the bowel (i.e., crescent sign or target sign). On ultrasound, an intussusception resembles a kidney in the sagittal plane and a doughnut-shaped appearance in the transverse plane.

Differential Diagnosis
- Appendicitis
- Meckel diverticulum

Discussion

Appendicitis can mimic several abdominal conditions, including intussusception. Symptoms usually include pain in the right lower quadrant of the abdomen with local and referred rebound tenderness, overlying muscle spasm, and cutaneous hyperesthesia. With progression, patients have worsening pain, vomiting, nausea, and anorexia. Patients (usually infants) with intussusception usually present with vomiting, abdominal pain, passage of blood and mucus, lethargy, and a palpable abdominal mass; these symptoms may be preceded by an upper respiratory infection. Meckel diverticulum, a common congenital abnormality of the small intestine, is caused by incomplete obliteration of the vitelline duct (i.e., omphalomesenteric duct). Meckel diverticulum can act as a lead point for an ileocolic or ileoileal intussusception.

Diagnosis

Intussusception

Suggested Readings

Daneman A, Navarro O: Intussusception, part 1: A review of diagnostic approaches. Pediatr Radiol 33:79-85, 2003.

Ko HS, Schenk JP, Tröger J, et al: Current radiological management of intussusception in children. Eur Radiol 17:2411-2421, 2007.

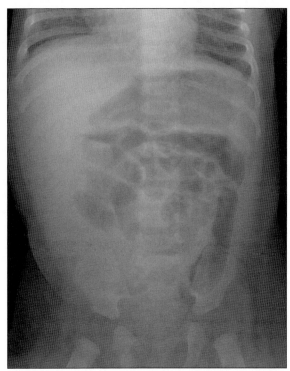

Figure 1. Supine radiograph of the abdomen reveals mildly dilated loops of small bowel. There is no air in the cecum.

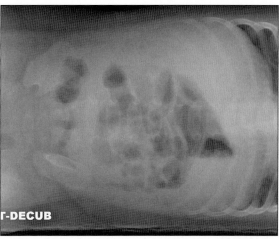

Figure 2. Left lateral decubitus radiograph of the abdomen shows multiple air-fluid levels in the bowel. There is no air in the cecum.

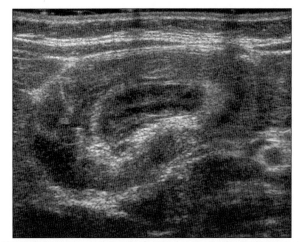

Figure 3. Sagittal ultrasound of right lower quadrant shows heterogeneous mass that resembles a kidney, consistent with an intussusception.

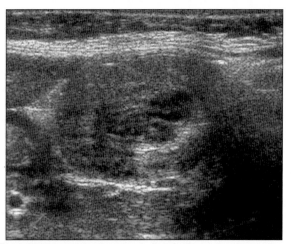

Figure 4. Transverse ultrasound of right lower quadrant shows mass with a target or doughnut shape, consistent with an intussusception.

Case 52

DEMOGRAPHICS/CLINICAL HISTORY

The patient is a 3-month-old infant with fullness in the left inguinal region.

FINDINGS

Longitudinal ultrasound in the left inguinal region (Fig. 1) shows a tubular, hypoechoic structure within the inguinal canal. Seconds later, the tubular structure appears to undergo peristalsis, changing its configuration (Fig. 2). A bowel wall signature is suggested, with alternating hypoechoic and hyperechoic bands. On color Doppler imaging (Fig. 3) seconds later, the structure shows vascularity within the wall and continues to change configuration, compatible with a bowel-containing inguinal hernia.

DISCUSSION

Definition/Background
Inguinal hernias can contain bowel or gonads, and they often are diagnosed by clinical examination.

Characteristic Clinical Features
Patients have fullness in the inguinal region, which is often reducible on examination.

Characteristic Radiologic Findings
Ultrasound, the imaging modality of choice, shows evidence of any viscera within the inguinal canal. Bowel should undergo peristalsis and show flow within the bowel wall. Evidence of inflammation, pain, and lack of peristalsis should raise suspicion for an incarcerated hernia.

Differential Diagnosis
■ Hydrocele of the spermatic cord or encysted hydrocele

Discussion
During the normal closure of the previously patent canal, fluid can be trapped within the canal, creating a tubular, hypoechoic structure, but it does not undergo peristalsis or have vascularity, and it does not communicate with the peritoneal cavity.

Diagnosis
Inguinal hernia

Suggested Reading
Graf JL, Caty MG, Martin DJ, Glick PL: Pediatric hernias. Semin Ultrasound CT MR 23:197-200, 2002.

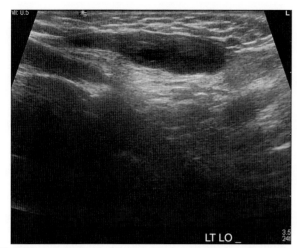

Figure 1. Longitudinal ultrasound in left inguinal region shows a tubular, hypoechoic structure within the inguinal canal.

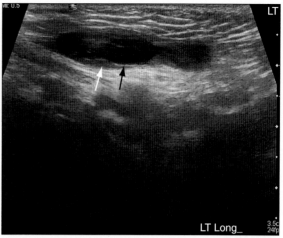

Figure 2. Seconds later, the tubular structure appears to undergo peristalsis, changing its configuration. A bowel wall signature is suggested, with alternating hypoechoic (*white arrow*) and hyperechoic (*black arrow*) bands.

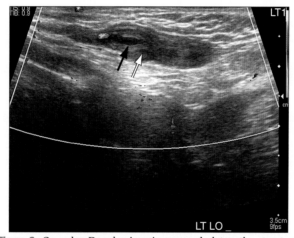

Figure 3. On color Doppler imaging seconds later, the structure shows vascularity within the wall (*black arrow*) and continues to change configuration (*white arrow*), compatible with a bowel-containing inguinal hernia.

Case 53

DEMOGRAPHICS/CLINICAL HISTORY

The diagnosis is a 9-day-old girl with persistent vomiting and failure to thrive.

FINDINGS

Anteroposterior (Fig. 1) and lateral (Fig. 2) fluoroscopic spot images from an upper gastrointestinal (GI) examination show contrast material in the stomach and the first through third portions of the duodenum, which are mildly dilated. There is an abrupt tapering of the duodenum at the third portion, and no contrast material was able to pass beyond this point.

DISCUSSION

Definition/Background

Congenital duodenal obstruction is the result of an embryologic defect in foregut development and is a common anomaly in infants. One third to one half of cases are associated with another congenital condition, such as a cardiac defect or Down syndrome.

Characteristic Clinical Features

Patients present soon after birth with symptoms of vomiting (usually bilious), failure to thrive, and potential electrolyte imbalances.

Characteristic Radiologic Findings

Upper GI examination is the imaging method of choice for diagnosis. Contrast material flows freely from the stomach to the duodenum, where the passage of contrast material abruptly terminates at the level of the obstruction. The duodenum is often dilated proximal to the obstruction.

Less Common Radiologic Manifestations

Plain radiographs may show a dilated stomach and proximal duodenum, with a paucity of gas in the distal bowel.

Differential Diagnosis
- Duodenal stenosis
- Annular pancreas
- Duodenal web

Discussion

Duodenal stenosis refers to conditions, including annular pancreas and duodenal web, in which there is a focal narrowing in the duodenum causing obstruction without complete atresia of the lumen. Annular pancreas refers to an abnormality of pancreatic development in which the pancreas completely encircles the duodenum and causes obstruction of the lumen. A duodenal web is a thin diaphragm that forms within the duodenal lumen, causing a characteristic windsock deformity and various degrees of obstruction.

Diagnosis

Duodenal atresia

Suggested Readings

Escobar MA, Ladd AP, Grosfeld JL, et al: Duodenal atresia and stenosis: Long-term follow-up over 30 years. J Pediatr Surg 39:867-871, 2004.

Mustafawi AR, Hassan ME: Congenital duodenal obstruction in children: A decade's experience. Eur J Pediatr Surg 18:93-97, 2008.

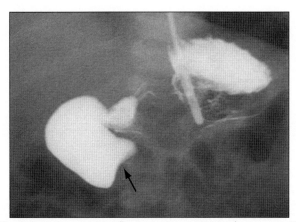

Figure 1. Anteroposterior fluoroscopic spot image from upper GI examination shows nasogastric tube in the stomach, which is decompressed. Contrast material outlines the stomach and the dilated first through third portions of the duodenum, with an abrupt tapering of the duodenum and complete obstruction to the passage of contrast material in the third portion (*arrow*).

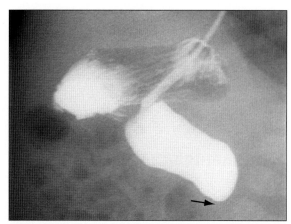

Figure 2. Right lateral fluoroscopic spot image from upper GI examination shows nasogastric tube in the stomach, which is decompressed. Contrast material outlines the stomach and the dilated first through third portions of the duodenum, with an abrupt tapering of the duodenum and complete obstruction to the passage of contrast material in the third portion (*arrow*).

Case 54

DEMOGRAPHICS/CLINICAL HISTORY

The patient is a newborn with copious oral secretions.

FINDINGS

A frontal radiograph of the chest and abdomen (Fig. 1) shows a coiled orogastric tube in the upper esophagus and a gasless abdomen. A frontal radiograph of the chest in another patient (Fig. 2) shows a coiled orogastric tube in a distended proximal esophageal pouch and gas in the stomach. A frontal radiograph of the abdomen (Fig. 3) confirms gas within the stomach and bowel, indicating the presence of a concomitant tracheoesophageal fistula.

DISCUSSION

Definition/Background

Esophageal atresia is commonly paired with a distal tracheoesophageal fistula, reflected by the presence of gas within the stomach and bowel. Esophageal atresia is often associated with other abnormalities, such as vertebral, cardiac, and radial anomalies.

Characteristic Clinical Features

The typical clinical history is increased secretions and inability to pass an orogastric tube.

Characteristic Radiologic Findings

Distention of the proximal esophagus and a coiled orogastric tube are the typical findings on radiography. If there is a tracheoesophageal fistula, gas is found in the stomach and bowel. If not, a gasless abdomen is noted. Associated anomalies can be seen, such as vertebral and radial anomalies.

Differential Diagnosis

■ Improper tube placement

Discussion

Although the coiling of an orogastric tube does not definitively indicate esophageal atresia, the clinical history usually includes several attempts at passage. Visualization of the dilated proximal esophageal pouch and lack of distal bowel gas lead to the correct diagnosis of esophageal atresia. If the diagnosis is in question, passage of the orogastric tube can be attempted under fluoroscopy.

Diagnosis

Esophageal atresia

Suggested Reading

Berrocal T, Madrid C, Novo S, et al: Congenital anomalies of the tracheobronchial tree, lung, and mediastinum: Embryology, radiology, and pathology. RadioGraphics 24:e17, 2004.

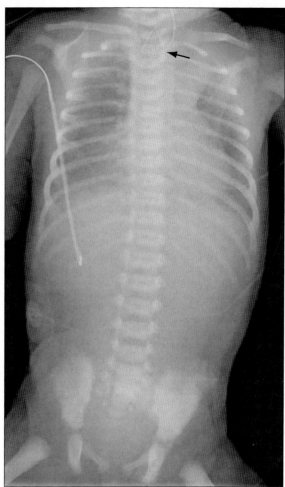

Figure 1. Frontal view of the chest and abdomen shows coiled oro-gastric tube (*arrow*) in upper esophagus and a gasless abdomen.

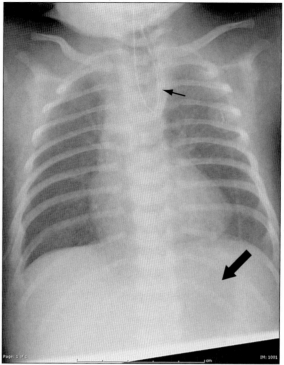

Figure 2. Frontal view of the chest in another patient shows coiled orogastric tube (*small arrow*) in a distended proximal esophageal pouch and gas in the stomach (*large arrow*).

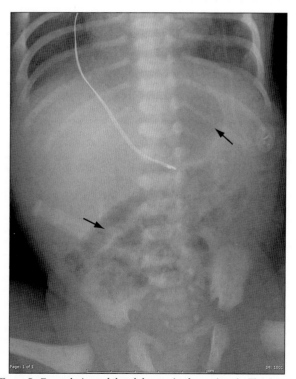

Figure 3. Frontal view of the abdomen in the patient in Fig. 2 con-firms gas within the stomach and bowel (*arrows*), indicating the presence of a concomitant tracheoesophageal fistula.

Case 55

DEMOGRAPHICS/CLINICAL HISTORY

The patient is a 1-day-old boy with abdominal distention and failure to pass meconium within 24 hours of birth.

FINDINGS

A supine radiograph (Fig. 1) shows dilated loops in the configuration of the colon. A supine view from a water-soluble contrast enema (Fig. 2) shows a redundant sigmoid colon, with a dilated proximal sigmoid colon and a narrow distal sigmoid and rectum. The transition point, in the mid-sigmoid colon, is not well opacified. A lateral view from the water-soluble contrast enema (Fig. 3) shows the corresponding appearance of the sigmoid, with a narrow distal sigmoid and rectum and dilated proximal sigmoid.

DISCUSSION

Definition/Background

Hirschsprung disease is a congenital partial or total colonic aganglionosis. Involvement of the colon is distal-to-proximal, and diagnosis is made by rectal biopsy.

Characteristic Clinical Features

Failure to pass meconium within the first 24 hours, abdominal distention, and constipation are common histories in Hirschsprung disease.

Characteristic Radiologic Findings

Radiographs may show dilated bowel. In partial colonic Hirschsprung disease, a contrast enema typically shows a normal-caliber or small-caliber distal colon and a dilated proximal colon, often to the region of the transition zone. In total colonic aganglionosis, the contrast enema may show a microcolon or a question-mark configuration, or may appear normal.

Differential Diagnosis

■ Small left colon syndrome (meconium plug syndrome)

Discussion

If the transition is near the splenic flexure, the contrast enema of small left colon syndrome can appear similar to Hirschsprung disease. If total colonic Hirschsprung disease is present, the contrast enema can show a false-negative result or mimic meconium ileus. Surgical rectal biopsy is diagnostic, determining the presence or absence of ganglion cells.

Diagnosis

Hirschsprung disease

Suggested Readings

Jamieson DH, Dundas SE, Belushi SA, et al: Does the transition zone reliably delineate aganglionic bowel in Hirschsprung's disease? Pediatr Radiol 34:811-815, 2004.

Stranzinger E, Dipietro MA, Teitelbaum DH, et al: Imaging of total colonic Hirschsprung disease. Pediatr Radiol 38:1162-1170, 2008.

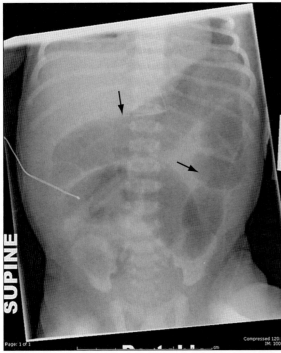

Figure 1. Supine radiograph shows dilated loops in the configuration of the colon (*arrows*).

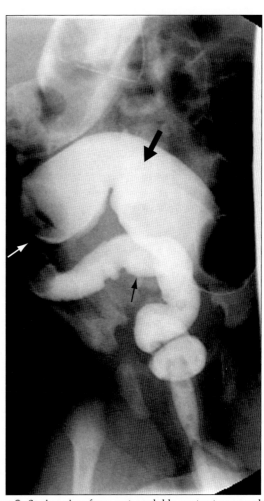

Figure 2. Supine view from water-soluble contrast enema shows redundant sigmoid colon, with dilated proximal sigmoid colon (*thick black arrow*) and narrow distal sigmoid and rectum (*thin black arrow*). The transition point (*white arrow*), in the mid-sigmoid colon, is not well opacified.

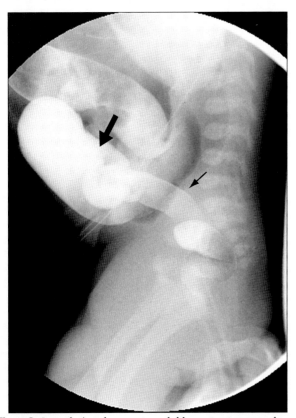

Figure 3. Lateral view from water-soluble contrast enema shows corresponding appearance of the distal colon, with a narrow distal sigmoid and rectum (*small arrow*) and dilated proximal sigmoid (*large arrow*).

Case 56

DEMOGRAPHICS/CLINICAL HISTORY

The patient is a newborn with dilated bowel suggested on prenatal ultrasound.

FINDINGS

Supine radiograph (Fig. 1) shows a few dilated loops of bowel, without evidence of distal bowel gas. Several areas of jejunal and ileal atresia were discovered at surgery.

DISCUSSION

Definition/Background

Jejunal atresias can occur along any portion of the jejunum and can be singular or multiple. Prenatal ischemic injury is the proposed mechanism.

Characteristic Clinical Features

Patients typically present in the newborn period with abdominal distention and feeding intolerance. Other patients are detected prenatally.

Characteristic Radiologic Findings

The presence of a few dilated proximal bowel loops in a neonate should suggest the diagnosis. Enema, if performed, shows a microcolon.

Less Common Radiologic Manifestations

A rare variant called "apple peel" jejunal atresia is associated with malrotation and has genetic implications. A contrast enema shows malrotation of the colon, suggesting the diagnosis.

Differential Diagnosis

- Ileal atresia
- Colonic atresia

Discussion

If many dilated loops are seen, the obstruction is more distal, suggesting ileal or colonic atresia.

Diagnosis

Jejunal atresia

Suggested Readings

Seashore JH, Collins FS, Markowitz RI, et al: Familial apple peel jejunal atresia: Surgical, genetic, and radiographic aspects. Pediatrics 80:540-544, 1987.

Wax JR, Hamilton T, Cartin A, et al: Congenital jejunal and ileal atresia: Natural prenatal sonographic history and association with neonatal outcome. J Ultrasound Med 25:337-342, 2006.

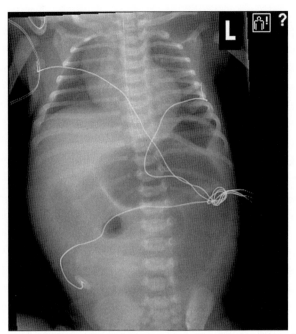

Figure 1. Supine radiograph shows a few dilated loops of bowel, without evidence of distal bowel gas.

Case 57

DEMOGRAPHICS/CLINICAL HISTORY

The patient is a 3-month-old boy with a cystic abdominal lesion noted on prenatal ultrasound examination.

FINDINGS

Ultrasound examination of the abdomen (Fig. 1) shows a round, hypoechoic mass in the right lower quadrant inferior to the lower pole of the right kidney and anterior to the psoas muscle. The mass has an outer hypoechoic layer and an inner hyperechoic layer consistent with gut signature and is intimately related to a loop of small bowel in the right lower quadrant (Fig. 2).

DISCUSSION

Definition/Background
A duplication cyst of the gastrointestinal tract most often occurs attached to the region of the ileum. It is usually a tubular or spherical structure lined with alimentary tract epithelium.

Characteristic Clinical Features
Children usually present within the first year of life with abdominal distention, vomiting, bleeding, pain, or palpable abdominal mass.

Characteristic Radiologic Findings
Characteristic ultrasound features of an ileal duplication cyst include an inner hypoechoic rim (representing mucosa or submucosa) and an outer hypoechoic layer (muscularis).

Less Common Radiologic Manifestations
Upper gastrointestinal (GI) examination with small bowel follow-through may reveal a submucosal mass extending into the lumen of the GI tract.

Differential Diagnosis
- Choledochal cyst
- Meckel diverticulum
- Mesenteric cyst

Discussion
A choledochal cyst is a congenital anomaly of the biliary tract often associated with an anomalous junction of the common bile duct with the pancreatic duct. Meckel diverticulum is a true bowel diverticulum that represents a vestigial remnant of the omphalomesenteric duct. It is located in the ileum and occurs in approximately 2% of the population. A mesenteric cyst can occur anywhere along the mesentery of the gastrointestinal tract and may be simple or complex. Mesenteric cysts most commonly occur in the small bowel mesentery on the mesenteric side of the bowel.

Diagnosis
Enteric duplication cyst

Suggested Readings
Hur J, Yoon CS, Kim MJ, et al: Imaging features of gastrointestinal tract duplications in infants and children: From oesophagus to rectum. Pediatr Radiol 37:691-699, 2007.

Macpherson RI: Gastrointestinal tract duplications: Clinical, pathologic, etiologic, and radiologic considerations. RadioGraphics 13:1063-1080, 1993.

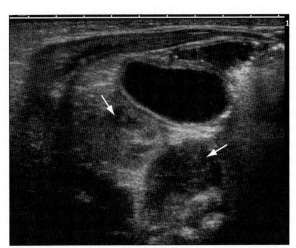

Figure 1. Ultrasound of the abdomen shows round, hypoechoic mass in right lower quadrant inferior to the lower pole of the right kidney (*white arrow*) and anterior to the psoas muscle (*arrow*).

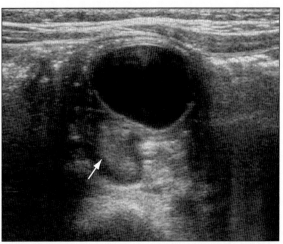

Figure 2. Ultrasound of right lower quadrant shows that mass has an outer hypoechoic layer and an inner hyperechoic layer consistent with gut signature and is intimately related to a loop of small bowel in the right lower quadrant (*arrow*).

Case 58

DEMOGRAPHICS/CLINICAL HISTORY

The patient is a 3-week-old infant with vomiting and weight loss.

FINDINGS

A spot film from an upper gastrointestinal (GI) series obtained in frontal projection (Fig. 1) shows dilation of the proximal duodenum and an abnormal course of the duodenal sweep. The sweep does not cross to the left of the left-sided pedicles of the vertebral body at the level of the duodenal bulb. A stored fluoroscopic image from the same upper GI series (Fig. 2) better shows the abnormal course and caliber of the duodenum. The sweep does not cross to the left of the left spinal pedicle. Surgery confirmed malrotation.

DISCUSSION

Definition/Background
Intestinal malrotation results from lack of rotation (non-rotation) or incomplete rotation of the fetal bowel. The condition can become life-threatening if the malrotated bowel twists on the short pedicle, causing a volvulus and potentially bowel ischemia.

Characteristic Clinical Features
Patients often present with bilious emesis or abdominal pain or both.

Characteristic Radiologic Findings
Upper GI series is the study of choice for evaluation. The normal duodenal sweep crosses from the right abdomen to the left abdomen (past the left pedicle of the spine) and ascends to the level of the duodenal bulb. Jejunal loops are typically seen in the left abdomen. In patients with malrotation, upper GI films show abnormal position of the ligament of Treitz (duodenum typically does not cross into the left abdomen and does not rise to the level of the bulb). Often, malrotated jejunal loops are in the right hemiabdomen. Lateral views in normal rotation show the retroperitoneal location of the duodenal sweep. Malrotated bowel may not preserve the entirely retroperitoneal location. In chronic malrotation, dilation of the proximal duodenum can be present.

Differential Diagnosis
- Normal ligament of Treitz

Discussion
If the stomach is distended or the duodenum is redundant, upper GI series can be difficult to interpret as normal.

Diagnosis
Malrotation

Suggested Reading
Applegate KE, Anderson JM, Klatte EC: Intestinal malrotation in children: A problem-solving approach to the upper gastrointestinal series. RadioGraphics 26:1485-1500, 2006.

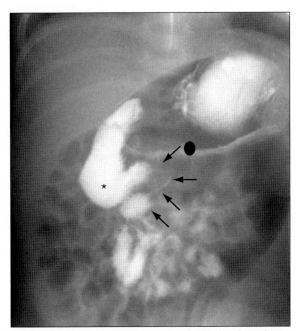

Figure 1. Spot film from upper GI series obtained in frontal projection shows dilation of the proximal duodenum (*asterisk*) and an abnormal course of the duodenal sweep (*arrows*). The sweep does not cross to the left of the left-sided pedicles (*oval*) of the vertebral body at the level of the duodenal bulb.

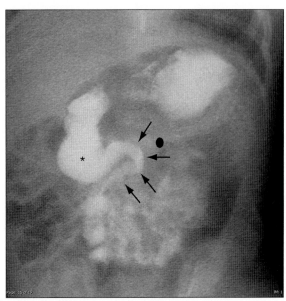

Figure 2. Stored fluoroscopic image from the same upper GI series shows the abnormal course (*arrows*) and caliber (*asterisk*) of the duodenum better. The sweep does not cross to the left of the left spinal pedicle (*oval*). Surgery confirmed malrotation.

Case 59

DEMOGRAPHICS/CLINICAL HISTORY

The patient is a 14-year-old girl with heartburn and intermittent dysphagia.

FINDINGS

Two fluoroscopic spot images from an upper gastrointestinal (GI) series with barium (Figs. 1 and 2) show normal positioning of the duodenal bulb and the descending (second) portion of the duodenum. The third portion of the duodenum, which is usually horizontal, ascends obliquely in a near-vertical orientation, and the fourth portion, which is usually vertical, appears horizontal. The duodenojejunal junction remains in a normal position to the left of midline at the level of the duodenal bulb, with no evidence of malrotation.

DISCUSSION

Definition/Background
Duodenum inversum is generally considered a normal variant with little clinical significance. In some patients, it is confused with malrotation because of the abnormal course of the duodenum.

Characteristic Clinical Features
Patients may present with dysphagia or bilious emesis that prompts an upper GI examination, although these symptoms are likely unrelated to the duodenum inversum. Delayed gastric emptying may also be present.

Characteristic Radiologic Findings
The duodenojejunal junction is in a normal location in the left upper quadrant at the level of the duodenal bulb; the third portion of the duodenum ascends to the level of the bulb to the right of the spine, and the fourth portion travels horizontally to the left of the spine.

Differential Diagnosis
■ Malrotation

Discussion
Malrotation is often difficult to diagnose on upper GI examination because many findings may simulate malrotation. Patients with malrotation nearly universally have an abnormally positioned duodenojejunal junction that is not situated at the level of the duodenal bulb to the left of the spine.

Diagnosis
Duodenum inversum

Suggested Readings
Applegate KE, Anderson JM, Klatte EC: Intestinal malrotation in children: A problem-solving approach to the upper gastrointestinal series. RadioGraphics 26:1485-1500, 2006.

Long FR, Kramer SS, Markowitz RI, et al: Intestinal malrotation in children: Tutorial on radiographic diagnosis in difficult cases. Radiology 198:775-780, 1996.

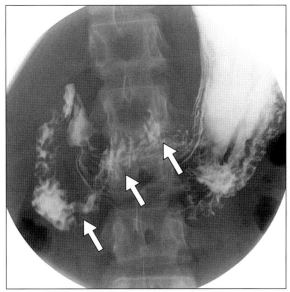

Figure 1. Fluoroscopic spot image from upper GI examination shows that the third portion of the duodenum, which is usually horizontal, ascends obliquely in a near-vertical orientation, and the fourth portion, which is usually vertical, appears horizontal (*arrows*).

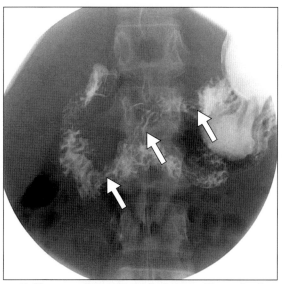

Figure 2. Fluoroscopic spot image from upper GI examination acquired several seconds after Fig. 1 shows that the third portion of the duodenum, which is usually horizontal, ascends obliquely in a near-vertical orientation, and the fourth portion, which is usually vertical, appears horizontal (*arrows*). The contrast agent has passed more distally on this image, and the duodenojejunal junction can be appreciated. The duodenojejunal junction remains in a normal position to the left of midline at the level of the duodenal bulb, with no evidence of malrotation.

Case 60

DEMOGRAPHICS/CLINICAL HISTORY

The patient is a 6-year-old child with relapsed Wilms tumor, status post–bone marrow transplant with a decrease in platelets and right upper quadrant pain.

FINDINGS

A transverse ultrasound scan of the upper abdomen (Fig. 1) shows a rounded heterogeneous mass at the level of the gallbladder. Curvilinear echogenicities represent the displaced and compressed duodenal mucosa. Computed tomography (CT) (Fig. 2) shows the duodenal hematoma displacing and compressing the duodenal lumen, with a small amount of adjacent stranding and fluid. Recurrent Wilms tumor is seen in the postsurgical bed. A coronal reconstruction of the CT scan (Fig. 3) shows the duodenal hematoma adjacent to the pancreas. Fluid is seen in the duodenum just proximal to the hematoma.

DISCUSSION

Definition/Background

Duodenal hematomas are usually post-traumatic in etiology; if no appropriate history is given, child abuse should be considered.

Characteristic Clinical Features

Abdominal pain and vomiting are typical features, along with a history of trauma.

Characteristic Radiologic Findings

Imaging shows the intramural location of the hematoma adjacent to the head of the pancreas. Mass effect from the hematoma causes partial or complete obstruction of the duodenal lumen, and can cause dilation of the pancreatic duct. Imaging characteristics of the hematoma depend on the age of the hematoma. Free fluid can be seen in the abdomen.

Less Common Radiologic Manifestations

In rarer cases of duodenal perforation, contrast extravasation or free air can indicate the perforation.

Differential Diagnosis

- Gastrointestinal stromal tumor (GIST)
- Lymphoma
- Pancreatic neoplasm

Discussion

Gastrointestinal stromal tumor, bowel lymphoma, or a pancreatic head neoplasm could possibly mimic the appearance of the duodenal mass. Gastrointestinal stromal tumor can be heterogeneous and intramural, but is not commonly at the characteristic location in the peripancreatic duodenum or does not have the characteristic history. Lymphoma involving the bowel has a homogeneous appearance, often does not narrow or obstruct the lumen, and is usually accompanied by lymphadenopathy. Pancreatic head neoplasms may have mass effect on, but are typically discernible as separate from, the duodenal wall.

Diagnosis

Duodenal hematoma

Suggested Readings

Guzman C, Bousvaros A, Buonomo C, Nurko S: Intraduodenal hematoma complicating intestinal biopsy: Case reports and review of the literature. Am J Gastroenterol 93:2547-2550, 1998.

Winthrop AL, Wesson DE, Filler RM: Traumatic duodenal hematoma in the pediatric patient. J Pediatr Surg 21:757-760, 1986.

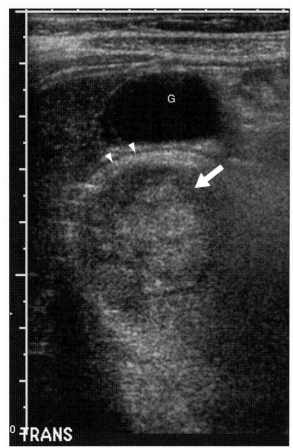

Figure 1. Transverse ultrasound of upper abdomen shows rounded heterogeneous mass (*arrow*) at the level of the gallbladder (*G*). Curvilinear echogenicities (*arrowheads*) represent the displaced and compressed duodenal mucosa.

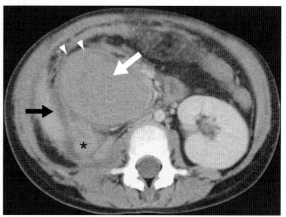

Figure 2. CT scan shows duodenal hematoma (*white arrow*) displacing and compressing duodenal lumen (*arrowheads*), with a small amount of adjacent stranding and fluid (*black arrow*). Recurrent Wilms tumor is seen in the postsurgical bed (*asterisk*).

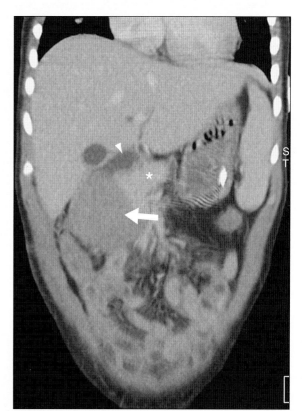

Figure 3. Coronal reconstruction of CT scan shows duodenal hematoma (*arrow*) adjacent to the pancreas (*asterisk*). Fluid is seen in the duodenum (*arrowhead*) just proximal to the hematoma.

Case 61

DEMOGRAPHICS/CLINICAL HISTORY

The patient is a 7-week-old infant with nonbilious emesis.

FINDINGS

A supine abdominal radiograph (Fig. 1) shows an elevated left hemidiaphragm, a markedly distended air-filled stomach, and a paucity of distal bowel gas. An image from an upper gastrointestinal (GI) series (Fig. 2) shows reversal of the normal orientation, with the pylorus located superiorly above the gastroesophageal junction, and the gastric fundus up into the thorax, beneath the elevated left hemidiaphragm. A lateral image (Fig. 3) shows the pylorus located superiorly above the gastroesophageal junction and the gastric fundus in the thorax, beneath the elevated left hemidiaphragm.

DISCUSSION

Definition/Background

Gastric volvulus is divided into two categories: organoaxial and mesenteroaxial. Diaphragmatic hernia, abdominal situs abnormality, and lax ligamental attachments are considered risk factors.

Characteristic Clinical Features

Common presentations of volvulus include nonbilious vomiting, pain, and abdominal (gastric) distention.

Characteristic Radiologic Findings

Gaseous distention of the stomach, paucity of distal bowel gas, and eventration of the left hemidiaphragm may be seen. On upper GI series, an organoaxial volvulus shows the greater curvature of the stomach located superior and to the right of the lesser curvature, with an inferior direction of the pylorus. On upper GI series, a mesenteroaxial volvulus shows the pylorus located superior to the gastroesophageal junction.

Differential Diagnosis

■ Mass effect from an abdominal mass

Discussion

A large abdominal mass could have mass effect on the greater curvature of the stomach, simulating an organoaxial volvulus, but clinical presentation, palpation, or ultrasound imaging can help differentiate the two.

Diagnosis

Gastric volvulus

Suggested Reading

Oh SK, Han BK, Levin TL, et al: Gastric volvulus in children: The twists and turns of an unusual entity. Pediatr Radiol 38:297-304, 2008.

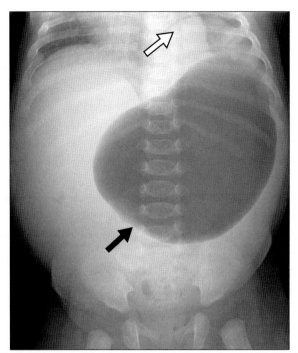

Figure 1. Supine abdominal radiograph shows elevated left hemidiaphragm (*white arrow*), a markedly distended air-filled stomach (*black arrow*), and a paucity of distal bowel gas.

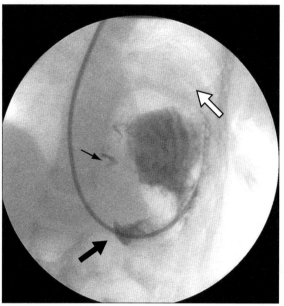

Figure 2. Image from upper GI series shows reversal of the normal orientation, with the pylorus (*small black arrow*) located superiorly above the gastroesophageal junction (*large black arrow*), and the gastric fundus up into the thorax, beneath the elevated left hemidiaphragm (*white arrow*).

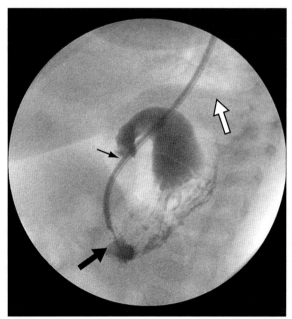

Figure 3. Lateral image shows pylorus (*small black arrow*) located superiorly above the gastroesophageal junction (*large black arrow*) and the gastric fundus in the thorax, beneath the elevated left hemidiaphragm (*white arrow*).

Case 62

DEMOGRAPHICS/CLINICAL HISTORY

The patient is a 5-month-old boy transferred from another hospital with concern for severe intestinal obstruction. An ileostomy has already been performed, although the level of obstruction is as yet unverified.

FINDINGS

A scout radiograph for a contrast enema (Fig. 1) shows multiple loops of mildly dilated bowel within the mid-abdomen. For the most part, the loops have been decompressed by the creation of a right lower quadrant ileostomy, which was performed at an outside hospital, although the site of obstruction was not identified. An anteroposterior abdominal radiograph during a contrast enema (Fig. 2) shows a small microcolon, with an abrupt cutoff to the passage of contrast agent past the level of the splenic flexure. This was later shown to represent the site of colonic stricture.

DISCUSSION

Definition/Background
Colonic atresia is one of the rarest causes of neonatal intestinal obstruction. Its etiology is as yet uncertain, although some series suggest it occurs secondary to an in utero mesenteric vascular accident.

Characteristic Clinical Features
Patients are typically full-term infants who present with abdominal distention and bilious emesis soon after birth.

Characteristic Radiologic Findings
Plain abdominal radiographs reveal multiple dilated loops of bowel with air-fluid levels.

Less Common Radiologic Manifestations
Contrast enema shows the presence of a microcolon, with no further passage of contrast agent proximal to the level of the atresia. The atresia is most often located within the right colon.

Differential Diagnosis
- Small left colon syndrome
- Ileal atresia
- Hirschsprung disease
- Meconium ileus

Discussion
Neonatal small left colon syndrome is an uncommon cause of intestinal obstruction; it is associated with a maternal history of gestational diabetes and characterized by an abrupt change in caliber of the colon around the level of the splenic flexure. Ileal atresia is a cause of neonatal intestinal obstruction where the level of the atresia occurs in the ileum. A microcolon is also typically present. Hirschsprung disease is another cause of neonatal intestinal obstruction; the etiology is abnormal, aganglionic bowel involving a small segment of the anus or rectum, but which can involve the entire colon. Meconium ileus is a cause of infantile bowel obstruction found in patients with cystic fibrosis associated with microcolon, multiple dilated loops of small bowel proximal to a functional obstruction most commonly at the level of the terminal ileum secondary to obstructing, inspissated meconium plugs.

Diagnosis
Colonic atresia

Suggested Readings
Etensel B, Temir G, Karkiner A, et al: Atresia of the colon. J Pediatr Surg 40:1258-1268, 2005.

Piper HG, Alesbury J, Waterford SD, et al: Intestinal atresias: Factors affecting clinical outcomes. J Pediatr Surg 43:1244-1248, 2008.

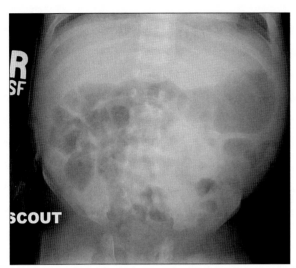

Figure 1. Scout radiograph for contrast enema shows multiple loops of mildly dilated bowel within the mid-abdomen. For the most part, the loops have been decompressed by the creation of a right lower quadrant ileostomy, although the site of obstruction was not identified at the time of surgery.

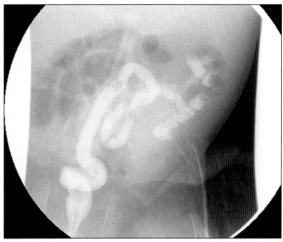

Figure 2. Anteroposterior abdominal radiograph during contrast enema shows a small microcolon, with an abrupt cutoff to the passage of contrast agent past the level of the splenic flexure. This was later shown to represent the site of colonic stricture.

Case 63

DEMOGRAPHICS/CLINICAL HISTORY

The patient is a 4-day-old girl with worsening abdominal distention.

FINDINGS

A supine, portable radiograph of the abdomen (Fig. 1) shows multiple dilated loops of bowel in the abdomen. An anteroposterior fluoroscopic spot film obtained during a contrast enema shows (Fig. 2) a small-caliber colon. Contrast agent refluxed into the terminal ileum shows the normal caliber of the distal small bowel (see Fig. 2). Contrast agent was unable to reflux any more proximally into the dilated bowel loops.

DISCUSSION

Definition/Background

Meconium ileus refers to the impaction of meconium in the small bowel and colon, causing obstruction. It most often occurs in patients with cystic fibrosis.

Characteristic Clinical Features

Infants present with abdominal distention and may fail to pass meconium in the first 24 to 48 hours of life.

Characteristic Radiologic Findings

Plain radiographs of the abdomen show multiple, dilated loops of bowel. Contrast enema reveals a microcolon. The key to the enema is to attempt to reflux contrast agent into the small bowel proximal to the point of obstruction to show the dilated small bowel with intraluminal filling defects (i.e., meconium), in contrast to ileal atresia, in which the contrast agent terminates at the point of atresia in a nondilated ileum.

Differential Diagnosis

- Hirschsprung disease
- Small left colon syndrome
- Ileal atresia
- Colonic atresia

Discussion

In Hirschsprung disease, an abnormally aganglionic section of bowel begins at the anus and may extend proximally for some length. The bowel proximal to the aganglionic segment becomes dilated because of a functional obstruction. Small left colon syndrome is frequently associated with maternal gestational diabetes. It is characterized by a caliber reduction in the sigmoid and descending colon. Ileal atresia refers to an imperforate ileal segment that leads to small bowel obstruction proximal to the level of the atresia. Patients usually have a microcolon identified during a contrast enema. Colonic atresia refers to an imperforate segment of colon, which may occur at any level of the colon. It is characterized by small and large bowel obstruction proximal to the level of the atresia.

Diagnosis

Meconium ileus

Suggested Readings

Berrocal T, Lamas M, Gutierrez J, et al: Congenital anomalies of the small intestine, colon, and rectum. RadioGraphics 19:1219-1236, 1999.

Johnson JF, Robinson LH: Localized bowel distention in the newborn: A review of the plain film analysis and differential diagnosis. Pediatrics 73:206-215, 1984.

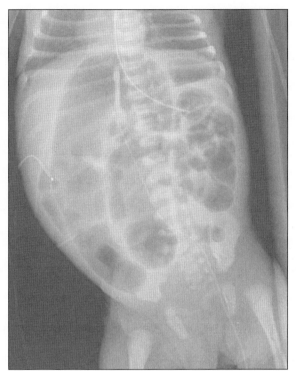

Figure 1. Supine, portable radiograph shows multiple, dilated loops of bowel in the abdomen. A nasogastric tube is in place.

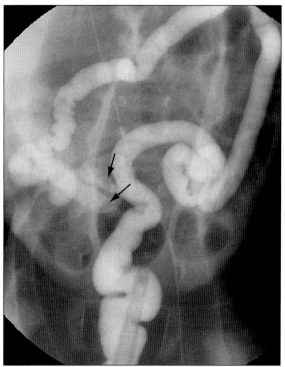

Figure 2. Anteroposterior fluoroscopic spot film obtained during a contrast enema shows a small-caliber colon. Contrast agent refluxed into the terminal ileum reveals the normal caliber of the distal small bowel and multiple intraluminal filling defects (*arrows*). Contrast agent was unable to reflux any more proximally into the dilated bowel loops in this patient.

Case 64

DEMOGRAPHICS/CLINICAL HISTORY

The patient is a 16-year-old with a history of chronic right lower quadrant pain and diarrhea.

FINDINGS

Radiographs obtained during a small bowel series show irregular narrowing of the terminal ileum without (Fig. 1) and with focal compression (Fig. 2). An axial image from a computed tomography (CT) scan (Fig. 3) in another patient with Crohn disease shows "creeping fat" appearance and "comb sign." Reconstructed coronal image from the same CT scan (Fig. 4) shows wall thickening and irregularity along the distal and terminal ileum.

DISCUSSION

Definition/Background

Crohn disease is an inflammatory process commonly affecting the terminal ileum that often manifests in late childhood or early adulthood with pain and diarrhea.

Characteristic Clinical Features

Abdominal pain, diarrhea, and weight loss are common presentations.

Characteristic Radiologic Findings

Although inflammation of the bowel wall can occur anywhere (or in multiple areas) along the digestive tract, the most common location is the terminal ileum. Narrowing, wall thickening, increased focal mesenteric fat ("creeping fat"), and prominent mesenteric vessels within focal fat ("comb sign") are often seen. Strictures, fistulas, and pseudosacculations can also be seen.

Differential Diagnosis
- Infectious enteritis
- Henoch-Schönlein purpura
- Ulcerative colitis

Discussion

Bowel wall thickening can be seen in other entities, including infectious enteritis and Henoch-Schönlein purpura. Clinical history and stool cultures can be helpful in the initial evaluation. When Crohn disease involves the entire colon without "skip lesions," ulcerative colitis is also in the differential diagnosis.

Diagnosis

Crohn disease

Suggested Readings

Gaca AM, Jaffe TA, Delaney S, et al: Radiation doses from small-bowel follow-through and abdomen/pelvis MDCT in pediatric Crohn disease. Pediatr Radiol 38:285-291, 2008.

Toma P, Granata C, Magnano G, Barabino A: CT and MRI of paediatric Crohn disease. Pediatr Radiol 37:1083-1092, 2007.

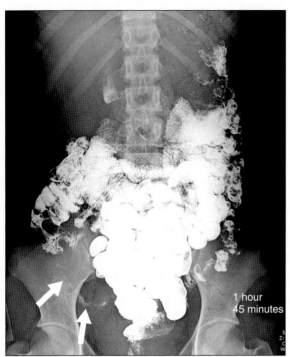

Figure 1. Radiograph during small bowel series shows irregular narrowing (*arrows*) of the terminal ileum without compression.

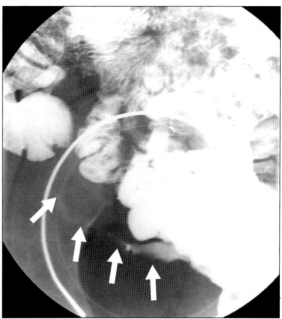

Figure 2. Spot film with compression during small bowel series also shows the irregularity of the lumen (*arrows*) and overall narrowing of the caliber.

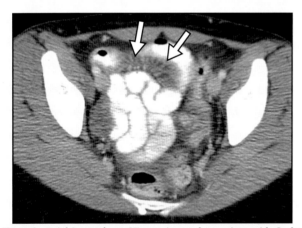

Figure 3. Axial image from CT scan in another patient with Crohn disease shows "creeping fat" appearance and "comb sign" (*arrows*).

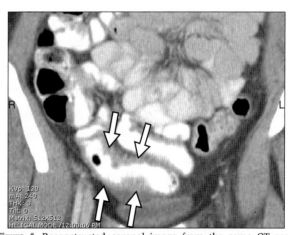

Figure 4. Reconstructed coronal image from the same CT scan shows wall thickening and irregularity along the distal and terminal ileum (*arrows*).

Case 65

DEMOGRAPHICS/CLINICAL HISTORY

The patient is a 15-year-old boy with several days of hematochezia, with dark, melenic stools, undergoing a Meckel scan.

FINDINGS

An anteroposterior projection from a Meckel scan (Fig. 1) reveals an abnormal focus of tracer uptake within the left lower quadrant.

DISCUSSION

Definition/Background
Meckel diverticulum is the most common congenital anomaly of the gastrointestinal (GI) tract; it occurs in 4% of the general population.

Characteristic Clinical Features
Most Meckel diverticula are asymptomatic, but when symptomatic, patients may present with GI bleeding or bowel obstruction. The patient in this case was taken to the operating room based on the positive results of the Meckel scan. At surgery, he was found to have a large Meckel diverticulum approximately 50 cm proximal to the ileocecal valve.

Characteristic Radiologic Findings
A Meckel scan in nuclear medicine (using intravenous technetium 99m (^{99m}Tc)–labeled pertechnetate) is the test of choice for diagnosis. No other imaging was performed in this patient.

Differential Diagnosis
- Appendicitis
- Crohn disease

Discussion
Acute appendicitis is a very common cause of right lower quadrant pain in children. The diagnosis is often confirmed with either ultrasound or computed tomography (CT) showing a dilated (> 6 mm) tubular, noncompressible bowel loop in the right lower quadrant arising from the cecum. Crohn disease is a form of inflammatory bowel disease that may manifest with diffuse abdominal pain or pain localized to the right lower quadrant. CT or upper GI examinations often suggest the diagnosis (which is ultimately confirmed at biopsy) by showing thickened loops of small or large bowel with surrounding mesenteric inflammation and ulceration of the bowel mucosa (best shown on upper GI study with small bowel follow-through), most severe in the terminal ileum.

Diagnosis
Meckel diverticulum

Suggested Readings

Connolly SA, Drubach LA, Connolly LP: Meckel's diverticulitis: Diagnosis with computed tomography and Tc-99m pertechnetate scintigraphy. Clin Nucl Med 29:823, 2004.

Elsayes KM, Menias CO, Harvin HJ, et al: Imaging manifestations of Meckel's diverticulum. AJR Am J Roentgenol 189:81, 2007.

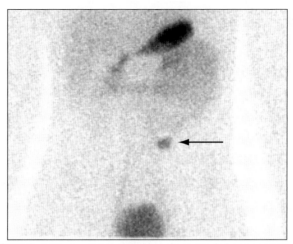

Figure 1. Anteroposterior projection from Meckel scan acquired after intravenous administration of radiolabeled pertechnetate shows normal tracer localization to the stomach and bladder, and an abnormal focus of tracer uptake in the lower abdomen just to the left of midline (*arrow*).

Case 66

DEMOGRAPHICS/CLINICAL HISTORY

The patient is a 3-year-old boy with colicky abdominal pain and diarrhea.

FINDINGS

Ultrasound evaluation of the abdomen shows multiple loops of small bowel in the right lower quadrant with circumferential bowel wall thickening (Fig. 1), and enlarged mesenteric lymph nodes (Fig. 2). Axial contrast-enhanced computed tomography (CT) scan of the abdomen and pelvis (Fig. 3) shows multifocal, circumferential bowel wall thickening in the right lower quadrant and vascular engorgement in the mesentery.

DISCUSSION

Definition/Background

Henoch-Schönlein purpura is a small vessel vasculitis that affects children more commonly than adults. It tends to involve many organ systems, including the skin, joints, gastrointestinal tract, and kidneys.

Characteristic Clinical Features

A common initial presenting complaint is colicky abdominal pain with or without nausea, vomiting, or diarrhea.

Characteristic Radiologic Findings

Ultrasound and CT evaluations of the bowel in patients with Henoch-Schönlein purpura show multifocal areas of circumferential bowel wall thickening with associated luminal narrowing and fold thickening. The jejunum and ileum are the most commonly involved portions of the bowel.

Less Common Radiologic Manifestations

CT may show evidence of mesenteric edema, lymphadenopathy, and vascular engorgement.

Differential Diagnosis

- Inflammatory bowel disease
- Small bowel hemorrhage
- Bowel ischemia

Discussion

Small bowel hemorrhage and small bowel ischemia may result from various underlying conditions, including systemic vasculitides.

Diagnosis

Henoch-Schönlein purpura

Suggested Readings

Jeong YK, Ha HK, Yoon CH, et al: Gastrointestinal involvement in Henoch-Schönlein syndrome: CT findings. AJR Am J Roentgenol 168:965-968, 1997.

Johnson PT, Horton KM, Fishman EK: Case 127: Henoch-Schönlein purpura. Radiology 245:909-913, 2007.

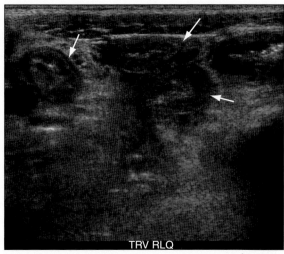

Figure 1. Ultrasound of the abdomen shows multiple loops of small bowel in the right lower quadrant with circumferential bowel wall thickening (*arrows*).

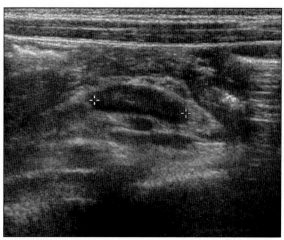

Figure 2. Ultrasound of the abdomen shows enlarged mesenteric lymph nodes.

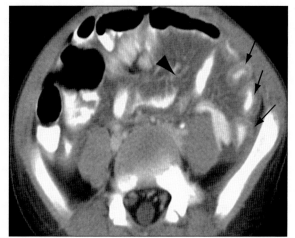

Figure 3. Axial contrast-enhanced CT of the abdomen and pelvis shows multifocal, circumferential bowel wall thickening in the right lower quadrant (*arrows*), and vascular engorgement in the mesentery (*arrowhead*).

Case 67

DEMOGRAPHICS/CLINICAL HISTORY

The patient is a 12-week-old girl with vomiting and abdominal distention.

FINDINGS

Anteroposterior (Fig. 1) and cross-table lateral (Fig. 2) radiographs of the abdomen show multiple dilated loops of small and large bowel, nearly filling the entire abdomen. Gas is noted to the level of the rectum. Axial image from a non–contrast-enhanced computed tomography (CT) scan of the abdomen and pelvis (Fig. 3) better shows the degree of diffuse bowel dilation throughout the abdomen without cause for obstruction. Postevacuation radiograph performed after a barium enema examination (Fig. 4) shows a dilated, capacious colon that was unable to be completely filled with barium during the examination secondary to the large capacity of the colon and has not evacuated the contrast agent effectively 20 minutes after the procedure.

DISCUSSION

Definition/Background

Intestinal pseudo-obstruction describes a chronic, recurring dilation of the intestines without known mechanical cause. The condition may be primary, neuropathic, or myopathic.

Characteristic Clinical Features

Nearly half of patients present within the first month of life. Patients present with vomiting, diarrhea, abdominal distention, and constipation.

Characteristic Radiologic Findings

Plain radiographs show multiple dilated loops of bowel, particularly the colon. The presence of air-fluid levels relates to the lack of peristalsis.

Less Common Radiologic Manifestations

Contrast enema often shows megacolon and poor bowel motility.

Differential Diagnosis

- Neuronal intestinal dysplasia
- Functional constipation

Discussion

Neuronal intestinal dysplasia is a disorder of intestinal innervation that manifests with constipation in children. Contrast enema typically reveals a flaccid megacolon and poor motor activity. Functional constipation usually manifests in slightly older children (i.e., > 2 years old). Radiographs show a significant volume of stool within the colon and rectum with secondary small bowel dilation.

Diagnosis

Intestinal pseudo-obstruction

Suggested Reading

Glassman M, Spivak W, Mininberg D, et al: Chronic idiopathic intestinal pseudo-obstruction: A commonly misdiagnosed disease in infants and children. Pediatrics 83:603, 1989.

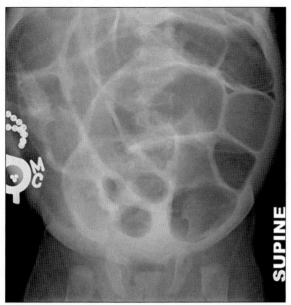

Figure 1. Anteroposterior radiograph of abdomen shows multiple dilated loops of small and large bowel, nearly filling the entire abdomen.

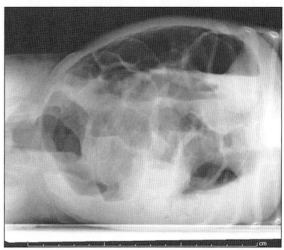

Figure 2. Cross-table lateral radiograph of abdomen shows multiple dilated loops of small and large bowel, nearly filling the entire abdomen. Gas is noted to the level of the rectum.

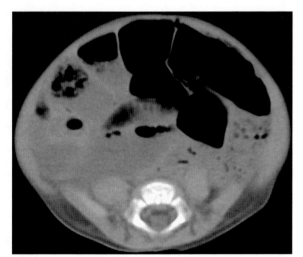

Figure 3. Axial image from non–contrast-enhanced CT scan of abdomen and pelvis better shows the degree of diffuse bowel dilation throughout the abdomen without cause for obstruction.

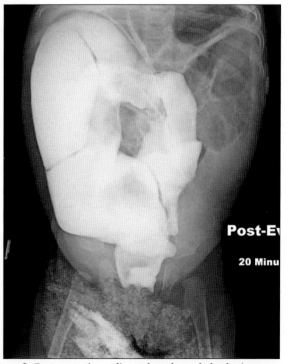

Figure 4. Postevacuation radiograph performed after barium enema examination shows dilated, capacious colon that was unable to be completely filled with barium during the examination secondary to the large capacity of the colon, with retention of a significant amount of contrast agent after the procedure.

Case 68

DEMOGRAPHICS/CLINICAL HISTORY

The patient is a 22-year-old woman with cystic fibrosis and abdominal distention.

FINDINGS

An upright view of the abdomen (Fig. 1) shows a debris-filled stomach. Upper gastrointestinal (GI) study via injection of the patient's gastrostomy tube (Fig. 2) shows the stomach filled with compacted debris. At surgery, a large bezoar was removed.

DISCUSSION

Definition/Background
A bezoar is a collection of debris that forms within the intestinal tract, typically the stomach. Bezoars can be composed of food or inorganic material. Common components are milk by-products, cellulose, and hair.

Characteristic Clinical Features
Common presenting symptoms include abdominal distention, fullness, and vomiting.

Characteristic Radiologic Findings
Radiographic studies show a filling defect within the stomach, signs of obstruction, and stomach distention.

Differential Diagnosis
- Gastric outlet obstruction

Discussion
If a patient has a gastric outlet obstruction, or another site of bowel obstruction, food particles and stasis can mimic a bezoar.

Diagnosis
Bezoar

Suggested Readings
Ciampa A, Moore BE, Listerud RG, et al: Giant trichophytobezoar in a pediatric patient with trichotillomania. Pediatr Radiol 33:219-220, 2003.
Graham RJ, Stein P: Gastric outlet obstruction in an infant: Lactobezoar. Am J Emerg Med 25:98-99, 2007.

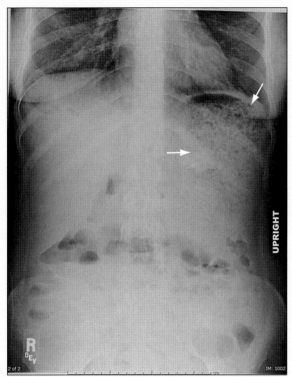

Figure 1. Upright view of abdomen shows debris-filled stomach (*arrows*).

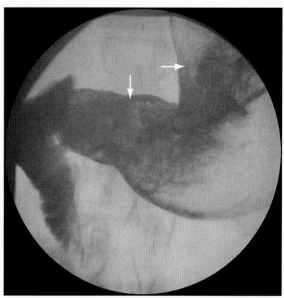

Figure 2. Upper GI via injection of patient's gastrostomy tube shows the stomach filled with compacted debris (*arrows*).

Case 69

DEMOGRAPHICS/CLINICAL HISTORY

The patient is a 4-year-old girl with dysphagia.

FINDINGS

A frontal view of the chest (Fig. 1) shows a round density projecting over the lower thoracic midline. The patient admitted to swallowing a coin.

DISCUSSION

Definition/Background

Foreign body ingestion is common in young children. Coins are the most common radiodense ingested foreign body in North America. More dangerous foreign body ingestions include swallowing of multiple magnets (due to pressure erosion and bowel perforation) and swallowing of batteries (can cause chemical erosion of the intestines and perforation).

Characteristic Clinical Features

Dysphagia, pain, drooling, and difficulty breathing all can be presenting symptoms of foreign body ingestion.

Characteristic Radiologic Findings

Foreign bodies that are radiodense can be seen. Radio-lucent foreign bodies may be suggested by surrounding esophageal edema, causing mass effect on the trachea. If the ingested foreign body is a battery, a small step-off along the edge may be seen.

Less Common Radiologic Manifestations

Distention of the proximal esophageal air column or evidence of esophageal perforation are less common.

Differential Diagnosis

■ Aspirated foreign body

Discussion

If the foreign body is in the proximal esophagus, it can be superimposed over the trachea, mimicking an aspirated foreign body. The lateral radiograph should clearly localize the esophageal foreign body posterior to the tracheal air column.

Diagnosis

Foreign body (coin) ingestion

Suggested Reading

Wahbeh G, Wyllie R, Kay M: Foreign body ingestion in infants and children: Location, location, location. Clin Pediatr (Phila) 41:633-640, 2002.

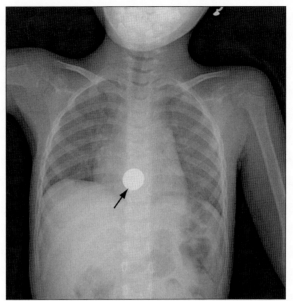

Figure 1. Frontal view of chest shows round density projecting over lower thoracic midline.

Case 70

DEMOGRAPHICS/CLINICAL HISTORY

The patient is a 5-year-old boy with congenital microgastria, diagnosed on prenatal imaging.

FINDINGS

Fluoroscopic spot images from a contrast study performed through an indwelling gastric tube (Figs. 1 and 2) show that the stomach lumen is abnormally small, and that contrast agent passes readily into the duodenum (which is normal).

DISCUSSION

Definition/Background

Congenital microgastria is a rare anomaly resulting from abnormal foregut development in utero and is usually accompanied by other anomalies, such as malrotation, asplenia, or the VACTERL (vertebral anomalies, anal atresia, cardiac abnormalities, tracheoesophageal fistula or esophageal atresia, renal agenesis and dysplasia, and limb defects) association of disorders.

Characteristic Clinical Features

Prenatal ultrasound may reveal a small or nonvisualized stomach, mimicking esophageal atresia. After birth, patients may present with postprandial vomiting or failure to thrive.

Characteristic Radiologic Findings

Upper gastrointestinal (GI) contrast examination shows the stomach is small, midline, and tubular-shaped. Gastroesophageal reflux and megaesophagus are often present as well.

Differential Diagnosis
- Esophageal atresia
- Pyloric stenosis
- Malrotation
- Prepyloric antral web

Discussion

In fetuses with esophageal atresia, a small or nonvisualized stomach often is revealed on prenatal ultrasound, which can mimic congenital microgastria. Infants with pyloric stenosis present with postprandial vomiting and failure to thrive because of gastric outlet obstruction. These clinical symptoms may mimic congenital microgastria. Infants with malrotation usually present within the first month of life with vomiting, although the emesis is typically bilious in nature. A prepyloric antral web is a rare anomaly that may cause symptoms of gastric outlet obstruction, similar to those in patients with microgastria.

Diagnosis

Microgastria

Suggested Readings

Kroes EJ, Festen C: Congenital microgastria: A case report and review of the literature. Pediatr Surg Int 13(5-6):416-418, 1998.

Ramos CT, Moss RL, Musemeche CA: Microgastria as an isolated anomaly. J Pediatr Surg 31:1445-1447, 1996.

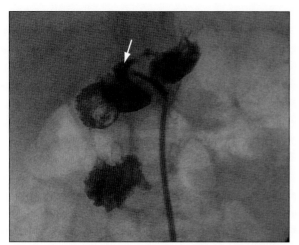

Figure 1. Fluoroscopic spot image from a contrast study performed through an indwelling gastric tube shows that the stomach lumen is abnormally small (*arrow*), and that contrast agent passes readily into the duodenum.

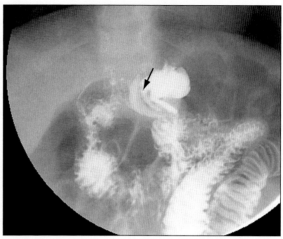

Figure 2. Fluoroscopic spot image from a contrast study performed through an indwelling gastric tube acquired several minutes after the image in Fig. 1 shows that the stomach lumen is abnormally small (*arrow*), and that the contrast-opacified duodenum and proximal jejunum are otherwise normal (no evidence of malrotation).

Case 71

DEMOGRAPHICS/CLINICAL HISTORY

The patient is a 14-year-old girl with MRCP, now presenting with abdominal distention and nonbilious vomiting.

FINDINGS

A left lateral decubitus abdominal radiograph (Fig. 1) shows a gastric tube in place. There is significant distention of the stomach and of the proximal duodenum with an air-fluid level. A fluoroscopic spot image from an upper gastrointestinal (GI) examination (Fig. 2) shows mild dilation of the first and second portions of the duodenum, mild mucosal fold thickening, and an abrupt change in caliber of the duodenum in the third portion as it crosses over the spine.

DISCUSSION

Definition/Background

SMA syndrome refers to vascular compression of the duodenum by the superior mesenteric artery (SMA), leading to bowel obstruction.

Characteristic Clinical Features

Patients present with abdominal distention and vomiting, which may occur secondary to a wasting disorder such as anorexia related to cancer, head trauma, spinal deformity, or postoperative state.

Characteristic Radiologic Findings

Upper GI contrast studies show dilation of the first and second portions of the duodenum, vertical and oblique compression of the mucosal folds of the duodenum, antiperistaltic flow of barium proximal to the obstruction, and delay in transit time through the duodenum.

Less Common Radiologic Manifestations

Computed tomography (CT) or CT angiography of the abdomen and pelvis may show a nearly vertical course of the proximal SMA as it arises from the abdominal aorta and as it subtends the third portion of the duodenum, with dilation of the first and second portions of the duodenum.

Differential Diagnosis

- Malrotation
- Duodenal web

Discussion

Malrotation is a congenital condition related to abnormal rotation of the bowel in utero, which leads to abnormal mobility of the bowel, which is not tethered appropriately by the mesentery. The most serious consequence of malrotation is midgut volvulus, in which the bowel twists around the root of the mesentery, producing bowel obstruction and ischemia. This is best diagnosed on upper GI, where an obstruction to the passage of contrast agent occurs at, usually, the second portion of the duodenum; any contrast agent that does pass through assumes a "corkscrew" configuration. A duodenal web is a thin membrane of tissue within the lumen of the duodenum that may cause partial or complete obstruction. The characteristic "windsock" deformity is shown on upper GI.

Diagnosis

SMA syndrome

Suggested Readings

Agrawal GA, Johnson PT, Fishman EK: J Clin Gastroenterol 41(1): 62-65, 2007.

Hines JR, Gore RM, Ballantyne GH: Superior mesenteric artery syndrome: Diagnostic criteria and therapeutic approaches. Am J Surg 148(5):630-632, 1984.

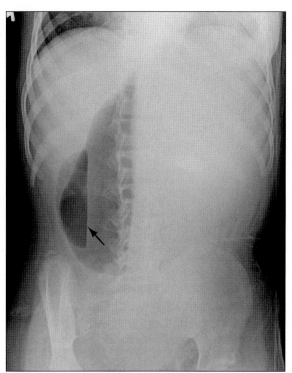

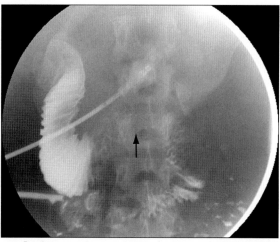

Figure 2. Fluoroscopic spot image from upper GI examination shows mild dilation of the first and second portions of the duodenum, mild mucosal fold thickening, and an abrupt change in caliber of the duodenum in the third portion as it crosses over the spine (*arrow*).

Figure 1. Left lateral decubitus abdominal radiograph shows gastric tube in place. There is significant distention of the stomach and of the proximal duodenum with an air-fluid level (*arrow*).

Case 72

DEMOGRAPHICS/CLINICAL HISTORY

The patient is a fetus whose prenatal sonogram showed an abnormal abdominal finding.

FINDINGS

A prenatal sonogram (Fig. 1) in a sagittal plane to the fetus shows a rounded protuberance along the anterior abdomen. A half-Fourier acquisition single shot turbo-spin echo (HASTE) sequence from fetal magnetic resonance imaging (MRI) in a sagittal plane to the fetus (Fig. 2) shows a large portion of the liver protruding out of the abdomen, completely covered, consistent with a large omphalocele. The midline insertion of the umbilical cord along the inferior aspect of the omphalocele is seen. An abdominal radiograph (Fig. 3) in a different newborn with an omphalocele shows the large omphalocele and insertion of the umbilical cord in a midline location along the inferior aspect of the omphalocele.

DISCUSSION

Definition/Background

Omphalocele is the most common abdominal wall defect in neonates and is commonly associated with other anomalies, including chromosomal abnormalities.

Characteristic Clinical Features

Omphalocele is typically diagnosed prenatally. At birth, the newborn is noted to have a sac covering extruded abdominal contents, particularly the liver.

Characteristic Radiologic Findings

Radiologic studies can show the extent of the abdominal organs contained within the thin sac, including liver, stomach, and bowel. Other abnormalities also can be visualized, such as ascites; heart abnormalities; other gastrointestinal abnormalities, particularly anal atresia; and genitourinary abnormalities, such as exstrophy.

Differential Diagnosis

- Abdominal wall laxity
- Gastroschisis
- Amniotic band syndrome

Discussion

Occasionally, the abdominal wall is so lax that the abdomen can allow the liver and intestines; however, the laxity is skin covered. Gastroschisis has multiple small bowel loops external to the patient without a normal skin cover.

Diagnosis

Omphalocele

Suggested Reading

Biard JM, Wilson RD, Johnson MP, et al: Prenatally diagnosed giant omphaloceles: Short- and long-term outcomes. Prenat Diagn 24: 434-439, 2004.

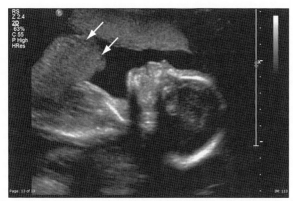

Figure 1. Prenatal sonogram in a sagittal plane to the fetus shows a rounded protuberance along the anterior abdomen (*arrows*).

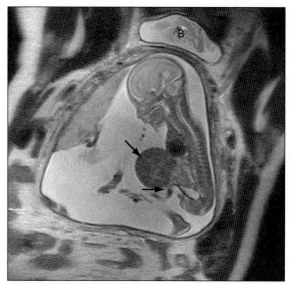

Figure 2. HASTE sequence from fetal MRI in a sagittal plane to the fetus shows a large portion of the liver protruding out of the abdomen, completely covered, consistent with a large omphalocele (*upper arrow*). The midline insertion of the umbilical cord along the inferior aspect of the omphalocele (*lower arrow*) is seen. This image has been rotated from its original acquisition, and the maternal bladder (B) is at the top of the image.

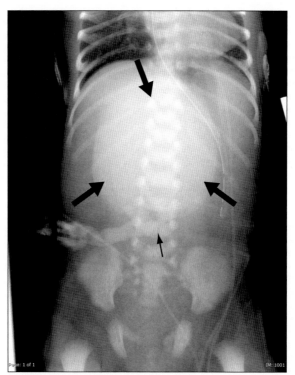

Figure 3. Abdominal radiograph in a different newborn with an omphalocele shows the large omphalocele (*thick arrows*) and insertion of the umbilical cord in a midline location (*thin arrow*) along the inferior aspect of the omphalocele.

Case 73

DEMOGRAPHICS/CLINICAL HISTORY

The patient is a 3-month-old infant with bilious emesis. The patient underwent Ladd procedure shortly after birth for duodenal web and malrotation.

FINDINGS

Fluoroscopic spot images from an upper gastrointestinal (GI) examination (Figs. 1 and 2) performed in the first few days of life show contrast agent within the stomach and dilated duodenum. The dilated duodenum abruptly tapers at the level of the duodenojejunal junction. The duodenojejunal junction is abnormally positioned consistent with malrotation. A small trickle of contrast agent passes through to decompressed loops of proximal small bowel. A plain radiograph of the abdomen performed 3 months later (Fig. 3) shows multiple dilated loops of small bowel consistent with bowel obstruction.

DISCUSSION

Definition/Background
Ladd bands are fibrous bands of peritoneal tissue that attach the cecum to the right abdominal wall, which may cause obstruction of the duodenum.

Characteristic Clinical Features
Patients present with bilious emesis secondary to bowel obstruction distal to the ampulla of Vater.

Characteristic Radiologic Findings
Plain radiographs of the abdomen reveal dilation of the proximal duodenum secondary to obstruction by Ladd bands. An upper GI study is the study of choice to evaluate for underlying malrotation.

Less Common Radiologic Manifestations
Patients often present after a Ladd procedure (which involves lysis of Ladd bands) with small bowel obstruction that occurs secondary to adhesions that develop as a consequence of surgery.

Differential Diagnosis
- Midgut volvulus
- Duodenal stenosis

Discussion
Midgut volvulus is a surgical emergency. This is a closed-loop obstruction related to the twisting of the bowel loops around the mesentery, which effectively causes infarction of the bowel secondary to vascular compromise. This condition occurs in patients with underlying malrotation. Duodenal stenosis is a narrowing, or sometimes complete atresia, of the duodenum, which may be secondary to a duodenal web or annular pancreas. Approximately 30% of patients with duodenal stenosis have Down syndrome.

Diagnosis
Ladd bands

Suggested Readings
Powell DM, Othersen HB, Smith CD: Malrotation of the intestines in children: The effect of age on presentation and therapy. J Pediatr Surg 24:777-780, 1989.

Torres AM, Ziegler MM: Malrotation of the intestine. World J Surg 17:326-331, 1993.

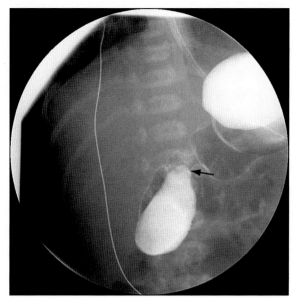

Figure 1. Fluoroscopic spot image from an upper GI examination performed in the first few days of life shows contrast agent within the stomach and dilated duodenum. There is a nasogastric tube in place. The dilated duodenum abruptly tapers at the level of the duodenojejunal junction (*arrow*). The duodenojejunal junction is abnormally positioned consistent with malrotation.

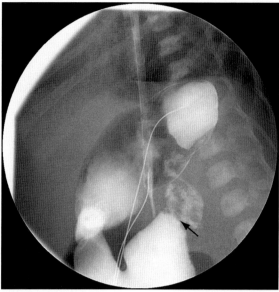

Figure 2. Fluoroscopic spot image from upper GI examination performed in the first few days of life shows contrast agent within the stomach and dilated duodenum. The dilated duodenum abruptly tapers at the level of the duodenojejunal junction (*arrow*). The duodenojejunal junction is abnormally positioned consistent with malrotation. A small trickle of contrast agent passes through to decompressed loops of proximal small bowel.

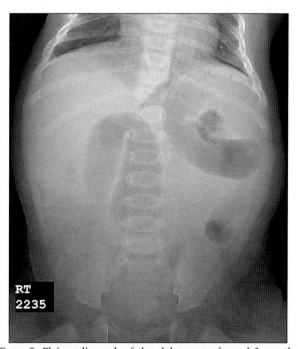

Figure 3. Plain radiograph of the abdomen performed 3 months later shows multiple dilated loops of small bowel consistent with bowel obstruction.

Case 74

DEMOGRAPHICS/CLINICAL HISTORY

The patient is a 19-year-old woman with dysphagia.

FINDINGS

Fluoroscopic spot image from a barium swallow (Fig. 1) shows barium in a dilated esophagus with a beaklike narrowing at the gastroesophageal junction. A chest radiograph performed 10 minutes after the procedure (Fig. 2) shows persistence of barium within the esophagus and delayed passage into the stomach, indicative of delayed peristalsis.

DISCUSSION

Definition/Background

Primary achalasia is an idiopathic condition characterized by incomplete relaxation of the lower esophageal sphincter and absent primary peristalsis.

Characteristic Clinical Features

Patients often present with long-standing dysphagia.

Characteristic Radiologic Findings

On barium studies, the esophagus shows a tapered, beaklike narrowing at the level of the gastroesophageal junction.

Differential Diagnosis

- Esophageal carcinoma

Diagnosis

Achalasia

Suggested Readings

Levine MS, Rubesin SE: Diseases of the esophagus: Diagnosis with esophagography. Radiology 237:414-427, 2005.

Noh HM, Fishman EK, Forastiere AA, et al: CT of the esophagus: Spectrum of disease with emphasis on esophageal carcinoma. RadioGraphics 15:1113-1134, 1995.

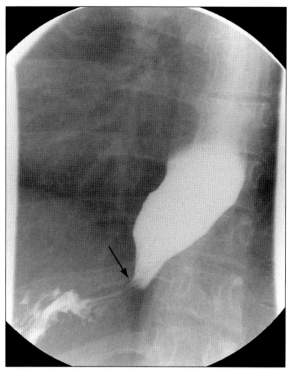

Figure 1. Fluoroscopic spot image from barium swallow examination shows dilated distal esophagus with a beaklike narrowing at the gastroesophageal junction (*arrow*).

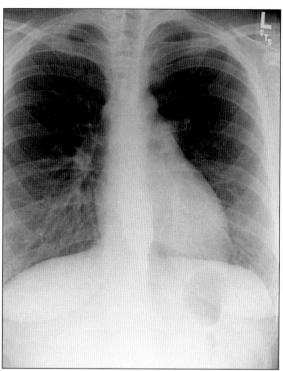

Figure 2. Delayed chest radiograph performed 10 minutes after the barium swallow in Fig. 1 shows persistent column of barium within the esophagus.

Case 75

DEMOGRAPHICS/CLINICAL HISTORY

The patient is a 19-year-old man with an abnormality noted on upper endoscopy, performed for treatment of an esophageal stricture.

FINDINGS

Spot fluoroscopic images acquired during an upper gastrointestinal (GI) examination (Figs. 1 and 2) reveal that the gastric rugae extend cephalad into the chest, indicating the presence of a hiatal hernia.

DISCUSSION

Definition/Background

Large hiatal hernias are uncommon in children.

Characteristic Clinical Features

Although small hiatal hernias are most often asymptomatic, larger hernias may be associated with symptoms of reflux and dysphagia. The patient in this case had an esophageal stricture most likely secondary to reflux.

Characteristic Radiologic Findings

A portion of the stomach is seen herniating into the chest on upper GI examination. Gastroesophageal reflux is commonly associated.

Less Common Radiologic Manifestations

On plain radiographs of the chest, a hiatal hernia sometimes can be appreciated as a round mass behind the heart with an air-fluid level.

Differential Diagnosis

- Congenital diaphragmatic hernia
- Bronchogenic cyst

Discussion

Congenital diaphragmatic hernia refers to herniation of abdominal contents through a defect in the diaphragm. Most commonly, the defect is posterolateral (foramen of Bochdalek) and on the left side. When the defect is severe, pulmonary hypoplasia also is present. A bronchogenic cyst can occur in the lung or mediastinum, but does not communicate with the airway. The cyst may cause compression of the tracheobronchial tree. Cross-sectional imaging reveals a fluid attenuation mass, which is often discovered incidentally.

Diagnosis

Hernia, hiatal

Suggested Readings

Arthur RJ, Ziervogel MA, Axmy AF: Barium meal examination of infants under 4 months of age presenting with vomiting: A review of 100 cases. Pediatr Radiol 14:84, 1984.

Simanovsky N, Buonomo C, Nurko S: The infant with chronic vomiting: The value of the upper GI series. Pediatr Radiol 32:549, 2002.

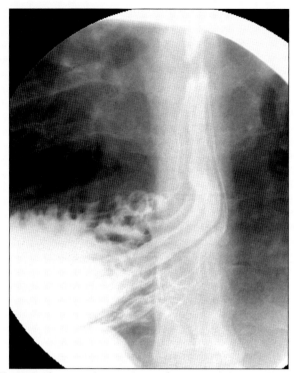

Figure 1. Fluoroscopic spot image from upper GI examination reveals gastric rugae outlined by orally ingested barium; the rugae extend into the lower chest.

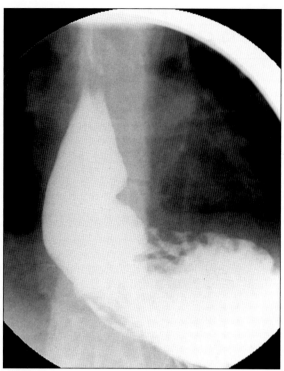

Figure 2. Fluoroscopic image from upper GI examination with the patient lying on the left side. Contrast material opacifies the gastric fundus, which has herniated into the lower chest.

Case 76

DEMOGRAPHICS/CLINICAL HISTORY

The patient is a 15-year-old boy, presenting after involvement in a high-speed motor vehicle accident.

FINDINGS

Contrast-enhanced computed tomography (CT) of the abdomen (Figs. 1 and 2) shows abnormal fluid and inflammation in the retroperitoneum surrounding the duodenum and pancreas and within the anterior pararenal space. There is extraluminal contrast material and extraluminal gas medial to the second portion of the duodenum secondary to a duodenal rupture.

DISCUSSION

Definition/Background
Bowel injuries are uncommon injuries after blunt abdominal trauma relative to other solid parenchymal organ injuries.

Characteristic Clinical Features
Patients are most often the victims of trauma (either blunt or perforating) and may have abdominal pain or abdominal contusions signaling an intra-abdominal injury. Many trauma patients are obtunded and unresponsive on arrival at an emergency department and are unable to verbalize symptoms; imaging is performed based on the mechanism of injury.

Characteristic Radiologic Findings
Bowel injuries may be difficult to detect on imaging studies because findings detectable on imaging may take several hours to develop after an injury. Common imaging findings of bowel rupture on CT examinations are extraluminal gas (highly specific for bowel injury), intraperitoneal or retroperitoneal free fluid, and extraluminal contrast material (if the patient was given oral contrast agent). Affected segments of the bowel may show wall thickening and hyperenhancement.

Differential Diagnosis
- Inflammatory bowel disease
- Henoch-Schönlein purpura
- Hypotension ("shock bowel")

Discussion
In the absence of a history of trauma, segmental bowel wall thickening and enhancement may be related to inflammatory bowel disease such as Crohn disease or ulcerative colitis. These conditions may also lead to bowel rupture in extreme cases. Henoch-Schönlein purpura also may manifest with areas of segmental bowel wall thickening as the result of intramural hemorrhage. Small bowel intussusception may also be present; bowel rupture is uncommon. Patients with profound hypotension who have been aggressively resuscitated may show diffuse bowel wall enhancement abnormalities that may mimic bowel injury.

Diagnosis
Bowel rupture

Suggested Readings

Brofman N, Atri M, Hanson JM, et al: Evaluation of bowel and mesenteric blunt trauma with multidetector CT. RadioGraphics 26:1119-1131, 2006.

Sivit CJ, Eichelberger MR, Taylor GA: CT in children with rupture of the bowel caused by blunt trauma: Diagnostic efficacy and comparison with hypoperfusion complex. AJR Am J Roentgenol 163:1195-1198, 1994.

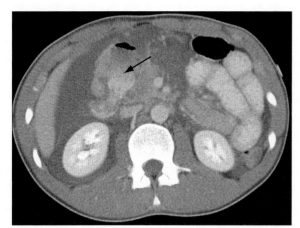

Figure 1. Axial image from contrast-enhanced CT scan of the abdomen shows abnormal fluid and inflammation in the retroperitoneum surrounding the duodenum and pancreas and within the anterior pararenal space. There is extraluminal contrast material and extraluminal gas medial to the second portion of the duodenum secondary to a duodenal rupture (*arrow*). Abnormal enhancement of the pancreatic head is secondary to a concomitant pancreatic laceration.

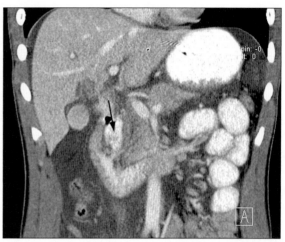

Figure 2. Coronal reformatted image from contrast-enhanced CT scan of the abdomen better shows extraluminal contrast material extravasating medial to the descending portion of the duodenum (*arrow*). Abnormal fluid is present within the right paracolic gutter.

Case 77

DEMOGRAPHICS/CLINICAL HISTORY

The patient is a 6-week-old girl with a hepatic cyst detected by a prenatal ultrasound scan.

FINDINGS

Ultrasound evaluation of the liver (Figs. 1 and 2) shows a large, anechoic fluid collection within the left lobe of the liver that is consistent with a simple cyst.

DISCUSSION

Definition/Background

Solitary cysts are uncommon in children. They are benign.

Characteristic Clinical Features

Hepatic cysts are often incidental findings on imaging performed for other reasons.

Characteristic Radiologic Findings

Ultrasound evaluation shows an anechoic, intrahepatic lesion that is sharply demarcated from the surrounding liver.

Differential Diagnosis

- Hepatic abscess
- Choledochal cyst (i.e., cystic dilation of the biliary tree)
- Foregut duplication cyst

Diagnosis

Hepatic cyst, neonatal

Suggested Readings

Charlesworth P, Ade-Ajayi N, Davenport M: Natural history and long-term follow-up of antenatally detected liver cysts. J Pediatr Surg 42:494-499, 2007.

Rogers TN, Woodley H, Ramsden W, et al: Solitary liver cysts in children: Not always so simple. J Pediatr Surg 42:333-339, 2007.

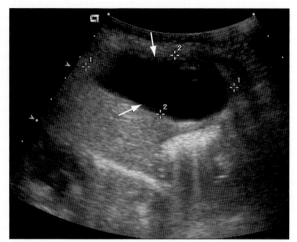

Figure 1. Longitudinal ultrasound through the liver shows large, well-defined, anechoic fluid collection within the left lobe of the liver (*arrows*).

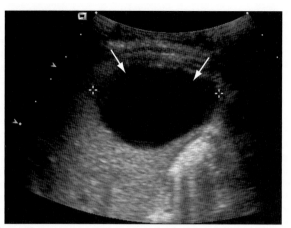

Figure 2. Transverse ultrasound study the liver shows large, well-defined, anechoic fluid collection within the left lobe of the liver (*arrows*).

Case 78

DEMOGRAPHICS/CLINICAL HISTORY

The patient is a 3-week-old infant (born premature at 29 weeks of gestation) with sepsis after umbilical venous catheter placement.

FINDINGS

Ultrasound evaluation of the liver (Figs. 1 and 2) in this premature neonate at the time of diagnosis revealed a large, heterogeneous collection in the right lobe of the liver, with echogenic foci representing gas. Several months later, ultrasound showed a decrease in size of the collection, which appeared as a dense, shadowing calcification (Fig. 3). Computed tomography (CT) performed several days later also (Fig. 4) shows the large, chunky calcification in the liver at the site of the previous abscess.

DISCUSSION

Definition/Background

Hepatic abscesses are rare in neonates and usually result from hematogenous spread of infection related to sepsis, umbilical line placement, or omphalitis. Other risk factors include chronic granulomatous disease, bone marrow transplantation, chemotherapy, and immunodeficiency disorder.

Characteristic Clinical Features

Infants with hepatic abscess most often present with symptoms of sepsis.

Characteristic Radiologic Findings

Ultrasound findings include a hypoechoic cystic mass with increased through-transmission, the presence of internal debris, and a surrounding hypoechoic rim of edema.

Less Common Radiologic Manifestations

CT findings include a low attenuation collection with an enhancing abscess wall and low attenuation surrounding edema.

Differential Diagnosis

- Hepatic cyst
- Fungal infection (e.g., *Aspergillus*)
- Hydatid cyst

Discussion

A hydatid cyst represents infestation by the larval form of the *Echinococcus* tapeworm. Humans are infected when they eat food or water contaminated with the fecal material from the definitive host (e.g., dogs, other carnivores).

Diagnosis

Hepatic abscess

Suggested Readings

Sharma S, Mohta A, Sharma P: Hepatic abscess in a preterm neonate. Indian Pediatr 44:226-228, 2007.

Tan NW, Sriram B, Tan-Kendrick AP, et al: Neonatal hepatic abscess in preterm infants: A rare entity? Ann Acad Med Singapore 34:558-564, 2005.

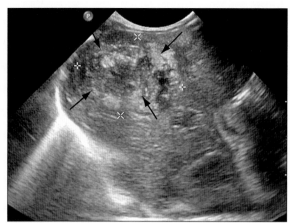

Figure 1. Longitudinal ultrasound of the liver shows a heterogeneous collection in the right lobe of the liver (*arrows*), with multiple echogenic foci representing gas.

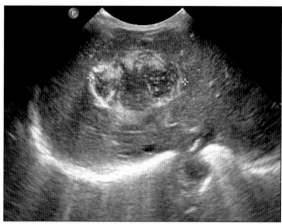

Figure 2. Transverse ultrasound of the liver shows a large, heterogeneous collection in the right lobe of the liver and echogenic foci.

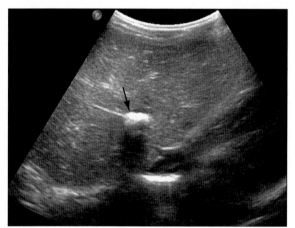

Figure 3. Transverse ultrasound study of the liver performed several months later shows interval decrease in the size of the collection, which consists of a dense, shadowing calcification (*arrow*).

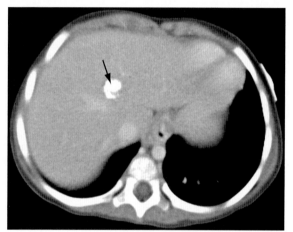

Figure 4. Axial, contrast-enhanced CT scan through the liver of the abdomen and pelvis shows dense calcification in the liver (*arrow*) at the site of a prior abscess.

Case 79

DEMOGRAPHICS/CLINICAL HISTORY

The patient is a 14-month-old boy with a palpable abdominal mass.

FINDINGS

Ultrasound of the abdomen (Fig. 1) reveals a large, cystic mass within the right upper quadrant and midline. The mass contains multiple septa and arises from the liver. Contrast-enhanced computed tomography (CT) of the abdomen (Figs. 2 and 3) shows a large, multicystic mass within the liver that extends into the left upper quadrant.

DISCUSSION

Definition/Background
Mesenchymal hamartoma is a rare, cystic, developmental anomaly that occurs mainly in infants. It is not a true tumor.

Characteristic Clinical Features
Patients usually present with diffuse abdominal enlargement or a palpable abdominal mass.

Characteristic Radiologic Findings
Ultrasound and CT are commonly employed to evaluate an abdominal mass. Mesenchymal hamartoma is a predominantly cystic mass that contains internal septa, and it usually can be seen arising from the liver.

Less Common Radiologic Manifestations
Ascites may rarely be present. Some portions of the mass may appear solid.

Differential Diagnosis
- Hepatic abscess
- Hepatoblastoma (cystic)
- Embryonal sarcoma

Discussion
Hepatic abscess manifests as a solitary lesion or multiple collections of pus within the liver as a result of infection by bacteria, protozoa, fungi, or other agents; polymicrobial involvement is common. CT and ultrasound are the best modalities for screening and for guiding percutaneous aspiration and drainage. On CT, the lesions are well-demarcated areas that are hypodense compared with surrounding hepatic parenchyma. Peripheral enhancement is seen after intravenous contrast agent is administered. Cystic hepatoblastomas and simple hepatic cysts have similar ultrasound characteristics, but the finding of internal septa can differentiate them, and the lesions are extremely sonolucent. Cystic hepatoblastoma may have malignant potential. Embryonal sarcoma is a malignant mesenchymal tumor of the liver that may have cystic spaces within it. These tumors usually occur in older children and young adults.

Diagnosis
Mesenchymal hamartoma

Suggested Readings
Ros PR, Goodman ZD, Ishak KG, et al: Mesenchymal hamartoma of the liver: Radiologic-pathologic correlation. Radiology 158:619-624, 1986.

Wooton-Gorges SL, Thomas KB, Harned RK, et al: Giant cystic abdominal masses in children. Pediatr Radiol 35:1277-1288, 2005.

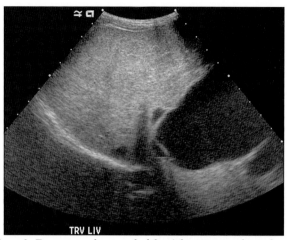

Figure 1. Transverse ultrasound of the right upper quadrant shows a large cystic mass that appears to arise from the left lobe of the liver.

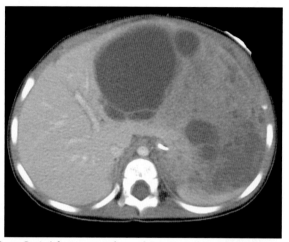

Figure 2. Axial contrast-enhanced CT scan of the abdomen reveals a multicystic mass with one large dominant cyst arising from the left lobe of the liver and extending into the left upper quadrant.

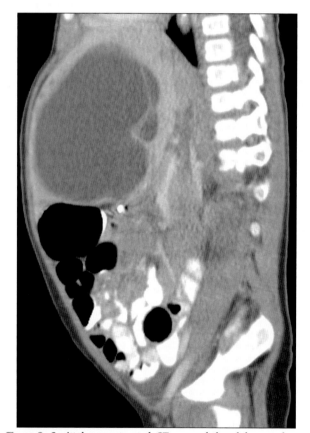

Figure 3. Sagittal reconstructed CT scan of the abdomen shows the dominant cyst replacing almost the entire left lobe of the liver.

Case 80

DEMOGRAPHICS/CLINICAL HISTORY

The patient is a newborn with liver failure and thrombocytopenia.

FINDINGS

Contrast-enhanced computed tomography (CT) of the liver (Figs. 1 and 2) shows a large, heterogeneously enhancing mass within the liver. The mass has a predominantly peripheral pattern of enhancement (see Fig. 2). The celiac axis and hepatic artery are enlarged, and the abdominal aorta distal to the celiac artery is markedly diminished in caliber (Fig. 3).

DISCUSSION

Definition/Background

Infantile hemangiomas are most common in white female patients.

Characteristic Clinical Features

Patients may present with abdominal distention, coagulopathy, or thrombocytopenia. The presence of high-flow arteriovenous shunting may lead to congestive heart failure or respiratory distress.

Characteristic Radiologic Findings

CT and magnetic resonance imaging (MRI) of the liver show well-defined, lobular liver masses, which avidly enhance after contrast agent administration, with enlarged feeding arteries and draining veins.

Less Common Radiologic Manifestations

Plain radiographs may reveal signs of congestive heart failure, including an enlarged heart and pulmonary edema.

Differential Diagnosis

- Metastatic neuroblastoma

Discussion

Although metastatic neuroblastoma can manifest with many enhancing liver lesions, the enlargement of the hepatic artery and the presence of arteriovenous shunting are more consistent with hepatic hemangioma, especially in a newborn.

Diagnosis

Hepatic hemangioma

Suggested Readings

Kassarjian A, Zurakowski D, Dubois J, et al: Infantile hepatic hemangiomas: Clinical and imaging findings and their correlation with therapy. AJR Am J Roentgenol 182:785-795, 2004.

Konez O, Burrows PE, Mulliken JB, et al: Angiographic features of rapidly involuting congenital hemangioma (RICH). Pediatr Radiol 33:15-19, 2003.

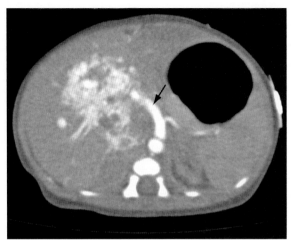

Figure 1. Axial contrast-enhanced CT scan through the abdomen shows an avidly, heterogeneously enhancing mass within the liver. The hepatic artery is markedly enlarged (*arrow*).

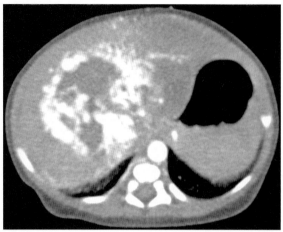

Figure 2. Axial contrast-enhanced CT scan through the abdomen reveals predominantly peripheral enhancement of the mass at this relatively early phase of contrast enhancement.

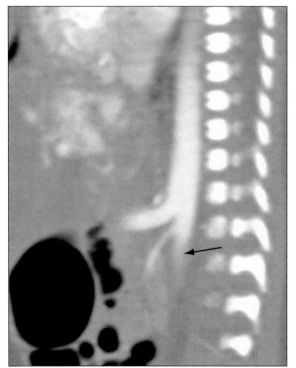

Figure 3. Sagittal reformatted contrast-enhanced CT scan through the abdomen shows an enlarged celiac axis. The caliber of the abdominal aorta inferior to the celiac axis is markedly diminished (*arrow*).

Case 81

DEMOGRAPHICS/CLINICAL HISTORY

The patient is an 8-month-old girl with an incidentally discovered liver mass.

FINDINGS

Computed tomography (CT) scanning through the liver after administration of intravenous contrast material (Figs. 1 and 2) shows a large lesion within the right lobe of the liver, which is nearly isoattenuating to the remainder of the normal liver parenchyma, but which has hyperenhancement on arterial phase imaging. Ultrasound examination of the right lobe of the liver (Fig. 3) shows a large, round lesion, which is slightly hyperechoic relative to the surrounding liver parenchyma without associated biliary dilation or central scarring or necrosis.

DISCUSSION

Definition/Background
Focal nodular hyperplasia (FNH) is a benign hepatic tumor that is uncommon in children. There is an increased incidence of FNH in children who have completed oncologic treatment compared with healthy children.

Characteristic Clinical Features
FNH lesions are often discovered incidentally on imaging performed for other indications. Larger lesions may manifest as an abdominal mass or hepatomegaly.

Characteristic Radiologic Findings
Contrast-enhanced CT of the abdomen classically reveals a hypoattenuating lesion on noncontrast phase imaging that is hyperenhancing on arterial phase imaging. A hypodense scar is shown in only one third of cases.

Less Common Radiologic Manifestations
On ultrasound, FNH is commonly hypoechoic or isoechoic to the normal hepatic parenchyma. A central feeding artery may be shown with Doppler ultrasound with a spoke-wheel pattern running from the central scar to fibrous septa.

Differential Diagnosis
- Hepatoblastoma
- Hepatocellular carcinoma
- Hemangioma

Discussion
Hepatoblastoma is a malignant hepatic neoplasm that occurs in patients younger than 5 years old. Hepatocellular carcinoma is a malignant hepatic neoplasm usually seen in children older than 5 years old or who have underlying hepatic disease. Hepatic hemangioma is a benign vascular neoplasm, which may be present in infancy, and which has a characteristic enhancement pattern on dynamic contrast-enhanced CT studies reflective of the vascular nature of the tumor.

Diagnosis
Focal nodular hyperplasia

Suggested Readings
Joyner BL Jr, Levin TL, Goyal RK, et al: Focal nodular hyperplasia of the liver: A sequela of tumor therapy. Pediatr Radiol 35:1234, 2005.
Vilgrain V: Focal nodular hyperplasia. Eur J Radiol 58:236, 2006.

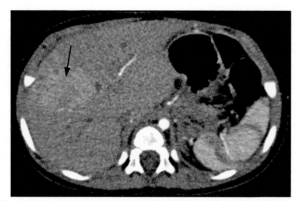

Figure 1. Axial CT image through the liver after administration of intravenous contrast material during arterial phase imaging shows large lesion within right lobe of the liver, which has hyperenhancement relative to normal hepatic parenchyma (*arrow*).

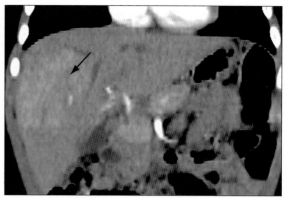

Figure 2. Coronal reformatted CT image through the liver after administration of intravenous contrast material shows large lesion within right lobe of the liver, which has hyperenhancement on arterial phase imaging (*arrow*).

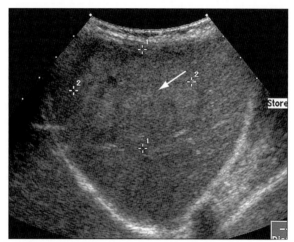

Figure 3. Ultrasound examination of right lobe of liver shows large, lobulated lesion (*arrow*), which is slightly hyperechoic relative to surrounding liver parenchyma without associated biliary dilation or central scarring or necrosis.

Case 82

DEMOGRAPHICS/CLINICAL HISTORY

The patient is a 5-month-old boy with a palpable abdominal mass.

FINDINGS

Ultrasound of the liver (Fig. 1) shows a large heterogeneous mass within the liver. Axial T2-weighted (Fig. 2) and coronal T2-weighted fat-saturated (Fig. 3) magnetic resonance imaging (MRI) shows the heterogeneous mass. Postcontrast T1-weighted fat-saturated MRI (Fig. 4) shows heterogeneous enhancement of the mass. The portal vein is seen displaced anteriorly and medially, but not invaded.

DISCUSSION

Definition/Background

Hepatoblastoma is the most common malignant pediatric hepatic neoplasm.

Characteristic Clinical Features

Patients with these tumors often present with a palpable mass.

Characteristic Radiologic Findings

Typically, a large heterogeneous intrahepatic mass is seen with heterogeneous enhancement. Mass effect on hepatic vessels is often seen as the result of the typically large tumor size, but tumor involvement or thrombus of the portal or hepatic venous systems can occur. Hepatoblastomas may metastasize within the liver and commonly metastasize to the lungs.

Less Common Radiologic Manifestations

Nodal metastases and peritoneal deposits are rare.

Differential Diagnosis

- Hemangioendothelioma/hemangioma

Discussion

Hemangiomas/hemangioendotheliomas are vascular neoplasms with intense enhancement, typically in a peripheral pattern with centripetal fill-in. Hepatic hemangiomas are common in patients with multiple cutaneous hemangiomas. Hemangioendotheliomas can be associated with coagulopathy (Kasabach-Merritt syndrome). Patients with hepatoblastomas typically have abnormal α-fetoprotein levels, which are not typically elevated in patients with hemangiomas and hemangioendotheliomas.

Diagnosis

Hepatoblastoma

Suggested Reading

Roebuck DJ, Olsen Ø, Pariente D: Radiological staging in children with hepatoblastoma. Pediatr Radiol 36:176-182, 2006.

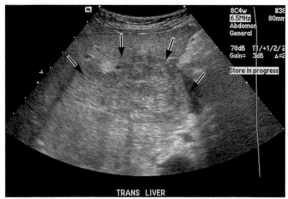

Figure 1. Ultrasound of the liver shows large heterogeneous mass (*arrows*) within the liver.

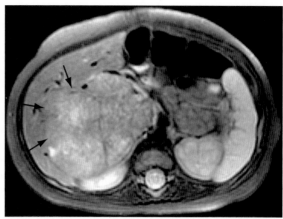

Figure 2. Axial T2-weighted MR image shows heterogeneous mass (*arrows*) displacing normal hepatic vessels.

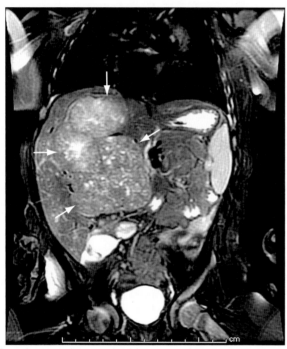

Figure 3. Coronal T2-weighted fat-saturated MR image shows large heterogeneous mass (*arrows*).

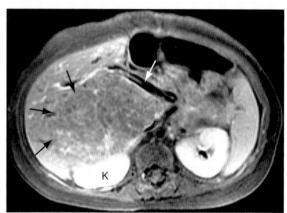

Figure 4. Postcontrast T1-weighted fat-saturated MR image shows heterogeneous enhancement of the mass (*black arrows*). The portal vein is seen displaced anteriorly and medially (*white arrow*), but not invaded. The right kidney (K) is seen posteriorly.

Case 83

DEMOGRAPHICS/CLINICAL HISTORY

The patient is a 3-year-old boy with decreased appetite.

FINDINGS

Axial and coronal reformatted images from a contrast-enhanced computed tomography (CT) examination of the abdomen (Figs. 1 and 2) show a large, heterogeneous, solid mass within the right and left lobes of the liver causing hepatomegaly. A transverse ultrasound image of the liver at a similar level to Fig. 1 shows that the masses appear relatively well defined and are hyperechoic and heterogeneous relative to normal liver parenchyma (Fig. 3).

DISCUSSION

Definition/Background

Hepatoblastoma is the most common malignant pediatric liver tumor. It is more common in boys.

Characteristic Clinical Features

Hepatoblastoma may manifest as an abdominal mass. Patients may present with anorexia, weight loss, emesis, and abdominal pain.

Characteristic Radiologic Findings

On ultrasound, hepatoblastoma appears as a solid, hyperechoic mass, most often in the right lobe of the liver.

Less Common Radiologic Manifestations

Hepatoblastoma is shown on CT as a hypoattenuating solid mass that may contain calcifications. CT is useful in showing the degree of vascular invasion and involvement of the tumor.

Differential Diagnosis

- Hepatocellular carcinoma
- Hemangioma
- Mesenchymal hamartoma
- Metastatic neuroblastoma

Discussion

Hepatocellular carcinoma is a malignant hepatic tumor that is more commonly seen in older patients or patients with underlying liver disease. Hemangioma is a vascular tumor of the liver that is seen in younger patients, including neonates. These lesions are highly vascular on contrast-enhanced CT or magnetic resonance imaging (MRI). Mesenchymal hamartoma is a benign, largely cystic tumor of the liver seen in children. Metastatic neuroblastoma may manifest with multiple liver lesions, rather than a single, dominant lesion.

Diagnosis

Hepatoblastoma

Suggested Readings

Emre S, McKenna GJ: Liver tumors in children. Pediatr Transplant 8:632, 2004.

Roebuck DJ, Olsen O, Pariente D: Radiological staging in children with hepatoblastoma. Pediatr Radiol 36:176, 2006.

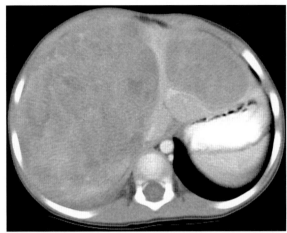

Figure 1. Axial contrast-enhanced CT image of abdomen shows large, heterogeneous, solid mass within right and left lobes of liver causing hepatomegaly.

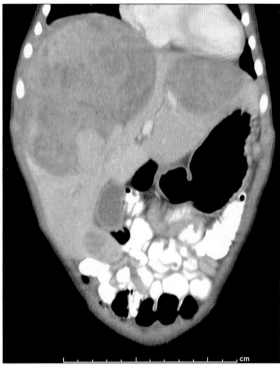

Figure 2. Coronal reformatted contrast-enhanced CT image of abdomen shows large, heterogeneous, solid mass within right and left lobes of liver causing hepatomegaly.

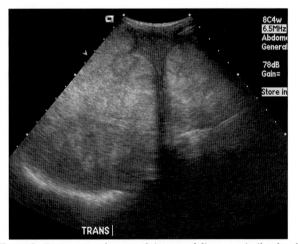

Figure 3. Transverse ultrasound image of liver at similar level to Fig. 1 shows that masses appear relatively well defined and are hyperechoic and heterogeneous relative to normal liver parenchyma.

Case 84

DEMOGRAPHICS/CLINICAL HISTORY

The patient is a 5-year-old girl with a known diagnosis of α_1-antitrypsin disease and liver disease.

FINDINGS

Ultrasound of the abdomen (Fig. 1) reveals diffusely coarsened and heterogeneous liver echotexture consistent with cirrhosis. Splenomegaly is present as well and is related to portal hypertension (Fig. 2). The patient also has recanalization of the umbilical vein secondary to portal hypertension (Fig. 3).

DISCUSSION

Definition/Background

α_1-antitrypsin disorder is an inherited condition associated with retention of the α_1-antitrypsin protein in the liver. It is more common in whites and rarely affects African-Americans or Asians.

Characteristic Clinical Features

Patients may present in the neonatal period with persistent jaundice and hepatomegaly, and may go on to develop chronic hepatitis, cirrhosis, and hepatocellular carcinoma. Destructive lung disease occurs later in life (third decade).

Characteristic Radiologic Findings

Ultrasound features of the disease are similar to features found in patients with liver disease and cirrhosis secondary to other etiologies. The liver appears coarsened and heterogeneous and may have a nodular surface contour. The gallbladder wall may appear thickened. Manifestations of portal hypertension include abnormal hepatofugal flow in the portal vein, monophasic flow in the hepatic veins, and splenomegaly. The umbilical vein may also be patent.

Differential Diagnosis
- Neonatal hepatitis
- Biliary atresia
- Alagille syndrome

Discussion

Neonatal hepatitis is an inflammation of the liver that occurs in infants from birth to 2 months. Often no inciting agent is identified. In approximately 20% of cases, it is caused by cytomegalovirus; rubella; or hepatitis A, B, or C viruses. Biliary atresia is an obliteration of the extrahepatic biliary system. Patients present in infancy with signs and symptoms of cholestasis. Alagille syndrome is an autosomal dominant condition associated with hepatic disease characterized by narrowed and malformed bile ducts.

Diagnosis

α_1-Antitrypsin deficiency

Suggested Readings

Perlmutter DH: Alpha-1-antitrypsin deficiency: Diagnosis and treatment. Clin Liver Dis 8:839-859, viii-ix, 2004.

Rosen HR: Liver disease associated with alpha1-antitrypsin deficiency. Clin Liver Dis 2:175-185, 1998.

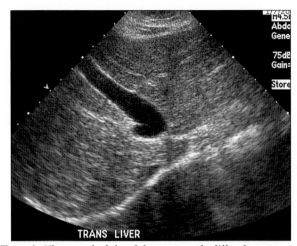

Figure 1. Ultrasound of the abdomen reveals diffusely coarsened and heterogeneous liver echotexture consistent with cirrhosis.

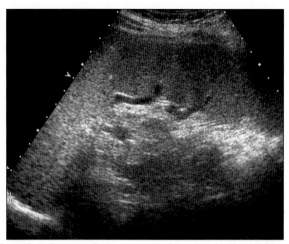

Figure 2. Splenomegaly is present and is related to portal hypertension.

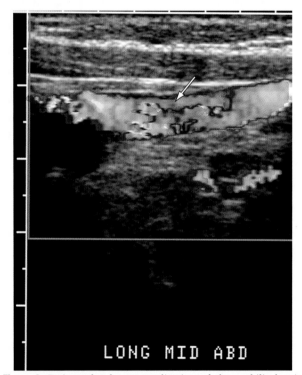

Figure 3. Patient also has recanalization of the umbilical vein secondary to portal hypertension (*arrow*).

Case 85

DEMOGRAPHICS/CLINICAL HISTORY

The patient is a 15-year-old boy after bone marrow transplant.

FINDINGS

Ultrasound images of the abdomen show a moderate amount of ascites (Fig. 1), diffuse circumferential gallbladder wall thickening (Fig. 2), and splenomegaly (Fig. 3).

DISCUSSION

Definition/Background

Hepatic veno-occlusive disease typically occurs within 20 days after bone marrow transplantation. It occurs in approximately half of all bone marrow transplant patients, and many cases resolve spontaneously.

Characteristic Clinical Features

Patients may present with jaundice, hepatomegaly, weight gain, and ascites.

Characteristic Radiologic Findings

Although there may be no imaging findings in some cases, classic ultrasound findings include ascites, gallbladder wall thickening, and hepatosplenomegaly. Reversed flow in the portal vein is another imaging finding consistent with the diagnosis.

Differential Diagnosis

- Graft-versus-host disease
- Cytomegalovirus (pediatric brain)
- Cholestasis
- Right heart failure

Discussion

Graft-versus-host disease occurs after bone marrow transplantation because of the transplantation of immunologically competent cells into an immunoincompetent host. It occurs within the first 100 days of transplantation, and patients may present with dermatitis, enteritis, and hepatitis. Cytomegalovirus is a herpesvirus infection that occurs in immunocompromised patients and that may cause hepatitis. Cholestasis is a condition, caused by a variety of different diseases, in which there is an obstruction to the flow of bile from the liver into the duodenum. Right heart failure can lead to an increase in the systemic venous pressures leading into the heart, which can lead to passive hepatic congestion.

Diagnosis

Veno-occlusive disease

Suggested Readings

McCarville MB, Hoffer FA, Howard SC, et al: Hepatic veno-occlusive disease in children undergoing bone-marrow transplantation: Usefulness of sonographic findings. Pediatr Radiol 31:102-105, 2001.
Teefey SA, Brink JA, Borson RA, et al: Diagnosis of venoocclusive disease of the liver after bone marrow transplantation: value of duplex sonography. AJR Am J Roentgenol 164:1397-1401, 1995.

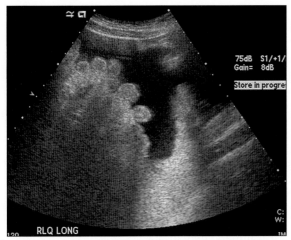

Figure 1. Transverse ultrasound of the abdomen in the right lower quadrant shows moderate amount of ascites.

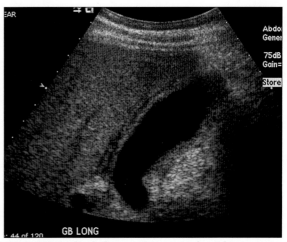

Figure 2. Longitudinal ultrasound image in the right upper quadrant shows distended gallbladder. There is diffuse circumferential gallbladder wall thickening.

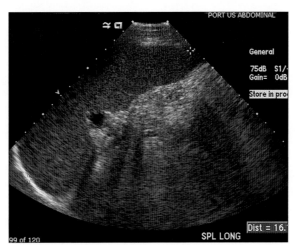

Figure 3. Longitudinal ultrasound image in the left upper quadrant shows splenomegaly (the spleen measures approximately 16 cm).

Case 86

DEMOGRAPHICS/CLINICAL HISTORY

The patient is a 5-year-old boy with an abdominal mass.

FINDINGS

An axial image from contrast-enhanced computed tomography (CT) scan of the abdomen (Fig. 1) shows a hypoattenuating lesion within the right lobe of the liver. Fluid-sensitive axial image from magnetic resonance imaging (MRI) of the abdomen (Fig. 2) shows that the lesion is bright in signal with multiple internal low signal septations, consistent with a complex cystic mass. Axial T1-weighted MRI through the abdomen with fat suppression after administration of intravenous contrast agent (Fig. 3) shows peripheral enhancement of the lesion without central enhancement.

DISCUSSION

Definition/Background

Embryonal sarcoma is a rare hepatic malignancy that occurs in children and young adults. Patients with this tumor usually have a poor prognosis.

Characteristic Clinical Features

Patients often present with abdominal pain or a palpable abdominal mass.

Characteristic Radiologic Findings

Most embryonal sarcomas show mostly water attenuation on CT with areas of intermediate soft tissue attenuation at the periphery of the lesion.

Less Common Radiologic Manifestations

MRI examination of embryonal sarcoma shows lesions that are predominantly bright signal on fluid-sensitive sequences and low in signal on T1-weighted images. After administration of contrast agent, the periphery of the lesion shows enhancement without significant internal enhancement.

Differential Diagnosis
- Mesenchymal hamartoma
- Echinococcal (hydatid) cyst
- Abscess
- Biliary cystadenoma
- Hepatocellular carcinoma
- Post-traumatic hematoma

Discussion

Mesenchymal hamartoma is a space-occupying lesion in the liver caused by hamartomatous growth of mesenchymal tissue of uncertain etiology. It is benign and is usually composed of multiple cysts of varying sizes. Echinococcal cysts of the liver are caused by infection with a small tapeworm (Echinococcus granulosus). These cysts are characterized by a thick-walled main cyst with multiple daughter cysts. Intrahepatic abscess may manifest as a thick-walled cystic lesion in the liver secondary to infection with various purulent organisms. Biliary cystadenoma is a benign hepatic neoplasm originating in the bile ducts that can appear as a unilocular or multilocular cystic intrahepatic mass. Hepatocellular carcinoma is a primary malignant tumor of the liver that is more common in adults with underlying liver disease (e.g., hepatitis, cirrhosis) and may show cystic areas when tumor necrosis has occurred. Post-traumatic hematoma is a complex cystic lesion within the liver that represents liquefying hematoma after traumatic hepatic injury.

Diagnosis

Sarcoma, embryonal

Suggested Readings

Buetow PC, Buck JL, Pantongrag-Brown L, et al: Undifferentiated (embryonal) sarcoma of the liver: Pathologic basis of imaging findings in 28 cases. Radiology 203:779-783, 1997.

Moon WK, Kim WS, Kim IO, et al: Undifferentiated embryonal sarcoma of the liver: US and CT findings. Pediatr Radiol 24:500-503, 1994.

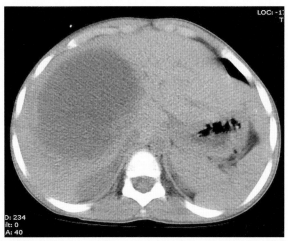

Figure 1. Axial image from contrast-enhanced CT scan of the abdomen shows large hypoattenuating lesion within the right lobe of the liver.

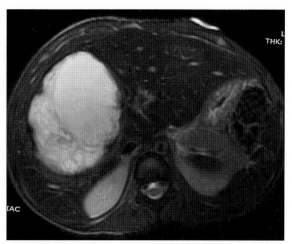

Figure 2. Fluid-sensitive axial image from MRI of the abdomen shows that lesion is bright in signal with multiple internal low signal septations, consistent with a complex cystic mass.

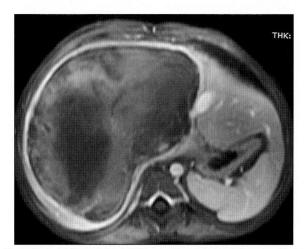

Figure 3. Axial T1-weighted MR image through the abdomen with fat suppression after administration of intravenous contrast agent shows peripheral enhancement of lesion without central enhancement.

Case 87

DEMOGRAPHICS/CLINICAL HISTORY

The patient is a 15-year-old girl with an incidental finding on computed tomography (CT) scan performed for evaluation of flank pain.

FINDINGS

CT scans of the abdomen and pelvis performed without administration of intravenous or oral contrast material (Figs. 1 and 2) show fusiform dilation of the common bile duct (CBD) throughout its entire course. A longitudinal image from an ultrasound study of the abdomen (Fig. 3) shows an anechoic structure in the right upper quadrant, which appears cystic and separate from the gallbladder. An anterior projection image (Fig. 4) acquired as part of a technetium 99m (^{99m}Tc)–labeled hepatobiliary iminodiacetic acid (HIDA) examination at 1 hour after injection shows accumulation of radiotracer into the cystic right upper quadrant structure.

DISCUSSION

Definition/Background

Choledochal cysts are congenital malformations of the bile ducts that usually manifest in childhood. There are several types of choledochal cyst; the most common is cystic dilation of the CBD (type 1), as in this patient.

Characteristic Clinical Features

Younger patients may present with jaundice, cholestasis, or pale-colored stools. Older children have a more insidious onset of right upper quadrant pain, jaundice, or cholangitis.

Characteristic Radiologic Findings

Ultrasound is the preferred modality to assess choledochal cysts. A type 1 choledochal cyst (as in this case) manifests as cystic dilation of the CBD.

Less Common Radiologic Manifestations

Type 2 cysts appear as a cystic lesion separate from the CBD. With type 3, there is cystic dilation of the distal CBD within the duodenal wall.

Differential Diagnosis

- Hepatic cyst
- Hepatic abscess
- Mesenchymal hamartoma

Discussion

Hepatic cyst is a simple cyst in the liver that is not connected to the biliary tree. Hepatic abscess manifests as a complex collection in the liver usually related to pyogenic infection, although uncommonly the result of parasitic infection. Mesenchymal hamartoma commonly manifests as a cystic mass in the liver and may rarely mimic a choledochal cyst.

Diagnosis

Choledochal cyst

Suggested Reading

Mishra A, Pant N, Chadha R, et al: Choledochal cysts in infancy and childhood. Indian J Pediatr 74:937, 2007.

Rha SY, Stovroff MC, Glick PL, et al: Choledochal cysts: A ten year experience. Am Surg 62:30, 1996.

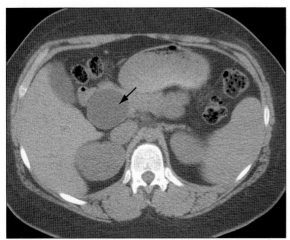

Figure 1. Axial image from CT scan of abdomen and pelvis performed without intravenous or oral contrast material shows fusiform dilation of CBD throughout its entire course (*arrow*).

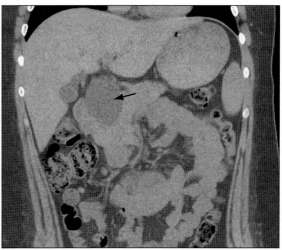

Figure 2. Coronal reformatted image from CT scan of abdomen and pelvis performed without intravenous or oral contrast material shows fusiform dilation of CBD throughout its entire course (*arrow*).

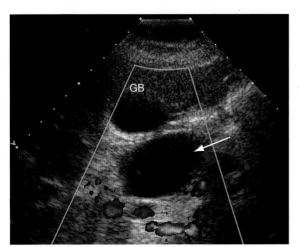

Figure 3. Longitudinal image from ultrasound of abdomen shows anechoic structure in right upper quadrant (*arrow*), which appears cystic, lacks color Doppler flow, and appears separate from gallbladder (GB).

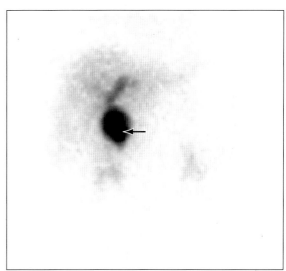

Figure 4. Anterior projection image acquired as part of ^{99m}Tc-labeled HIDA examination at 1 hour after injection shows accumulation of radiotracer in cystic right upper quadrant structure (*arrow*).

Case 88

The patient is a 1-year-old boy with jaundice of 3 days' duration and pruritus for 1 month.

FINDINGS

Ultrasound of the liver (Fig. 1) shows a tubular anechoic structure at the porta hepatis, separate from the gallbladder. Color Doppler (Fig. 2) of this structure shows no vascular flow within the structure. Coronal T2-weighted MRI (Fig. 3) shows a dilated extrahepatic biliary system, a dilated gallbladder, and a tiny stone within the cystic duct that was also seen on ultrasound (not shown). Coronal magnetic resonance cholangiopancreatography (MRCP) reconstruction (Fig. 4) shows mild intrahepatic biliary dilation, fusiform extrahepatic biliary ductal dilation, and distended gallbladder. At surgery, this was confirmed to be a type 1 choledochal cyst, and the intrahepatic dilation resolved after resection of the choledochal cyst.

DISCUSSION

Definition/Background
Choledochal cysts are classified (Todani classification) by the portions of the biliary system that are involved (intrahepatic or extrahepatic or both), the presence of a choledochocele, and by the type of dilation (fusiform or saccular). The most common type is type 1—dilation of the common bile duct.

Characteristic Clinical Features
Presentation may be the result of cholestasis with jaundice, pruritus, and acholic stools. A right upper quadrant mass or pain may also be present.

Characteristic Radiologic Findings
Dilation of the extrahepatic biliary ductal system is most commonly seen. Intrahepatic ductal dilation may be present either as part of the abnormal choledochal cyst or as the result of stasis. Small stones resulting from chronic stasis may be seen within the biliary system.

Differential Diagnosis
- Obstructing gallstones

Discussion
If an obstructing gallstone is causing cholestasis and dilation of the biliary system, it typically can be seen on MRCP (if not seen on ultrasound). In these cases, other gallstones are typically seen.

Diagnosis
Choledochal cyst

Suggested Reading
Fitoz S, Erden A, Boruban S: Magnetic resonance cholangiopancreatography of biliary system abnormalities in children. Clin Imaging 31:93-101, 2007.

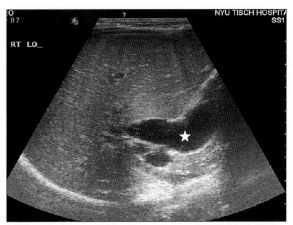

Figure 1. Ultrasound of the liver shows tubular anechoic structure (*star*) at the porta hepatis, separate from the gallbladder (not shown).

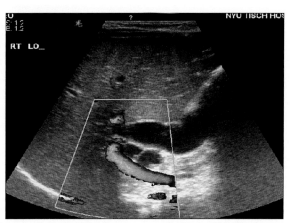

Figure 2. Color Doppler shows no vascular flow within the structure.

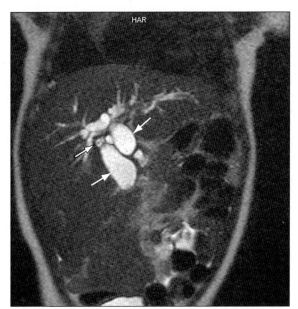

Figure 3. Coronal T2-weighted MRI shows dilated extrahepatic biliary system (*right arrow*), a dilated gallbladder (*left lower arrow*), and a tiny stone within the cystic duct (*left upper arrow*) that was also seen on ultrasound (not shown).

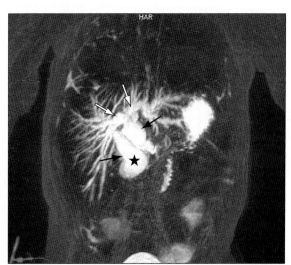

Figure 4. Coronal MRCP reconstruction shows mild intrahepatic biliary dilation (*white arrows*), fusiform extrahepatic biliary ductal dilation (*black arrow*), and distended gallbladder (*star*).

Case 89

DEMOGRAPHICS/CLINICAL HISTORY

The patient is an 8-year-old boy with abdominal pain.

FINDINGS

Axial (Fig. 1) and coronal (Fig. 2) T2-weighted images from magnetic resonance imaging (MRI) of the abdomen show fusiform enlargement of the main, right, and left hepatic ducts and of a portion of the common bile duct (CBD). A reconstructed maximum intensity projection (MIP) image in the coronal plane of the biliary system shows the same findings. The pancreatic duct is normal (Fig. 3).

DISCUSSION

Definition/Background

Choledochal cysts are congenital malformations of the bile ducts that usually manifest in childhood. There are several types of choledochal cyst; the most common is cystic dilation of the CBD (type 1), as in this patient.

Characteristic Clinical Features

Younger patients may present with jaundice, cholestasis, or pale-colored stools. Older children have a more insidious onset of right upper quadrant pain, jaundice, or cholangitis.

Characteristic Radiologic Findings

Ultrasound is the preferred modality to assess choledochal cysts. A type 1 choledochal cyst (as in this case) manifests as cystic dilation of the CBD.

Less Common Radiologic Manifestations

Type 2 cysts appear as cystic lesions separate from the CBD. A type 3 cyst is a cystic dilation of the distal CBD within the duodenal wall.

Differential Diagnosis

- Hepatic cyst
- Hepatic abscess
- Mesenchymal hamartoma

Discussion

Hepatic cyst is a simple cyst in the liver that is not connected to the biliary tree. Hepatic abscess manifests as a complex collection in the liver, usually related to pyogenic infection, although uncommonly the result of parasitic infection. Mesenchymal hamartoma commonly manifests as a cystic mass in the liver and may rarely mimic a choledochal cyst.

Diagnosis

Choledochal cyst

Suggested Readings

Mishra A, Pant N, Chadha R, et al: Choledochal cysts in infancy and childhood. Indian J Pediatr 74:937-943, 2007.

Rha SY, Stovroff MC, Glick PL, et al: Choledochal cysts: A ten year experience. Am Surg 62:30-34, 1996.

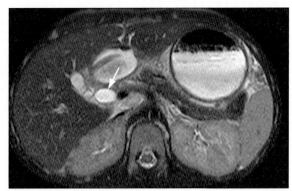

Figure 1. Axial T2-weighted MR image of the abdomen shows fusiform enlargement of the main, right, and left hepatic ducts and a portion of the CBD (*arrow*).

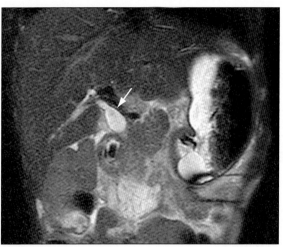

Figure 2. Coronal T2-weighted MR image of the abdomen shows fusiform enlargement of the main, right, and left hepatic ducts and a portion of the CBD (*arrow*).

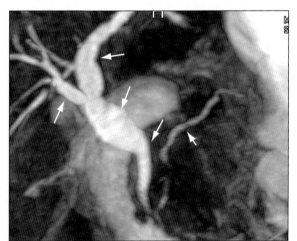

Figure 3. Reconstructed MIP image in the coronal plane of the biliary system shows the same findings (*long arrows*). The pancreatic duct is normal (*short arrow*).

Case 90

DEMOGRAPHICS/CLINICAL HISTORY

The patient is a newborn with elevated liver function test results.

FINDINGS

A hepatobiliary scan using iminodiacetic acid (IDA) radiopharmaceuticals shows prompt hepatic uptake of tracer over time (Fig. 1). After 24 hours, there is no evidence of contrast material within the bile ducts or bowel (Fig. 2).

DISCUSSION

Definition/Background

Biliary atresia consists of obliteration of the extrahepatic biliary system, which results in obstruction of the flow of bile.

Characteristic Clinical Features

The disorder manifests in the neonatal period with jaundice, dark urine, and light stools.

Characteristic Radiologic Findings

Hepatobiliary imaging is diagnostic by showing no excretion of radiolabeled tracer into the extrahepatic biliary system.

Less Common Radiologic Manifestations

Ultrasound of the liver and right upper quadrant shows absence of the gallbladder.

Differential Diagnosis
- Neonatal hepatitis
- Choledochal cyst

Diagnosis

Biliary atresia

Suggested Readings

Nadel HR: Hepatobiliary scintigraphy in children. Semin Nucl Med 26:25-42, 1996.

Sevilla A, Howman-Giles R, Saleh H, et al: Hepatobiliary scintigraphy with SPECT in infancy. Clin Nucl Med 32:16-23, 2007.

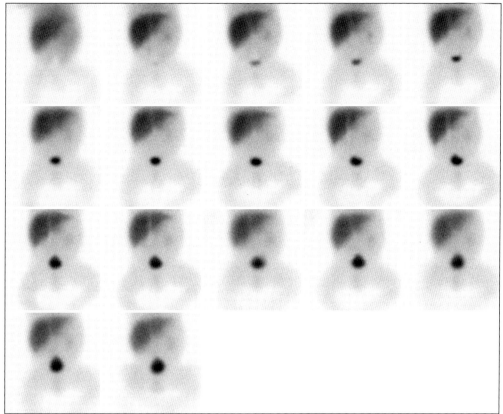

Figure 1. Anterior planar images obtained over the course of 1 hour from technetium 99m (^{99m}Tc)–labeled IDA scan reveals prompt liver uptake of tracer without excretion into the biliary system or bowel. There is urinary excretion of tracer.

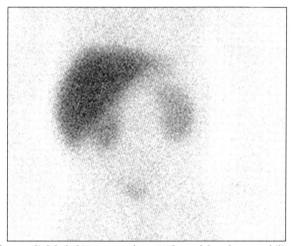

Figure 2. Static anterior planar image from radiolabeled IDA scan after a 24-hour delay shows no biliary excretion of tracer. There is contrast material within the kidneys and bladder.

Case 91

DEMOGRAPHICS/CLINICAL HISTORY

The patient is a 3-year-old girl with chronic renal failure resulting from hemolytic uremic syndrome and with multiple episodes of right upper quadrant pain.

FINDINGS

Longitudinal (Fig. 1) and transverse (Fig. 2) ultrasound images of the right upper quadrant show a distended gallbladder with multiple, layering, echogenic gallstones with posterior acoustic shadowing.

DISCUSSION

Definition/Background
Gallstones are far less common in children than in adults and tend to occur in patients with underlying medical problems, such as chronic infection, hemolytic disease, parenteral nutrition, and prior ileal resection.

Characteristic Clinical Features
Gallstones may lead to gallstone pancreatitis. Patients present with recurrent abdominal pain and jaundice.

Characteristic Radiologic Findings
Ultrasound is the diagnostic method of choice to identify gallstones because it can detect stones (e.g., echogenic, shadowing foci within the gallbladder); biliary duct dilation; secondary signs of cholecystitis (e.g., gallbladder wall thickening, pericholecystic fluid); and other complications, such as pancreatitis.

Less Common Radiologic Manifestations
Plain radiographs rarely show gallstones in children because the stones are rarely calcified.

Differential Diagnosis
- Biliary sludge

Discussion
Biliary sludge describes a mixture of particulate matter in the bile without discrete gallstone formation. In some cases, the bile may be very viscous and simulate a tumor (i.e., tumefactive sludge).

Diagnosis
Cholelithiasis

Suggested Readings
Akel S, Khalifeh M: Makhlouf Akel M: Gallstone pancreatitis in children: Atypical presentation and review. Eur J Pediatr 164:482-485, 2005.
Albu E, Buiumsohn A, Lopez R, et al: Gallstone pancreatitis in adolescents. J Pediatr Surg 22:960-962, 1987.

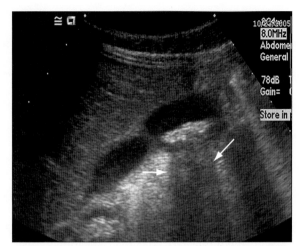

Figure 1. Longitudinal ultrasound image of right upper quadrant shows distended gallbladder with multiple, layering, echogenic gallstones with posterior acoustic shadowing (*arrows*).

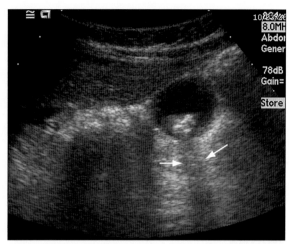

Figure 2. Transverse ultrasound image of right upper quadrant shows distended gallbladder with multiple, layering, echogenic gallstones with posterior acoustic shadowing (*arrows*).

Case 92

DEMOGRAPHICS/CLINICAL HISTORY

The patient is a newborn boy with a history of congenital diaphragmatic hernia.

FINDINGS

A plain radiograph of the abdomen (Fig. 1) shows a feeding tube coursing into a right-sided stomach. Contrast-enhanced computed tomography (CT) scan of the abdomen (Fig. 2) shows a central liver, a right-sided stomach, and asplenia. The inferior vena cava and aorta are positioned on the left side of the abdomen.

DISCUSSION

Definition/Background

The heterotaxy syndromes consist of abnormalities of visceral situs and occur sporadically, affecting 1 in 6000 to 20,000 live births.

Characteristic Clinical Features

Heterotaxy syndrome with asplenia consists of bilateral trilobed lungs, bilateral systemic atria, central liver, malrotated bowel, indeterminate stomach, asplenia, and cardiac anomalies. Heterotaxy syndrome with polysplenia consists of bilateral bilobed lungs, bilateral pulmonary atria, central liver, indeterminate stomach, malrotated bowel, multiple spleens, and cardiac anomalies, which are less common and less severe than in patients with asplenia.

Characteristic Radiologic Findings

Radiographic features depend on the nature of the disorder. On abdominal CT, the liver position is usually abnormal, the stomach may be right-sided, the spleen may be absent or there may be multiple spleens, and the position of the inferior vena cava may be abnormal.

Differential Diagnosis

- Situs inversus

Discussion

Situs inversus is the mirror image of normal visceral anatomy. There is a slightly higher incidence of congenital heart disease among patients with situs inversus compared with the normal population.

Diagnosis

Abdominal heterotaxy

Suggested Readings

Applegate KE, Goske MJ, Pierce G, et al: Situs revisited: Imaging of the heterotaxy syndrome. RadioGraphics 19:837-852, 1999.

Tonkin IL, Tonkin AK: Visceroatrial situs abnormalities: Sonographic and computed tomographic appearance. AJR Am J Roentgenol 138:509-515, 1982.

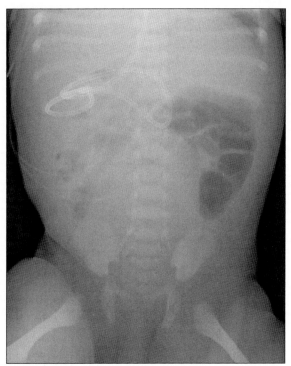

Figure 1. Anteroposterior radiograph of the abdomen shows a feeding tube coursing into a right-sided stomach.

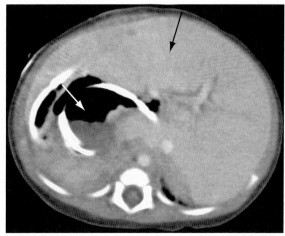

Figure 2. Axial contrast-enhanced CT scan of the abdomen shows a central liver (*black arrow*), a right-sided stomach (*white arrow*), and asplenia. The inferior vena cava and the aorta are located to the left of the vertebral column.

Case 93

DEMOGRAPHICS/CLINICAL HISTORY

The patient is a 7-week-old girl with increasing creatinine levels and abdominal distention.

FINDINGS

Contrast-enhanced computed tomography (CT) of the abdomen (Figs. 1-3) shows tapering of the abdominal aorta and hypoenhancement of the kidneys.

DISCUSSION

Definition/Background
Middle aortic syndrome is an acquired disorder.

Characteristic Clinical Features
Patients commonly present in the second decade of life with hypertension.

Characteristic Radiologic Findings
Imaging studies may include CT, magnetic resonance imaging (MRI), or angiography. Studies show diffuse narrowing of the thoracoabdominal aorta and major branch vessels.

Differential Diagnosis
- Takayasu arteritis

Discussion
Takayasu arteritis is an inflammatory arteritis that causes stenosis of major vessels, predominantly the vessels arising from the aortic arch.

Diagnosis
Middle aortic syndrome

Suggested Readings
Adams WM, John PR: US demonstration and diagnosis of the midaortic syndrome. Pediatr Radiol 28:461-463, 1998.
Lewis VD 3rd, Meranze SG, McLean GK, et al: The midaortic syndrome: Diagnosis and treatment. Radiology 167:111-113, 1988.

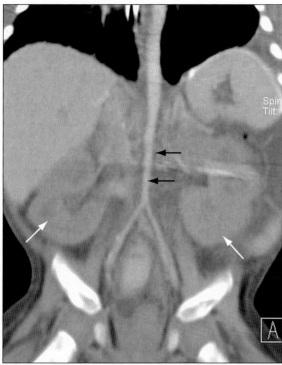

Figure 1. Coronal reformatted contrast-enhanced CT image of the abdomen shows smooth tapering of a long segment of the abdominal aorta (*black arrows*). Perfusion is compromised to both kidneys (*white arrows*).

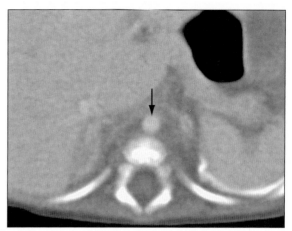

Figure 2. Axial contrast-enhanced CT image of the abdomen at the level of the spleen shows normal-caliber aorta (*arrow*).

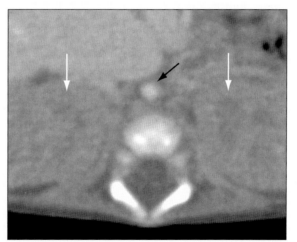

Figure 3. Axial contrast-enhanced CT image of the abdomen at the level of the kidneys shows small-caliber aorta (*black arrow*) and hypoperfused kidneys (*white arrows*).

Case 94

DEMOGRAPHICS/CLINICAL HISTORY

The patient is a 15-year-old girl presenting after a motor vehicle accident.

FINDINGS

A contrast-enhanced computed tomography (CT) scan of the abdomen (Fig. 1) shows a linear focus of hypoattenuation at the pancreatic body and tail junction that is consistent with a laceration; there is also peripancreatic fluid. A contrast-enhanced CT scan obtained 2 weeks later (Fig. 2) shows evolving complex retroperitoneal fluid collections, consistent with developing pseudocysts.

DISCUSSION

Definition/Background

Pancreatic lacerations are uncommon injuries in children and are most often caused by bicycle handlebar injuries.

Characteristic Clinical Features

Patients present with a history of abdominal trauma. Pancreatic enzyme levels may be elevated, but in some cases, there are no laboratory abnormalities at the time of presentation.

Characteristic Radiologic Findings

Fluid between the pancreas and splenic vein is an indicator of pancreatic injury. Other signs of pancreatic injury include enlargement of the pancreas, stranding of the adjacent mesenteric or retroperitoneal fat, and a visible hypoattenuating defect within the gland.

Differential Diagnosis

- Pancreatitis

Discussion

Pancreatitis is rare in children and is often related to prior trauma, anatomic abnormalities, metabolic disorders, and medications.

Diagnosis

Pancreatic laceration

Suggested Readings

Lane MJ, Mindelzun RE, Sandhu JS, et al: CT diagnosis of blunt pancreatic trauma: Importance of detecting fluid between the pancreas and the splenic vein. AJR Am J Roentgenol 163:833-835, 1994.

Sivit CJ, Eichelberger MR, Taylor GA, et al: Blunt pancreatic trauma in children: CT diagnosis. AJR Am J Roentgenol 158:1097-1100, 1992.

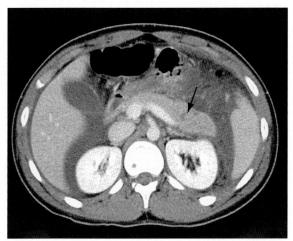

Figure 1. Axial contrast-enhanced CT of the abdomen shows transverse laceration through the body and tail of the pancreas (*arrow*) and surrounding peripancreatic fluid.

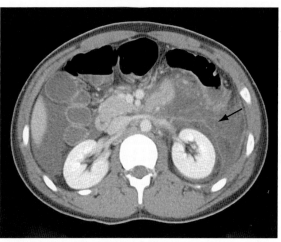

Figure 2. Axial contrast-enhanced CT of the abdomen performed 2 weeks later reveals evolving retroperitoneal fluid collections (*arrow*), which later evolved into infected pseudocysts. There is persistent free fluid in the abdomen.

Case 95

DEMOGRAPHICS/CLINICAL HISTORY

The patient is a 12-year-old boy with hypoglycemia.

FINDINGS

An axial image from a contrast-enhanced computed tomography (CT) scan of the abdomen (Fig. 1) shows a hyperenhancing lesion within the head of the pancreas. An intraoperative ultrasound examination (Fig. 2) shows a well-defined, hypoechoic lesion in the head of the pancreas.

DISCUSSION

Definition/Background

Insulinoma is the most common islet cell tumor of the pancreas in children.

Characteristic Clinical Features

Patients present with hypoglycemia, which may manifest as erratic behavior or seizure activity in children.

Characteristic Radiologic Findings

Insulinomas are round or oval and are hypervascular. Contrast-enhanced CT scans show marked hyperattenuation of these lesions after administration of contrast agent.

Less Common Radiologic Manifestations

On ultrasound, insulinomas are often hypoechoic relative to the remainder of the pancreatic parenchyma.

Differential Diagnosis

- Solid-cystic papillary tumor
- Pancreaticoblastoma
- Islet cell tumor

Discussion

Solid-cystic papillary tumor is most often seen in girls and manifests as a large, well-defined solid mass with cystic components. Pancreaticoblastoma is a tumor arising from the acinar cells of the pancreas, is more common in boys, and manifests as a hypodense mass in the pancreas on CT. Islet cell tumors are hormonally active tumors in the pancreas, and include insulinoma, VIPomas, glucagonomas, and gastrinomas.

Diagnosis

Insulinoma

Suggested Readings

Kumbasar B, Kamel IR, Tekes A, et al: Imaging of neuroendocrine tumors: accuracy of helical CT versus SRS. Abdom Imaging 29:696, 2004.

Rha SE, Jung SE, Lee KH, et al: CT and MR imaging findings of endocrine tumor of the pancreas according to WHO classification. Eur J Radiol 62:371, 2007.

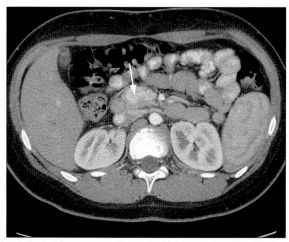

Figure 1. Axial contrast-enhanced CT image of abdomen shows hyperenhancing lesion within head of the pancreas (*arrow*).

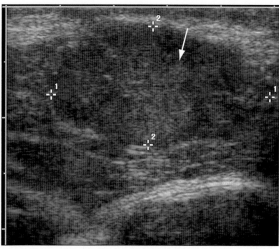

Figure 2. Intraoperative ultrasound shows well-defined, hypoechoic lesion in head of the pancreas (*arrow*).

Case 96

DEMOGRAPHICS/CLINICAL HISTORY

The patient is a 14-year-old girl with epigastric pain.

FINDINGS

Transverse ultrasound through the mid-abdomen (Fig. 1) at the level of the aortic takeoff of the superior mesenteric artery and portal venous confluence shows a large heterogeneous mass in the expected region of the head of the pancreas. An axial image from a subsequent contrast-enhanced computed tomography (CT) scan (Fig. 2) shows a large mass arising from the pancreas. An axial CT image, slightly more superior (Fig. 3), shows the mass and mild dilation of the pancreatic duct.

DISCUSSION

Definition/Background

Solid pseudopapillary tumor (SPT) is a tumor of the pancreas that occurs typically in adolescents, more commonly girls. This entity is known by a few other names, such as solid and cystic papillary neoplasm, solid and papillary epithelial neoplasm (SPEN), and Frantz tumor.

Characteristic Clinical Features

Abdominal pain and jaundice can be presenting features. Solid pseudopapillary tumor is more common in adolescent girls and young women.

Characteristic Radiologic Findings

A mass within the pancreas can be heterogeneous in appearance, particularly if large. These tumors are often large at diagnosis because of late manifestation of symptoms. Dilation of the pancreatic duct is often seen distal to large tumors. Dilation of the biliary system can be present if mass effect on the common bile duct causes biliary obstruction. Although reportedly more common in the body and tail of the pancreas, the tumor can be found in any location within the pancreas.

Differential Diagnosis
- Pancreatoblastoma
- Lymphoma

Discussion

Pancreatoblastoma is a rare primary pancreatic tumor typically seen in younger children. Imaging features can be identical to solid pseudopapillary tumor of the pancreas. Lymphoma can involve the pancreas and manifest as focal masses within the pancreas. Often other signs of systemic lymphoma are present, such as lymphadenopathy or other organ involvement.

Diagnosis

Solid pseudopapillary tumor of the pancreas

Suggested Readings

Jaksic T, Yaman M, Thorner P, et al: A 20-year review of pediatric pancreatic tumors. J Pediatr Surg 27:1315-1317, 1992.
Nijs E, Callahan MJ, Taylor GA: Disorders of the pediatric pancreas: Imaging features. Pediatr Radiol 35:358-373, 2005.
Vaughn DD, Jabra AA, Fishman EK: Pancreatic disease in children and young adults: Evaluation with CT. RadioGraphics 18:1171-1187, 1998.

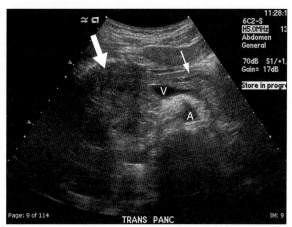

Figure 1. Transverse ultrasound through the mid-abdomen at the level of the aortic (A) takeoff of the superior mesenteric artery and portal venous confluence (V) shows large heterogeneous mass in the expected region of the head of the pancreas (*large arrow*). Mild dilation of the pancreatic duct is seen (*small arrow*).

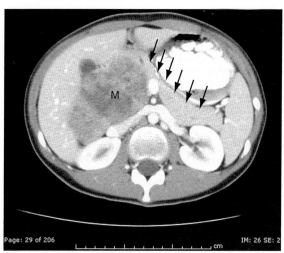

Figure 2. Axial image from subsequent contrast-enhanced CT scan shows large mass (M) arising from the pancreas (*arrows*).

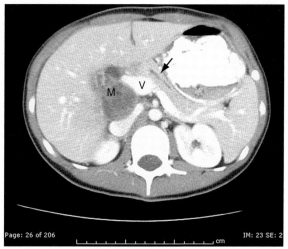

Figure 3. Axial CT image, slightly more superior than Figure 2, shows the mass (M) and mild dilation of the pancreatic duct (*arrow*) at the level of the portal venous confluence (V).

Case 97

DEMOGRAPHICS/CLINICAL HISTORY

The patient is an 11-year-old boy with a 2-week history of epigastric pain.

FINDINGS

Ultrasound evaluation of the pancreas (Fig. 1) shows that the pancreas is enlarged, bulky, and hypoechoic. Contrast-enhanced computed tomography (CT) through the abdomen (Fig. 2) shows that the body of the pancreas is enlarged, appears heterogeneous, and appears hypoattenuating relative to the more normal-appearing distal pancreatic tail. A gallium scan (nuclear medicine) (Fig. 3) shows increased radiotracer uptake in the region of the pancreatic mass in the mid-abdomen.

DISCUSSION

Definition/Background
Burkitt lymphoma is a type of non-Hodgkin, B cell lymphoma that usually occurs in the abdomen.

Characteristic Clinical Features
Patients present with various symptoms, including nausea, vomiting, abdominal pain, and gastrointestinal bleeding.

Characteristic Radiologic Findings
Burkitt lymphoma commonly involves the small bowel and manifests as circumferential bowel wall thickening on cross-sectional imaging.

Less Common Radiologic Manifestations
CT may reveal a discrete abdominal mass or a mass that involves other abdominal and retroperitoneal organs, as in this case.

Differential Diagnosis
- Pancreatitis
- Solid, papillary epithelial neoplasm

Discussion
Solid, papillary epithelial neoplasm is a rare, low-grade pancreatic malignancy that tends to occur in female patients.

Diagnosis
Burkitt lymphoma

Suggested Readings
Kamona AA, El-Khatib MA, Swaiden MY, et al: Pediatric Burkitt's lymphoma: CT findings. Abdom Imaging 32:381-386, 2007.
Karmazyn B, Ash S, Goshen Y, et al: Significance of residual abdominal masses in children with abdominal Burkitt's lymphoma. Pediatr Radiol 31:801-805, 2001.

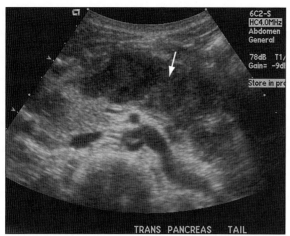

Figure 1. Transverse ultrasound image through the pancreas reveals enlarged, hypoechoic, nodular pancreas (*arrow*).

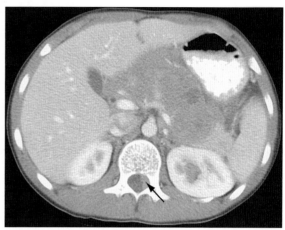

Figure 2. Axial contrast-enhanced CT scan through the abdomen reveals large, hypoattenuating mass within the pancreas. There is abnormal soft tissue density within the spinal canal that is consistent with metastasis (*arrow*).

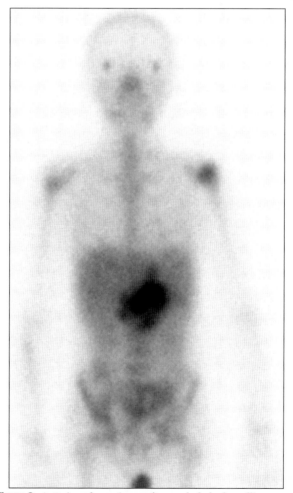

Figure 3. Anterior planar image from whole-body gallium scan shows increased radiotracer uptake in mid-epigastric region in the location of pancreatic mass.

Case 98

DEMOGRAPHICS/CLINICAL HISTORY

The patient is a 9-year-old boy with intermittent stridor and dyspnea.

FINDINGS

Posteroanterior chest radiograph (Fig. 1) shows a round mass along the right paratracheal stripe. Computed tomography (CT) of the chest (Figs. 2 and 3) shows a well-circumscribed, right paratracheal mass with avid contrast enhancement and no invasion into adjacent structures.

DISCUSSION

Definition/Background

Castleman disease, also known as angiofollicular lymph node hyperplasia, is an uncommon, benign lymphoproliferative disorder. It can occur at any age, but has a peak incidence in the third to fourth decades.

Characteristic Clinical Features

The mass is often completely asymptomatic and discovered incidentally during imaging performed for other reasons.

Characteristic Radiologic Findings

On chest radiographs, Castleman disease manifests as a round, solitary mass in the mediastinum or hilum. On CT, Castleman disease usually is visible as a solitary, noninvasive mass with avid, homogeneous contrast enhancement.

Less Common Radiologic Manifestations

Rarely, Castleman disease may arise from the pleura, pericardium, or other costal spaces, including the lung.

Differential Diagnosis

- Lymphoma
- Sarcoid

Discussion

Lymphoma is a solid neoplastic disorder that originates in the lymphatic system and often manifests with lymphadenopathy. Sarcoid is a disorder of the immune system that is characterized by noncaseating granulomas and lymphadenopathy.

Diagnosis

Castleman disease

Suggested Readings

Kaufman RA, Ball WS Jr, Han BK, et al: Pediatric case of the day: Angiomatous lymphoid hamartoma (Castleman's disease). RadioGraphics 8:997-1000, 1988.

Ko SF, Hsieh MJ, Ng SH, et al: Imaging spectrum of Castleman's disease. AJR Am J Roentgenol 182:769-775, 2004.

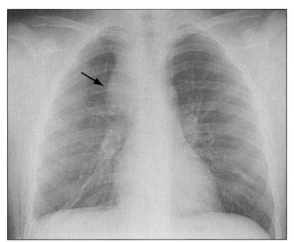

Figure 1. Posteroanterior chest radiograph shows well-circumscribed, round, soft tissue mass adjacent to right paratracheal stripe (*arrow*).

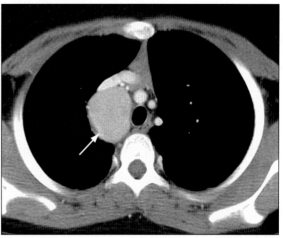

Figure 2. Axial contrast-enhanced CT scan of the chest at a level just above the bifurcation of the trachea shows round, well-defined, enhancing, soft tissue mass along right lateral aspect of the trachea (*arrow*).

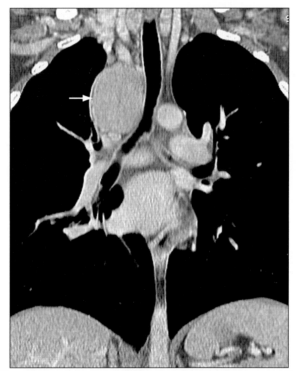

Figure 3. Coronal, reformatted, contrast-enhanced CT scan of the chest shows round, well-defined, enhancing, soft tissue mass along right lateral aspect of the trachea (*arrow*).

Case 99

DEMOGRAPHICS/CLINICAL HISTORY

The patient is a 10-year-old girl with abdominal distention.

FINDINGS

Axial contrast-enhanced computed tomography (CT) through the upper abdomen (Fig. 1) shows numerous varices around the stomach and spleen and a large amount of ascites. At the level of the porta hepatis (Fig. 2), no portal vein is shown, and multiple small collateral vessels are seen in the expected region of the portal vein. Thin curvilinear hypodensity in this area likely represents the chronically thrombosed portal vein.

DISCUSSION

Definition/Background

The term *cavernous transformation of the portal vein* is used for the collateral vessels that occur secondary to stenosis or chronic thrombosis of the portal vein.

Characteristic Clinical Features

Patients may present with symptoms secondary to liver damage, such as jaundice or ascites.

Characteristic Radiologic Findings

Imaging modalities show absence of a normal portal vein. In the porta hepatis, multiple small, tortuous venous collaterals are seen in the periportal region.

Portal hypertension may be reflected in the development of other collateral vessels adjacent to the esophagus, stomach, and spleen. Ascites may be present if there is liver damage.

Less Common Radiologic Manifestations

If liver damage is severe, and fibrosis or cirrhosis occurs, the liver appears heterogeneous with nodularity.

Differential Diagnosis

■ Vascular anomaly

Discussion

Vascular anomalies, such as venous malformations, may occur intra-abdominally and manifest as multiple serpiginous vessels, but the portal vein should still be present.

Diagnosis

Cavernous transformation of the portal vein

Suggested Readings

Corness JA, McHugh K, Roebuck DJ, et al: The portal vein in children: Radiological review of congenital anomalies and acquired abnormalities. Pediatr Radiol 36:87-96, 2006.

Wang L, Li ZS, Lu JP, et al: Cavernous transformation of the portal vein: Three-dimensional dynamic contrast-enhanced MR angiography. Abdom Imaging 33:463-468, 2008.

Zhang LJ, Yang GF, Jiang B, et al: Cavernous transformation of portal vein: 16-slice CT portography and correlation with surgical procedure of orthotopic liver transplantation. Abdom Imaging 33:529-535, 2008.

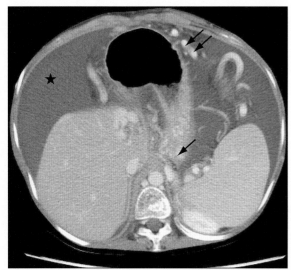

Figure 1. Axial contrast-enhanced CT image through the upper abdomen shows numerous varices around the stomach and spleen (*arrows*) and a large amount of ascites (*star*).

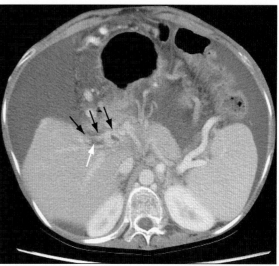

Figure 2. On CT image at the level of the porta hepatis, no portal vein is shown, and multiple small collateral vessels (*black arrows*) are seen in the expected region of the portal vein. Thin linear hypodensity (*white arrow*) in this area may represent a chronically thrombosed portal vein.

Case 100

DEMOGRAPHICS/CLINICAL HISTORY

The patient is a teenager with abdominal pain, no fever, and no elevated white blood cell count.

FINDINGS

Ultrasound (Fig. 1) shows a large amount of peritoneal fluid. Coronal T1-weighted fat-saturated postcontrast magnetic resonance imaging (MRI) (Fig. 2) shows diffuse peritoneal enhancement with focal areas of peritoneal thickening and a large amount of ascites. These findings are confirmed by axial T1-weighted fat-saturated postcontrast MRI (Fig. 3). A chest radiograph obtained later (Fig. 4) shows left hilar lymphadenopathy. The diagnosis of tuberculous peritonitis was confirmed by pathologic examination of fluid and thickened peritoneum.

DISCUSSION

Definition/Background
Tuberculous peritonitis can be a manifestation of *Mycobacterium tuberculosis* infection.

Characteristic Clinical Features
Patients with tuberculous peritonitis may present with abdominal pain, distention, and fever.

Characteristic Radiologic Findings
Radiologic findings include enhancement of the peritoneum and focal nodular areas of peritoneal and omental thickening. Typically, patients have a large amount of ascites. Abdominal tuberculosis is associated with enlarged mesenteric lymph nodes, solid organ involvement, and ileocecal involvement by the infection.

Less Common Radiologic Manifestations
Less commonly, fibrous, thick peritoneal adhesions are seen without a large amount of ascites.

Differential Diagnosis
- Metastatic disease
- Infections other than *M. tuberculosis*

Discussion
The absence of a primary tumor or foreign body (e.g., ventriculoperitoneal shunt) and evidence for pulmonary tuberculosis can be helpful, but biopsy typically is needed for the diagnosis.

Diagnosis
Tuberculous peritonitis

Suggested Readings
Ablin DS, Jain KA, Azouz EM: Abdominal tuberculosis in children. Pediatr Radiol 24:473-477, 1994.
Pereira JM, Madureira AJ, Vieira A, Ramos I: Abdominal tuberculosis: Imaging features. Eur J Radiol 55:173-180, 2005.

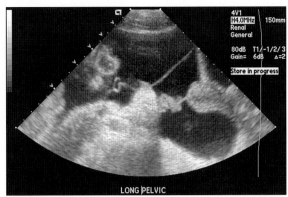

Figure 1. Ultrasound shows a large amount of peritoneal fluid.

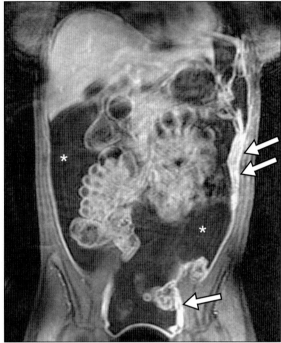

Figure 2. Coronal T1-weighted postcontrast MR image shows diffuse peritoneal enhancement with focal areas of peritoneal thickening (*arrows*) and a large amount of ascites (*asterisks*).

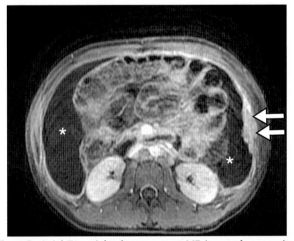

Figure 3. Axial T1-weighted postcontrast MR image shows peritoneal enhancement, focal thickening (*arrows*), and a large amount of ascites (*asterisks*).

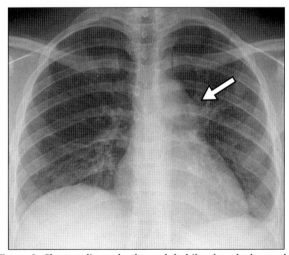

Figure 4. Chest radiograph shows left hilar lymphadenopathy (*arrow*).

Case 101

DEMOGRAPHICS/CLINICAL HISTORY

The patient is a 21-day-old boy with cystic fibrosis and cough.

FINDINGS

A frontal view of the chest (Fig. 1) shows curvilinear densities overlying the liver and spleen, representing the calcifications as sequelae from meconium peritonitis.

DISCUSSION

Definition/Background

Meconium peritonitis occurs as the result of spillage of bowel contents into the peritoneum, with resultant inflammation, and is often diagnosed by the presence of dystrophic peritoneal and intra-abdominal calcifications. The most common etiology of meconium peritonitis is bowel perforation, from causes such as bowel atresias and meconium ileus, resulting from cystic fibrosis.

Characteristic Clinical Features

Patients with cystic fibrosis may present with failure to pass meconium or abdominal distention.

Characteristic Radiologic Findings

Meconium peritonitis appears as small, curvilinear intra-peritoneal calcifications. Intra-abdominal meconium cysts can also be seen. In patients with failure to pass meconium, contrast enema may diagnose an atresia or may diagnose and possibly treat meconium ileus in a patient with cystic fibrosis.

Differential Diagnosis

- Neuroblastoma
- Adrenal hemorrhage
- Hemangioendothelioma

Discussion

Calcifications in the abdomen can be caused by abdominal tumors or prior adrenal hemorrhage. Ultrasound can be performed if the calcifications, physical examination, or history is concerning for an abdominal mass.

Diagnosis

Meconium peritonitis

Suggested Readings

Chan KL, Tang MH, Tse HY, et al: Meconium peritonitis: Prenatal diagnosis, postnatal management and outcome. Prenat Diagn 25:676-682, 2005.

Estroff JA, Bromley B, Benacerraf BR: Fetal meconium peritonitis without sequelae. Pediatr Radiol 22:277-278, 1992.

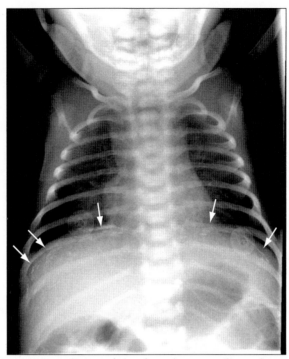

Figure 1. Frontal view of the chest shows curvilinear densities (*arrows*) overlying the liver and spleen, representing calcifications as sequelae from meconium peritonitis.

Case 102

DEMOGRAPHICS/CLINICAL HISTORY

The patient is a 21-day-old boy who is asymptomatic.

FINDINGS

Anteroposterior (Fig. 1) and lateral (Fig. 2) radiographs of the chest show coarse, linear calcifications overlying right and left hemidiaphragms along the peritoneal surface. There is no free intraperitoneal air, and the visualized bowel loops appear mildly dilated.

DISCUSSION

Definition/Background

Meconium peritonitis is secondary to a sterile chemical reaction that results from an in utero bowel perforation. It occurs in 1 of 35,000 live births, and 86% of cases have intra-abdominal calcifications.

Characteristic Clinical Features

Patients may be entirely asymptomatic, especially if the in utero gastrointestinal perforation healed early on, or may present with symptoms of bowel obstruction related to the underlying bowel disease that caused the perforation.

Characteristic Radiologic Findings

On abdominal radiographs, meconium peritonitis appears as linear or coarse calcifications in the abdomen or scrotum. Patients may also present with bowel obstruction and may have bowel atresia.

Less Common Radiologic Manifestations

Ultrasound features include diffuse hyperechoic punctate foci of increased echogenicity within the abdomen, along the hepatic surface, or within the scrotal sac. Ascites may be present.

Differential Diagnosis

- Neuroblastoma
- Adrenal hemorrhage
- Congenital cytomegalovirus

Discussion

Abdominal calcifications in a newborn may be seen in the setting of neuroblastoma. Coarse calcifications in the region of the adrenal glands may be secondary to prior adrenal hemorrhage. Patients with congenital cytomegalovirus may present with intra-abdominal calcifications that are intraparenchymal (i.e., within the liver or spleen).

Diagnosis

Meconium peritonitis

Suggested Readings

Foster MA, Nyberg DA, Mahoney BS, et al: Meconium peritonitis: Prenatal sonographic findings and their clinical significance. Radiology 165:661-665, 1987.

Zangheri G, Andreani M, Ciriello E, et al: Fetal intra-abdominal calcifications from meconium peritonitis: Sonographic predictors of postnatal surgery. Prenatal Diagn 27:960-963, 2007.

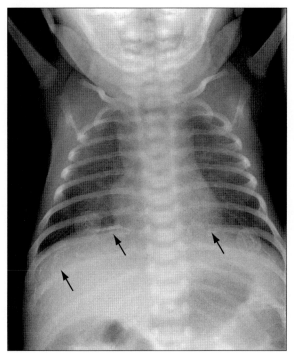

Figure 1. Anteroposterior radiograph of the chest shows coarse calcifications overlying right and left hemidiaphragms along the peritoneal surface (*arrows*). There is no free intraperitoneal air, and the visualized bowel loops appear mildly dilated.

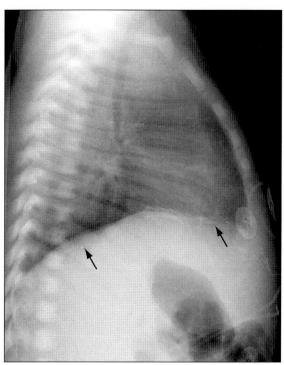

Figure 2. Lateral radiograph of the chest shows coarse calcifications overlying the diaphragm along the peritoneal surface (*arrows*).

Case 103

DEMOGRAPHICS/CLINICAL HISTORY

The patient is a 16-year-old girl with left upper quadrant pain.

FINDINGS

Longitudinal ultrasound of the left upper quadrant (Fig. 1) shows a round mass (measured) inseparable from the spleen. The mass is partly anechoic with layering isoechoic material dependently. Color Doppler (Fig. 2) does not show any vascularity within the mass. Axial computed tomography (CT) image (Fig. 3) shows the fluid density mass within the spleen. Coronal reconstruction (Fig. 4) confirms the location of the mass, and the left kidney is distinctly seen separately.

DISCUSSION

Definition/Background

Splenic cystic lesions are uncommon. Congenital cyst and post-traumatic pseudocyst are two of the most common lesions.

Characteristic Clinical Features

Splenic cyst may be an incidental finding. Pain may be a symptom if the cyst is large, hemorrhagic, or superinfected.

Characteristic Radiologic Findings

The most common appearance is a simple unilocular cystic lesion. If the cyst is superinfected or hemorrhagic, internal debris can be seen. Usually there is no vascularity within or around the cyst.

Less Common Radiologic Manifestations

Hyperemia and a thick ring may be seen if the cyst is superinfected.

Differential Diagnosis

- Abscess
- Parasitic cyst
- Post-traumatic pseudocyst
- Lymphatic malformation

Discussion

Although some imaging findings can suggest the other diagnoses, sometimes pathology may be necessary to distinguish between entities. Infections may have an irregular rind, surrounding hypervascularity. Lymphatic malformations may be multilocular.

Diagnosis

Splenic cyst

Suggested Reading

Hilmes MA, Strouse PJ: The pediatric spleen. Semin Ultrasound CT MR 28:3-11, 2007.

Urrutia M, Mergo PJ, Ros LH, et al: Cystic masses of the spleen: Radiologic-pathologic correlation. RadioGraphics 16:107-129, 1996.

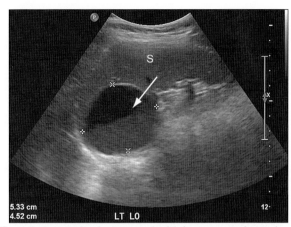

Figure 1. Longitudinal ultrasound of left upper quadrant shows round mass (measured) inseparable from the spleen (S). The mass is partly anechoic with layering (*arrow*) isoechoic material dependently.

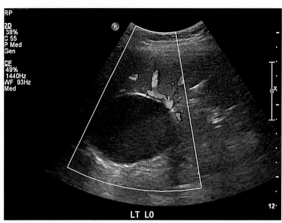

Figure 2. Color Doppler does not show any vascularity within the mass.

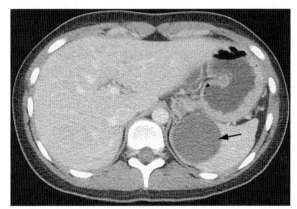

Figure 3. Axial CT image shows fluid density mass (*arrow*) within the spleen.

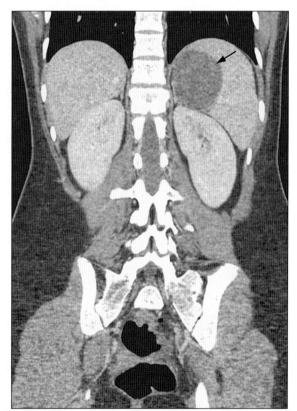

Figure 4. Coronal reconstruction confirms the splenic location of low-density mass (*arrow*), and the left kidney is distinctly seen separately.

Case 104

DEMOGRAPHICS/CLINICAL HISTORY

The patient is a 12-year-old girl presenting after ortho-topic heart transplant.

FINDINGS

An axial image from a contrast-enhanced computed tomography (CT) scan through the abdomen (Fig. 1) shows innumerable low attenuation lesions throughout the spleen, which is enlarged. A coronal reformatted image from a contrast-enhanced CT scan through the chest (Fig. 2) shows multiple, enlarged mediastinal and right hilar lymph nodes. A reformatted image from a contrast-enhanced CT scan of the abdomen and pelvis (Fig. 3) shows multiple, enlarged mesenteric lymph nodes along the para-aortic and parailiac chains. A whole-body image from ^{18}F-fluorodeoxyglucose posi-tron emission tomography (FDG-PET) scan (Fig. 4) shows multiple foci of abnormal uptake in the neck, chest, abdomen, and pelvis corresponding to enlarged lymph nodes noted on prior CT examination.

DISCUSSION

Definition/Background

Post-transplant lymphoproliferative disorder is a compli-cation of solid organ and allogeneic bone marrow trans-plantation usually associated with Ebstein-Barr virus infection of B cells.

Characteristic Clinical Features

Patients present with fever, lymphadenopathy, gastroin-testinal complaints, and infectious symptoms that simu-late infectious mononucleosis.

Characteristic Radiologic Findings

Because lymph nodes are the most common site of involvement, CT most often shows enlarged lymph nodes at various stations throughout the body. Associ-ated findings include hepatosplenomegaly or an abnor-mal mass lesion.

Differential Diagnosis

- Lymphoma
- Infectious mononucleosis

Discussion

Lymphoma is a neoplasm that originates in the lym-phocytes and may manifest as multiple, enlarged lymph nodes or as an abnormal nodal mass. Infectious mono-nucleosis is caused by Epstein-Barr virus and is charac-terized by fever, sore throat, and fatigue. Patients may develop splenomegaly or hepatomegaly or both.

Diagnosis

Lymphoproliferative disorder, post-transplant

Suggested Readings

Carbone A, Gloghini A, Dotti G: EBV-associated lymphoproliferative disorders: Classification and treatment. Oncologist 3:577-585, 2008.

Fernandez MC, Bes D, De Davila M, et al: Post-transplant lymphopro-liferative disorder after pediatric liver transplantation: Characteris-tics and outcome. Pediatr Transplant 13:307-310, 2009.

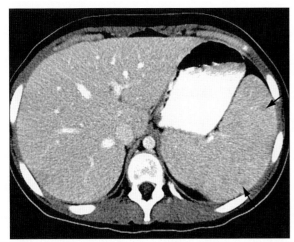

Figure 1. Axial image from contrast-enhanced CT scan through the abdomen shows innumerable low attenuation lesions throughout the spleen (*arrows*), which is enlarged.

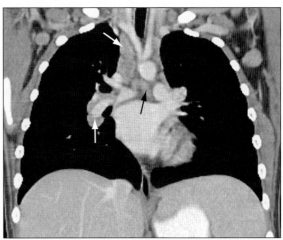

Figure 2. Coronal reformatted image from contrast-enhanced CT scan through the chest shows multiple, enlarged mediastinal and right hilar lymph nodes (*arrows*).

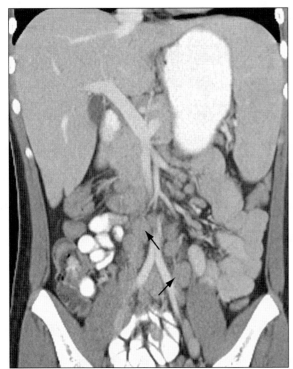

Figure 3. Reformatted image from contrast-enhanced CT scan of the abdomen and pelvis shows multiple, enlarged mesenteric lymph nodes along the para-aortic and para-iliac chains (*arrows*).

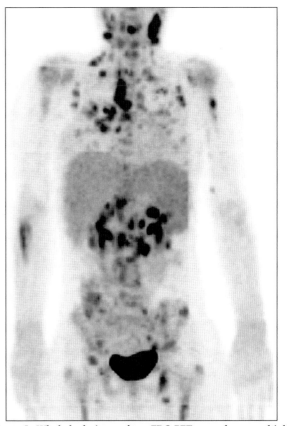

Figure 4. Whole-body image from FDG-PET scan shows multiple foci of abnormal uptake in the neck, chest, abdomen, and pelvis corresponding to enlarged lymph nodes noted on prior CT examination.

Case 105

DEMOGRAPHICS/CLINICAL HISTORY

The patient is an 11-month-old boy with protuberant abdomen and irritability.

FINDINGS

A plain radiograph of the abdomen (Fig. 1) shows a soft tissue mass in the left hemiabdomen that is displacing bowel loops. Axial (Fig. 2) and sagittal (Fig. 3) reformatted images from a contrast-enhanced computed tomography (CT) scan of the abdomen show a large, amorphous, heterogeneously enhancing soft tissue mass that is primarily retroperitoneal, and that is encasing the aorta and its major branches (celiac artery and superior mesenteric artery).

DISCUSSION

Definition/Background

Neuroblastoma is the third most common pediatric malignancy (behind leukemia and central nervous system tumors), and the second most common abdominal neoplasm in children (behind Wilms tumor).

Characteristic Clinical Features

Patients often present with nonspecific constitutional symptoms that mimic a viral illness. Other symptoms related to mass effect depend on tumor location.

Characteristic Radiologic Findings

Plain radiographs show a soft tissue mass only if it is causing significant displacement of organs or eroding into adjacent vertebral bodies. Ultrasound features of neuroblastoma include a heterogeneous, primarily hyperechoic mass that may contain discrete foci of calcification.

Less Common Radiologic Manifestations

CT is useful as a supplement to ultrasound. Nearly all abdominal neuroblastomas show calcification on CT. The mass appears lobular and without a discrete capsule, and may invade the psoas muscle or neural foramina.

Differential Diagnosis

- Wilms tumor
- Lymphoma

Discussion

Wilms tumor is a malignant neoplasm that arises from the kidney. In contrast to neuroblastoma, a "claw" of normal renal tissue can often be visualized splayed around the mass. Lymphoma is a malignant neoplasm of lymphocytes that manifests with enlarged lymph nodes in the abdomen. In contrast to neuroblastoma, lymphoma often displaces vessels without encasing them.

Diagnosis

Neuroblastoma

Suggested Readings

Hiorns MP, Owens CM: Radiology of neuroblastoma in children. Eur Radiol 11:2071-2081, 2001.
Papaioannou G, McHugh K: Neuroblastoma in childhood: Review and radiological findings. Cancer Imaging 5:116-127, 2005.

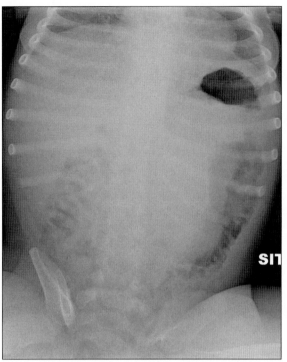

Figure 1. Plain radiograph of the abdomen shows a soft tissue mass in the left hemiabdomen that is displacing bowel loops.

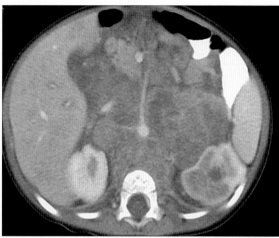

Figure 2. Axial image from a contrast-enhanced CT scan of the abdomen shows large, amorphous, heterogeneously enhancing soft tissue mass that is primarily retroperitoneal, and that is encasing the aorta and its major branches (celiac artery and superior mesenteric artery), which appear elongated and attenuated.

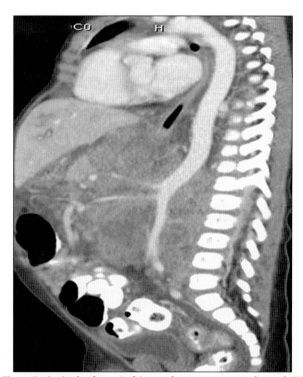

Figure 3. Sagittal reformatted image from a contrast-enhanced CT scan of the abdomen shows large, amorphous, heterogeneously enhancing soft tissue mass that is primarily retroperitoneal, and that is encasing the aorta and its major branches (celiac artery and superior mesenteric artery). The aorta is displaced anteriorly by the mass.

Case 106

DEMOGRAPHICS/CLINICAL HISTORY

The patient is a 20-month-old child with subcutaneous masses that are increasing in size.

FINDINGS

Axial postcontrast computed tomography (CT) (Fig. 1) shows bilateral adrenal masses with focal calcifications. Coronal postcontrast CT (Fig. 2) shows the suprarenal locations of the masses and heterogeneous appearance of the left adrenal mass. Iodine 131–metaiodobenzylguanidine (^{131}I-MIBG) scan (Fig. 3) shows uptake in the primary left adrenal mass and many subcutaneous and intramuscular metastases. Pathologic examination of the surgical specimen identified the mass as a neuroblastoma. A contrast-enhanced CT image (Fig. 4) of another patient with neuroblastoma shows a large, left adrenal mass with anterior displacement of the aorta, scattered calcifications, and narrowing and encasement of the vessels.

DISCUSSION

Definition/Background
Neuroblastoma is the second most common pediatric abdominal neoplasm, after Wilms tumor.

Characteristic Clinical Features
Patients typically present with an abdominal mass. Clinical presentations can also include symptoms from metastatic disease or direct extension into the neural foramina and spinal canal.

Characteristic Radiologic Findings
CT shows calcifications in more than 90% of patients with neuroblastoma, and it can show the encasement and narrowing of the aorta, inferior vena cava, and adjacent vessels. Metastases classically involve the osseous structures and the liver. Magnetic resonance imaging (MRI) is excellent for evaluation of the paraspinal components and invasion of the spinal canal through the neural foramina. MRI can also be used for evaluation of metastatic disease, particularly in the musculoskeletal system and orbits. ^{131}I-MIBG scanning can show the primary tumor and metastases. A bone scan can show additional bone metastases.

Differential Diagnosis
- Ganglioneuroblastoma
- Ganglioneuroma (pediatric)
- Wilms tumor

Discussion
Differentiating neuroblastoma from the less aggressive ganglioneuroblastoma and the benign ganglioneuroma can be difficult, and resection is usually necessary. Wilms tumor originates in the renal parenchyma, and often imaging in the coronal or sagittal plane can help localize the organ of origin.

Diagnosis
Neuroblastoma

Suggested Readings
Lonergan GJ, Schwab CM, Suarez ES, Carlson CL: Neuroblastoma, ganglioneuroblastoma, and ganglioneuroma: Radiologic-pathologic correlation. RadioGraphics 22:911-934, 2002.

Shulkin BL, Shapiro B, Hutchinson RJ: Iodine-131-metaiodobenzylguanidine and bone scintigraphy for the detection of neuroblastoma. J Nucl Med 33:1735-1740, 1992.

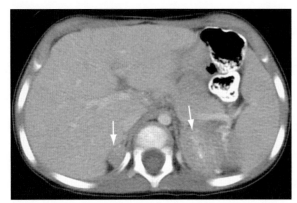

Figure 1. Axial postcontrast CT shows bilateral adrenal masses (*arrows*) with focal calcification in the left adrenal mass.

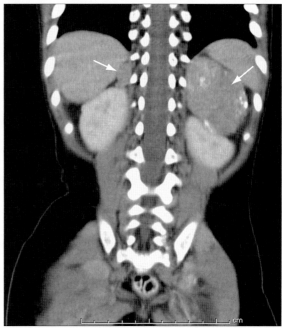

Figure 2. Coronal postcontrast CT shows suprarenal locations of the masses (*arrows*) and heterogeneous appearance of the left adrenal mass.

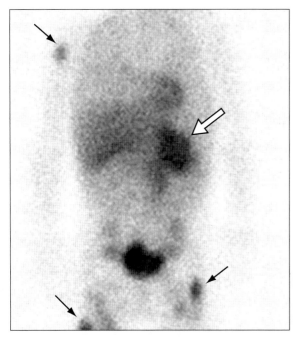

Anterior abdomen

Figure 3. ^{131}I-MIBG scan shows uptake in primary left adrenal mass (*white arrow*) and several subcutaneous and intramuscular metastases (*black arrows*). Pathologic examination of the surgical specimen confirmed the diagnosis of neuroblastoma.

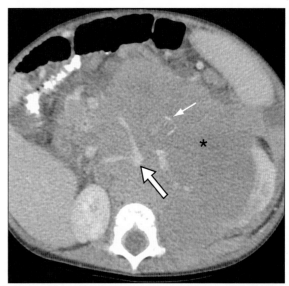

Figure 4. In another patient with neuroblastoma, contrast-enhanced CT shows large, left adrenal mass (*asterisk*) with anterior displacement of aorta (*large arrow*), scattered calcifications (*small arrow*), and narrowing and encasement of vessels.

Case 107

DEMOGRAPHICS/CLINICAL HISTORY

The patient is a 6-week-old boy with an incidental adrenal mass found on ultrasound to evaluate for pyloric stenosis.

FINDINGS

Longitudinal ultrasound of the abdomen (Fig. 1) shows a mass superior to the left kidney. Coronal T2-weighted fat-saturated magnetic resonance imaging (MRI) (Fig. 2) shows a heterogeneous mass in the expected location of the left adrenal gland. Coronal T1-weighted MRI (Fig. 3) shows the mass to be isointense and mildly heterogeneous. Postcontrast T1-weighted fat-saturated MRI (Fig. 4) shows heterogeneous enhancement of the left adrenal mass and normal appearance of the contralateral adrenal gland.

DISCUSSION

Definition/Background
Neuroblastoma is the second most common pediatric abdominal neoplasm after Wilms' tumor.

Characteristic Clinical Features
Patients can present with an abdominal mass or symptoms from metastatic disease or direct extension of disease (particularly into the spinal canal).

Characteristic Radiologic Findings
Computed tomography (CT) shows calcifications (present in > 90% of patients with neuroblastoma) and can show the encasement and narrowing of the aorta, inferior vena cava, and adjacent vessels. Bony disease can be seen in the visualized osseous structures. MRI is excellent for evaluation of the paraspinal components and invasion of the spinal canal via the neural foramina. MRI can also be used for evaluation of metastatic disease, particularly in the musculoskeletal system and orbits. Iodine 131–metaiodobenzylguanidine (^{131}I-MIBG) scanning can show the primary tumor and metastases. Bone scan can be helpful to show additional bone metastases.

Less Common Radiologic Manifestations
In diffuse disease, lung metastases may be seen, but they are less common than skeletal and hepatic metastases.

Differential Diagnosis
- Ganglioneuroblastoma/ganglioneuroma
- Adrenal cortical adenoma/carcinoma
- Adrenal hemorrhage

Discussion
Differentiating neuroblastoma from the less aggressive ganglioneuroblastoma and benign ganglioneuroma can be difficult and resection is usually necessary. Adrenal cortical tumors may be functional and are much rarer in children. Small intra-adrenal neuroblastomas are difficult to differentiate from adrenal cortical tumors. Adrenal hemorrhage can be found commonly in neonates, and the lack of internal flow/enhancement and decrease in size/resolution on follow-up imaging are expected.

Diagnosis
Neuroblastoma

Suggested Readings
Lonergan GJ, Schwab CM, Suarez ES: Neuroblastoma, ganglioneuroblastoma, and ganglioneuroma: Radiologic-pathologic correlation. RadioGraphics 22:911-934, 2002.

Shulkin BL, Shapiro B, Hutchinson RJ: Iodine-131-metaiodobenzylguanidine and bone scintigraphy for the detection of neuroblastoma. J Nucl Med 33:1735-1740, 1992.

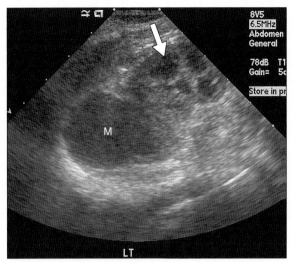

Figure 1. Longitudinal ultrasound of the abdomen shows mass (M) superior to the left kidney (*arrow*).

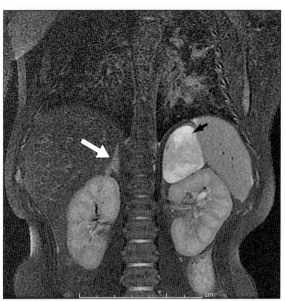

Figure 2. Coronal T2-weighted fat-saturated MR image shows heterogeneous mass (*black arrow*) in the expected location of the left adrenal gland. The normal-appearing right adrenal gland is seen (*white arrow*).

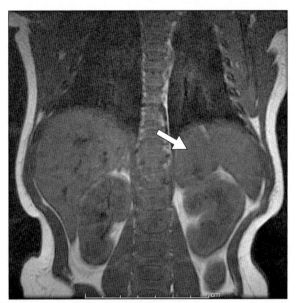

Figure 3. Coronal T1-weighted MR image shows mass (*arrow*) to be isointense and mildly heterogeneous.

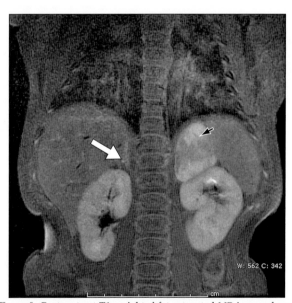

Figure 4. Postcontrast T1-weighted fat-saturated MR image shows heterogeneous enhancement of left adrenal mass (*black arrow*) and normal appearance of the contralateral adrenal gland (*white arrow*).

Case 108

DEMOGRAPHICS/CLINICAL HISTORY

The patient is a 5-month-old child with orbital swelling.

FINDINGS

Axial computed tomography (CT) image (Fig. 1) shows an orbital mass centered in the lateral orbital osseous structures. Another axial CT image (Fig. 2) shows a second lesion in the right frontal bone. Axial postcontrast T1-weighted magnetic resonance imaging (MRI) (Fig. 3) shows the enhancing mass in the left lateral orbital wall with soft tissue extension and a small second mass in the right lateral orbital wall. Bilateral adrenal masses are seen on abdominal CT (Fig. 4), as is a hepatic metastasis.

DISCUSSION

Definition/Background

Neuroblastoma has a predilection for metastasizing to the bones and liver. Involvement of the orbital bones, which are relatively superficial osseous structures, can be the presenting clinical finding leading to the discovery of the underlying neuroblastoma.

Characteristic Clinical Features

Periorbital involvement of metastatic neuroblastoma can lead to proptosis, a palpable mass, or ecchymosis ("raccoon eye").

Characteristic Radiologic Findings

Osseous destruction with enhancing soft tissue extension is the characteristic appearance of neuroblastoma metastatic to the orbit. The metastatic disease is often bilateral and asymmetric.

Less Common Radiologic Manifestations

Because of the proximity to the epidural surface of the brain, intracranial extension can be seen.

Differential Diagnosis

- Langerhans cell histiocytosis

Discussion

Langerhans cell histiocytosis can have an aggressive appearance, be multifocal, and have a soft tissue component. Additional imaging (e.g., abdominal ultrasound, chest radiograph) can help identify a primary neuroblastoma, but biopsy may be necessary for definitive diagnosis.

Diagnosis

Metastatic neuroblastoma

Suggested Readings

Khanna G, Sato Y, Smith RJ, et al: Causes of facial swelling in pediatric patients: Correlation of clinical and radiologic findings. RadioGraphics 26:157-171, 2006.

Lonergan GJ, Schwab CM, Suarez ES, Carlson CL: Neuroblastoma, ganglioneuroblastoma, and ganglioneuroma: Radiologic-pathologic correlation. RadioGraphics 22:911-934, 2002.

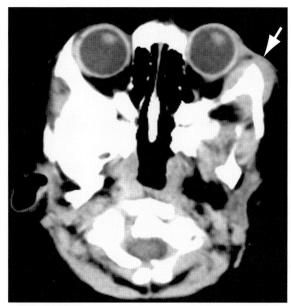

Figure 1. Axial CT shows an orbital mass (*arrow*) centered in the lateral orbital osseous structures.

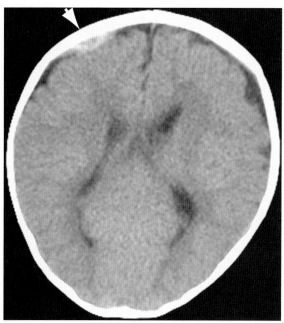

Figure 2. Axial CT shows a second lesion in the right frontal bone (*arrow*).

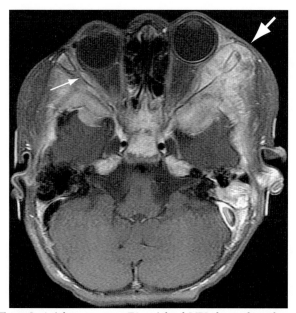

Figure 3. Axial postcontrast T1-weighted MRI shows the enhancing mass (*large arrow*) in the left lateral orbital wall with soft tissue extension and a small second mass (*small arrow*) in the right lateral orbital wall.

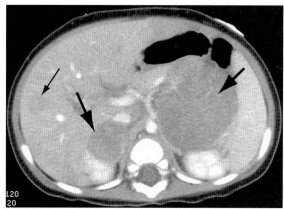

Figure 4. Bilateral adrenal masses (*large arrows*) are seen on contrast-enhanced abdominal CT, as is a hepatic metastasis (*small arrow*).

Case 109

DEMOGRAPHICS/CLINICAL HISTORY

The patient is a 3-year-old child with left upper quadrant pain.

FINDINGS

Axial contrast-enhanced computed tomography (CT) (Fig. 1) shows a large, heterogeneous mass replacing the upper pole of the left kidney. Coronal reformatted CT (Fig. 2) shows the large mass within the left kidney and the patency of the left renal vein. Another coronal reformatted CT image (Fig. 3) shows a normal-appearing right kidney.

DISCUSSION

Definition/Background
Wilms tumor is the most common pediatric renal neoplasm.

Characteristic Clinical Features
Presenting clinical features of Wilms tumor include a palpable abdominal mass, pain, and, less commonly, hematuria.

Characteristic Radiologic Findings
Ultrasound, CT, and magnetic resonance imaging (MRI) typically show a large, heterogeneous mass arising from the kidney. Heterogeneous contrast enhancement is seen. Invasion or thrombosis of the renal vein is common. Metastases to the lungs are common, and chest CT is routine in staging.

Less Common Radiologic Manifestations
Wilms tumors can be seen bilaterally in 5% to 10% of patients, particularly in patients with predisposing conditions, such as nephroblastomatosis, WAGR (Wilms tumor, aniridia, genitourinary anomalies, and mental retardation) syndrome, Beckwith-Wiedemann syndrome, and hemihypertrophy syndrome.

Differential Diagnosis
- Renal cell carcinoma
- Mesoblastic nephroma

Discussion
Renal cell carcinoma is much less common than Wilms tumor, and it occurs in older children. Mesoblastic nephroma typically presents in infancy.

Diagnosis
Wilms tumor

Suggested Readings

McHugh K: Renal and adrenal tumours in children. Cancer Imaging 7:41-51, 2007.

Riccabona M: Imaging of renal tumours in infancy and childhood. Eur Radiol 13(Suppl 4):L116-L129, 2003.

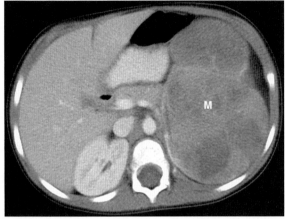

Figure 1. Axial, contrast-enhanced CT shows large, heterogeneous mass (M) replacing the upper pole of the left kidney.

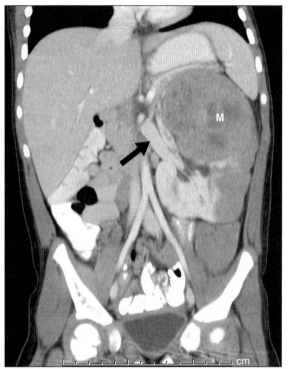

Figure 2. Coronal, reformatted CT shows large mass (M) within the left kidney and patency of the left renal vein (*arrow*).

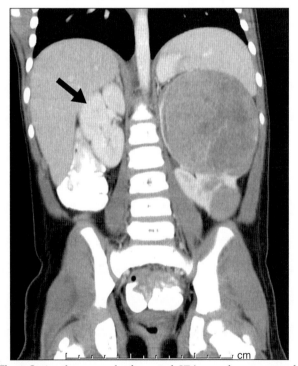

Figure 3. Another coronal reformatted CT image shows a normal-appearing right kidney (*arrow*).

Case 110

DEMOGRAPHICS/CLINICAL HISTORY

The patient is a 3-year-old child with abdominal pain.

FINDINGS

Longitudinal ultrasound of the left kidney (Fig. 1) shows a large mass in the left kidney. Axial contrast-enhanced Computed tomography (CT) image (Fig. 2) shows a large left renal mass. The renal vein is seen with a suggestion of nonocclusive thrombus. Coronal reconstructed CT image (Fig. 3) shows the mass within the kidney and the surrounding renal parenchyma.

DISCUSSION

Definition/Background

Wilms tumor is the most common pediatric renal neoplasm.

Characteristic Clinical Features

The presenting clinical features include palpable abdominal mass, pain, and, less commonly, hematuria.

Characteristic Radiologic Findings

Ultrasound, CT, and MRI typically show a large heterogeneous mass arising from the kidney. The "claw sign" refers to the presence of the normal solid organ tissue surrounding portions of the mass and is commonly seen in renal tumors. Heterogeneous contrast enhancement is seen. Invasion and thrombosis of the renal vein are common. Metastases to the lungs are commonly seen, and chest CT is routine in staging.

Less Common Radiologic Manifestations

Wilms tumors can be seen bilaterally in 5% to 10% of patients, particularly in patients with predisposing conditions, such as nephroblastomatosis, WAGR (*W*ilms tumor, *a*niridia, *g*enitourinary anomalies, and mental *r*etardation) syndrome, Beckwith-Wiedemann syndrome, and hemihypertrophy syndrome.

Differential Diagnosis

- Renal cell carcinoma
- Mesoblastic nephroma

Discussion

Renal cell carcinoma is much less common than Wilms tumor and occurs in older children. Mesoblastic nephroma occurs in a younger age group, usually manifesting in infancy.

Diagnosis

Wilms tumor

Suggested Readings

McHugh K: Renal and adrenal tumours in children. Cancer Imaging 7:41-51, 2007.

Riccabona M: Imaging of renal tumours in infancy and childhood. Eur Radiol 13(Suppl 4):L116-L129, 2003.

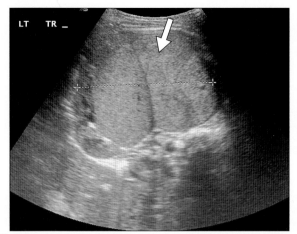

Figure 1. Longitudinal ultrasound of the left kidney shows large mass (*arrow*) in the left kidney.

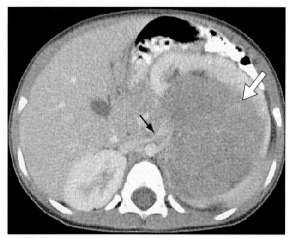

Figure 2. Axial contrast-enhanced CT image shows large left renal mass (*white arrow*). The renal vein is seen with a suggestion of nonocclusive thrombus (*black arrow*).

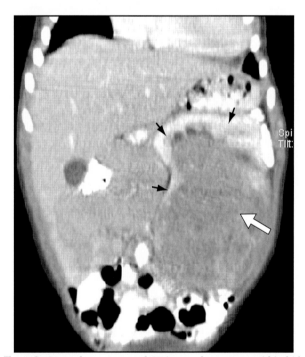

Figure 3. Coronal reconstructed CT image shows mass within kidney (*white arrow*) and the surrounding renal parenchyma (*black arrows*).

Case 111

DEMOGRAPHICS/CLINICAL HISTORY

The patient is a 9-year-old boy with back pain.

FINDINGS

Axial (Fig. 1) and coronal reformatted (Fig. 2) contrast-enhanced computed tomography (CT) images of the abdomen show multiple, low attenuation lesions in the kidneys. Sagittal reformatted CT image through the lumbar spine (Fig. 3) viewed with bone window settings shows a mixed lytic and sclerotic lesion involving the L5 vertebral body with an associated compression fracture of the vertebral body.

DISCUSSION

Definition/Background

CT reveals renal involvement by lymphoma in approximately 5% to 8% of patients with lymphoma.

Characteristic Clinical Features

Renal dysfunction occurs only late in the disease; more often, patients present with a mass effect resulting from lesions elsewhere in the body.

Characteristic Radiologic Findings

On contrast-enhanced CT, renal lymphoma may manifest as bilateral, enlarged, nonenhancing kidneys; a solitary renal mass; multiple, bilateral intraparenchymal lesions; or perirenal infiltration.

Differential Diagnosis
- Leukemia
- Multiple angiomyolipomas
- Fungal infection

Discussion

Acute leukemia may manifest with bilateral renal enlargement, which may be indistinguishable from lymphoma. Multiple angiomyolipomas in the kidneys may be seen in patients with tuberous sclerosis. Typically, these lesions contain fat. A diffuse parenchymal fungal infection may affect the kidneys in patients who are immunocompromised and manifest as multiple, low attenuation renal lesions.

Diagnosis

Renal lymphoma

Suggested Readings

Chepuri NB, Strouse PJ, Yanik GA, et al: CT of renal lymphoma in children. AJR Am J Roentgenol 180:429-431, 2003.

El-Sharkawy MS, Siddiqui N, Aleem A, et al: Renal involvement in lymphoma: Prevalence and various patterns of involvement on abdominal CT. Int Urol Nephrol 39:929-933, 2007.

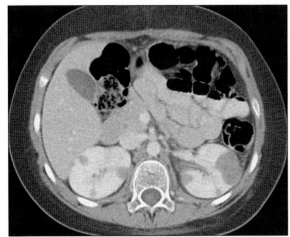

Figure 1. Axial contrast-enhanced CT of the abdomen shows multiple, low attenuation lesions in kidneys.

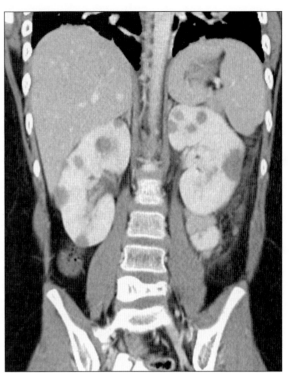

Figure 2. Coronal reformatted contrast-enhanced CT of the abdomen shows multiple, low attenuation lesions in kidneys.

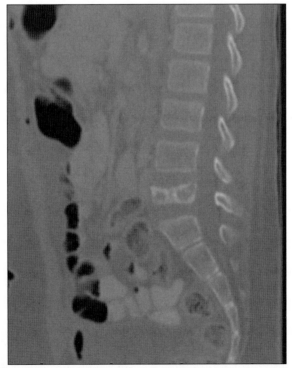

Figure 3. Sagittal reformatted CT through the lumbar spine using bone window settings shows mixed lytic and sclerotic lesion involving the L5 vertebral body with associated compression fracture of the vertebral body.

Case 112

DEMOGRAPHICS/CLINICAL HISTORY

The patient is a newborn with an abnormality seen on prenatal ultrasound.

FINDINGS

Axial contrast-enhanced computed tomography (CT) (Fig. 1) shows a hypodense mass within and expanding the right renal parenchyma. Coronal reconstructed CT (Fig. 2) shows the extent of involvement within the upper and lower poles of the right kidney. A normal contralateral kidney is seen.

DISCUSSION

Definition/Background
Mesonephric blastoma is the most common solid renal tumor in neonates.

Characteristic Clinical Features
Mesoblastic nephroma is sometimes detected on prenatal ultrasound or can be palpated as an abdominal mass. Less frequently, hematuria can be a presenting feature.

Characteristic Radiologic Findings
Mesoblastic nephromas typically are large, solid tumors within the renal parenchyma. No specific radiographic findings can differentiate mesoblastic nephromas from other histologic renal tumors.

Less Common Radiologic Manifestations
Mesoblastic nephroma can recur if incompletely resected, and it rarely metastasizes.

Differential Diagnosis
- Wilms tumor
- Renal abscess

Discussion
The age of presentation is the most common discriminating factor between Wilms tumor and mesoblastic nephroma; mesoblastic nephroma is much more common in children younger than 6 months. Renal abscess has a different clinical presentation, typically manifesting with fever and a history of urinary tract infection, and it does not typically look like a solid mass on imaging.

Diagnosis
Mesoblastic nephroma

Suggested Reading
Lowe LH, Isuani BH, Heller RM, et al: Pediatric renal masses: Wilms tumor and beyond. RadioGraphics 20:1585-1603, 2000.

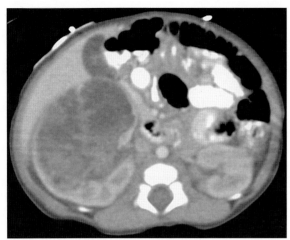

Figure 1. Axial contrast-enhanced CT shows hypodense mass within and expanding the right renal parenchyma.

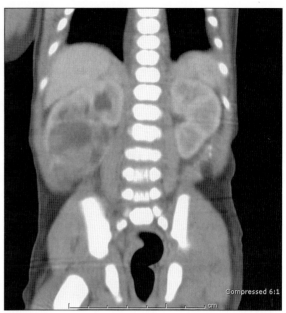

Figure 2. Coronal reconstructed CT shows extent of involvement within upper and lower poles of the right kidney. A normal contralateral kidney is seen.

Case 113

DEMOGRAPHICS/CLINICAL HISTORY

The patient is an 11-year-old child with tuberous sclerosis.

FINDINGS

Longitudinal ultrasound of the right kidney (Fig. 1) shows multiple hyperechoic areas within the renal cortex. Longitudinal ultrasound of the left kidney (Fig. 2) shows similar hyperechogenic areas within the left kidney. Axial T1-weighted in-phase magnetic resonance imaging (MRI) (Fig. 3) shows multiple hyperintense foci within both kidneys. Axial T1-weighted out-of-phase MRI (Fig. 4) shows India ink artifacts around the hyperintense foci, consistent with a macroscopic fat-water interface.

DISCUSSION

Definition/Background

Angiomyelolipomas (i.e., angiomyolipomas) are vascular, lipid-containing tumors. In pediatric patients, they are typically associated with tuberous sclerosis. They also are associated with neurofibromatosis and von Hippel-Lindau disease.

Characteristic Clinical Features

Angiomyelolipomas can spontaneously hemorrhage, particularly larger angiomyelolipomas (> 4 cm).

Characteristic Radiologic Findings

Angiomyelolipomas are characteristically located in the kidneys. Because of their fatty content, ultrasonography shows echogenic foci within the parenchyma. On MRI, these lesions are hyperintense on T1-weighted imaging, typically showing India ink artifacts around the lesions on chemical shift T1-weighted imaging, or signal dropout on frequency-selective, fat-suppressed images. Computed tomography (CT) shows that the lesions contain fatty attenuation (Hounsfield units < 0). Because of vascular elements, enhancement can be seen with administration of MRI or CT contrast agents.

Less Common Radiologic Manifestations

Angiomyelolipomas can be found in the liver, with imaging characteristics similar to lesions in other locations.

Differential Diagnosis

- Clear cell sarcoma

Discussion

Typically, angiomyelolipomas in children are associated with a condition or syndrome, such as tuberous sclerosis. Clear cell sarcoma is rare and solitary, and it can have some loss of signal on opposed-phase imaging, but it does not contain macroscopic fat and should not lose signal on frequency-selective, fat-suppressed T1-weighted MRI.

Diagnosis

Angiomyolipoma

Suggested Readings

Lowe LH, Isuani BH, Heller RM, et al: Pediatric renal masses: Wilms tumor and beyond. RadioGraphics 20:1585-1603, 2000.

Zhang J, Israel GM, Krinsky GA, Lee VS: Masses and pseudomasses of the kidney: Imaging spectrum on MR. J Comput Assist Tomogr 28:588-595, 2004.

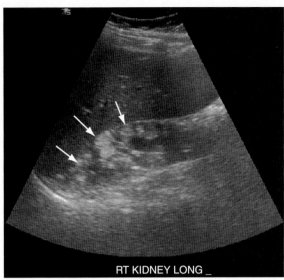

Figure 1. Longitudinal ultrasound of right kidney shows multiple hyperechoic areas within renal cortex (*arrows*).

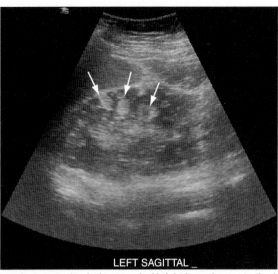

Figure 2. Longitudinal ultrasound of left kidney shows similar hyperechogenic areas within left kidney (*arrows*).

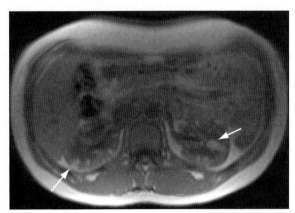

Figure 3. Axial T1-weighted in-phase MR image shows multiple hyperintense foci within both kidneys (*arrows*).

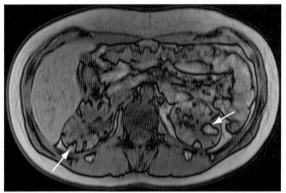

Figure 4. Axial T1-weighted out-of-phase MR image shows India ink artifacts around hyperintense foci (*arrows*), consistent with a macroscopic fat-water interface.

Case 114

DEMOGRAPHICS/CLINICAL HISTORY

The patient is a 15-year-old adolescent with hypertension.

FINDINGS

Coronal, reformatted image from a contrast-enhanced computed tomography (CT) (Fig. 1) shows an enhancing mass just below the iliac bifurcation. T2-weighted magnetic resonance imaging (MRI) (Fig. 2) shows a hyperintense mass adjacent to the left iliac vessels. Postcontrast, T1-weighted MRI (Fig. 3) shows small flow voids within the enhancing mass. Iodine 131–metaiodobenzylguanidine (^{131}I-MIBG) scintigraphy (Fig. 4) shows increased uptake within the mass.

DISCUSSION

Characteristic Clinical Features

Hypertension (typically sustained rather than paroxysmal), headaches, sweating, nausea, and vomiting can be symptoms of pheochromocytoma. Symptoms and laboratory values for increased plasma and urinary catecholamine levels and their metabolites (e.g., urinary epinephrine, metanephrine, homovanillic acid, vanillylmandelic acid) suggest the diagnosis.

Characteristic Radiologic Findings

^{131}I-MIBG scintigraphy and ultrasonography are often the first-line imaging modalities after the diagnosis has been suggested by laboratory values. Ultrasound appearance is nonspecific, with homogeneous or heterogeneous echotexture. CT or MRI is used for further evaluation and surgical planning. Nonionic contrast–enhanced CT can be performed safely without the need for adrenergic blockade to prevent a hypertensive crisis. Noncontrast CT can show areas of hemorrhage, and contrast-enhanced CT can show variable patterns of enhancement. On MRI, most pheochromocytomas typically show intense enhancement and slow washout after administration of contrast agent. The lesions are characteristically markedly hyperintense on T2-weighted MRI. Both adrenal glands and the sympathetic chain should be assessed because pheochromocytomas are commonly bilateral in children and can be extra-adrenal. Because pheochromocytomas can be seen in patients with multiple endocrine neoplasia (MEN) syndrome, von Hippel-Lindau disease, and neurofibromatosis, radiologic findings of these syndromes may be seen.

Less Common Radiologic Manifestations

There are reports of pheochromocytomas with early washout characteristics. Because of hemorrhage, pheochromocytomas occasionally can have calcifications.

Differential Diagnosis

- Neuroblastoma
- Ganglioneuroblastoma
- Ganglioneuroma
- Adrenocortical carcinoma

Discussion

Pheochromocytomas are much less likely to have calcifications than neuroblastomas. Evaluation for catecholamines and their by-products should be performed with any adrenal tumor. Pathologic examination of a specimen may be the only way to differentiate these tumors.

Diagnosis

Pheochromocytoma

Suggested Readings

McHugh K: Renal and adrenal tumours in children. Cancer Imaging 7:41-51, 2007.

Ross JH: Pheochromocytoma: Special considerations in children. Urol Clin North Am 27:393-402, 2000.

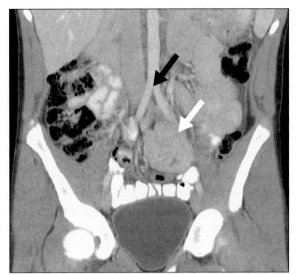

Figure 1. Coronal reformatted contrast-enhanced CT scan shows enhancing mass (*white arrow*) just below the iliac bifurcation (*black arrow*).

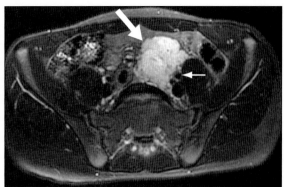

Figure 2. Axial T2 fat-saturated MRI shows hyperintense mass (*large arrow*) adjacent to left iliac vessels (*small arrow*).

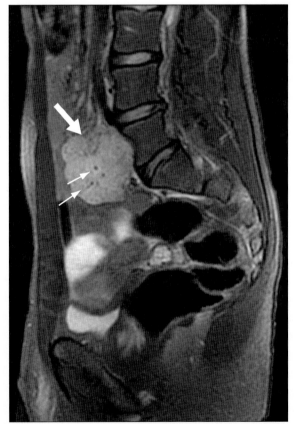

Figure 3. Postcontrast T1-weighted MR image shows small flow voids (*small arrows*) within enhancing mass (*large arrow*).

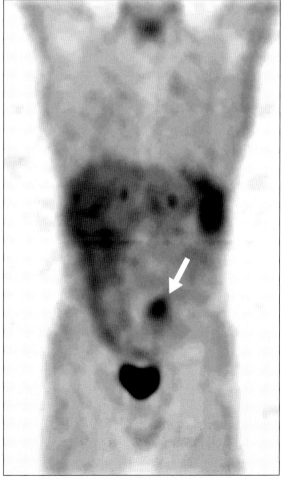

Figure 4. ^{131}I-MIBG scintigraphy shows increased uptake within mass (*arrow*).

Case 115

DEMOGRAPHICS/CLINICAL HISTORY

The patient is a newborn with ambiguous genitalia.

FINDINGS

An oblique view from a voiding cystourethrogram (VCUG) (Fig. 1) shows contrast in the bladder, vagina, and uterine cavity. The connection between the distal vagina and the urethra can be seen. Longitudinal ultrasound of the left adrenal gland (Fig. 2) shows that it is enlarged, curvilinear, and elongated. The appearance of the right adrenal gland was similar.

DISCUSSION

Definition/Background

Congenital adrenal hyperplasia is most commonly caused by 21-hydroxylase deficiency. It manifests more obviously in girls, who present with signs of virilization.

Characteristic Clinical Features

Patients may have ambiguous genitalia (in some girls), vomiting because of salt wasting, precocious or delayed puberty, and virilization.

Characteristic Radiologic Findings

Ultrasound shows elongated adrenal glands with a cerebriform pattern. A dilated vagina also may be seen on ultrasound. VCUG typically shows the distal vagina inserting into the urethra, a sign of incomplete migration of the vagina because of virilization.

Differential Diagnosis

- Urogenital sinus anomaly

Discussion

VCUG findings are similar for urogenital sinus anomaly and congenital adrenal hyperplasia. Patients with urogenital sinus anomalies do not have abnormal adrenal glands or hormonal levels.

Diagnosis

Congenital adrenal hyperplasia

Suggested Reading

Avni EF, Rypens F, Smet MH, Galetty E: Sonographic demonstration of congenital adrenal hyperplasia in the neonate: The cerebriform pattern. Pediatr Radiol 23:88-90, 1993.

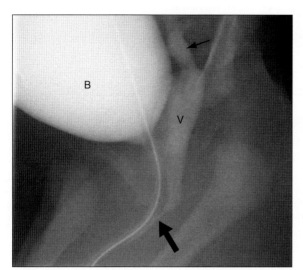

Figure 1. Oblique VCUG shows contrast in the bladder (B), vagina (V), and uterine cavity (*small arrow*). The connection between the distal vagina and the urethra (*large arrow*) can be seen.

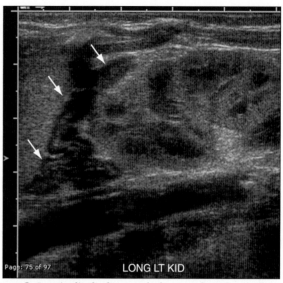

Figure 2. Longitudinal ultrasound shows enlarged, curvilinear, and elongated left adrenal gland (*arrows*). The appearance of the right adrenal gland was similar.

Case 116

DEMOGRAPHICS/CLINICAL HISTORY

The patient is a 22-year-old woman with abdominal and pelvic distention.

FINDINGS

Ultrasound examination of the abdomen and pelvis (Figs. 1 and 2) shows a large, complex mass occupying nearly the entire pelvis and much of the abdomen, which has solid and cystic components. Although the precise source of the mass is difficult to ascertain because of its large size, the right ovary was never identified separate from the mass. Axial images from a contrast-enhanced computed tomography (CT) scan of the abdomen and pelvis (Figs. 3 and 4) also show a large, complex mass with a dominant cystic component and a moderate amount of intra-abdominal ascites.

DISCUSSION

Definition/Background
Granulosa cell tumors account for a small percentage of ovarian neoplasms. There are adult and juvenile types of granulosa cell tumors. The tumors commonly produce estrogen.

Characteristic Clinical Features
Patients often present with symptoms of excess estrogen stimulation, increasing abdominal girth, or abdominal pain. Ascites is present in approximately 10% of patients.

Characteristic Radiologic Findings
On ultrasound, many granulosa cell tumors are large, complex cystic and solid masses, which may also contain hemorrhagic components. Ascites may be present in approximately 10%.

Differential Diagnosis
- Ovarian cystadenoma/cystadenocarcinoma
- Germ cell tumor of the ovary
- Hemorrhagic ovarian cyst

Discussion
Ovarian cystadenocarcinoma is an epithelial tumor and is the most common type of ovarian cancer. It typically occurs in adults and is uncommon in young girls. Ovarian germ cell tumors include teratoma and dermoids, which are most often benign masses, although uncommonly a malignant germ cell tumor may occur. Hemorrhagic ovarian cysts often have a complex appearance on ultrasound because of the evolution of hemorrhagic components, although there is no solid mass associated with these lesions.

Diagnosis
Granulosa cell tumor

Suggested Readings
Kim SH, Kim SH: Granulosa cell tumor of the ovary: Common findings and unusual appearances on CT and MR. J Comput Assist Tomogr 26:756, 2002.

Van Holsbeke C, Domali E, Holland TK, et al: Imaging of gynecological disease (3): Clinical and ultrasound characteristics of granulosa cell tumors of the ovary. Ultrasound Obstet Gynecol 31:450, 2008.

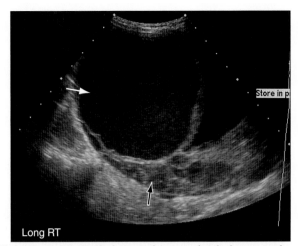

Figure 1. Longitudinal ultrasound image of right lower quadrant of abdomen shows large, complex mass occupying nearly the entire pelvis and much of the abdomen, which has solid (*white arrow*) and cystic (*black arrow*) components.

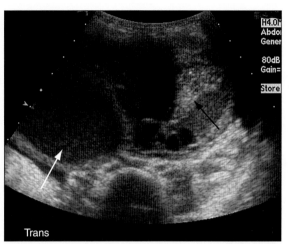

Figure 2. Transverse ultrasound image from examination of abdomen and pelvis shows large, complex mass occupying nearly the entire pelvis and much of the abdomen, which has solid (*white arrow*) and cystic (*black arrow*) components.

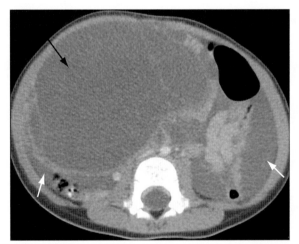

Figure 3. Axial image of abdomen from contrast-enhanced CT scan of abdomen and pelvis shows large, complex mass with dominant cystic component (*black arrow*), and moderate amount of intra-abdominal ascites (*white arrows*).

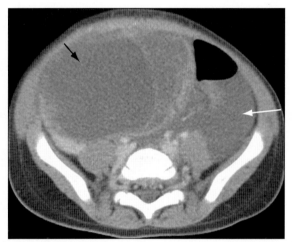

Figure 4. Axial image of pelvis from contrast-enhanced CT scan of abdomen and pelvis shows large, complex mass with dominant cystic component (*black arrow*), and moderate amount of intra-abdominal ascites (*white arrow*). The mass appears to originate from pelvis.

Case 117

DEMOGRAPHICS/CLINICAL HISTORY

The patient is a 6-year-old girl with anemia and low-grade fever.

FINDINGS

Transverse ultrasound of the abdomen (Fig. 1) shows a large, heterogeneous mass within the abdomen and pelvis. Contrast-enhanced computed tomography (CT) (Fig. 2) shows the heterogeneous mass and hydronephrosis of the right kidney caused by ureteral compression. Sagittal reconstructed CT (Fig. 3) shows the large size of the mass and its heterogeneity, including a focus of calcification. Pathologic examination revealed the tumor to be of mixed germ cell lineage, with a large teratoma component.

DISCUSSION

Definition/Background
The occurrence of ovarian germ cell tumors peaks in the middle to late teen years. Prognosis and treatment are dictated by the elements that characterize the tumor.

Characteristic Clinical Features
The masses grow slowly and often are palpated when they are quite large. Symptoms may result from the secondary mass effect of the tumor.

Characteristic Radiologic Findings
Ovarian germ cell tumors often are quite large when diagnosed, and the mass typically extends into the abdomen. The mass has a heterogeneous appearance, and elements of fat and calcium occasionally can be identified within the mass. Imaging with administration of contrast agent can show heterogeneous enhancement. Imaging for metastatic disease and peritoneal seeding should be evaluated.

Differential Diagnosis
- Stromal tumors

Discussion
In a female patient, large lower abdominal or pelvic masses often have an ovarian origin. If calcification and fat are seen within the mass, the diagnosis likely is a germ cell tumor. Considerations for secondary tumors and other causes should be reviewed carefully, and surgical resection and exploration can yield a definitive diagnosis.

Diagnosis
Ovarian germ cell tumor

Suggested Reading
Jung SE, Lee JM, Rha SE, et al: CT and MR imaging of ovarian tumors with emphasis on differential diagnosis. RadioGraphics 22:1305-1325, 2002.

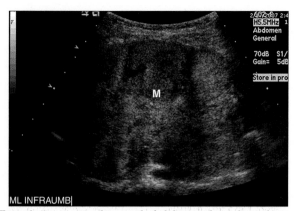

Figure 1. Transverse ultrasound of abdomen shows large, heterogeneous mass (M) within abdomen and pelvis.

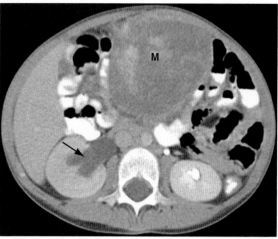

Figure 2. Contrast-enhanced CT shows heterogeneous mass (M) and hydronephrosis of right kidney (*arrow*) caused by ureteral compression.

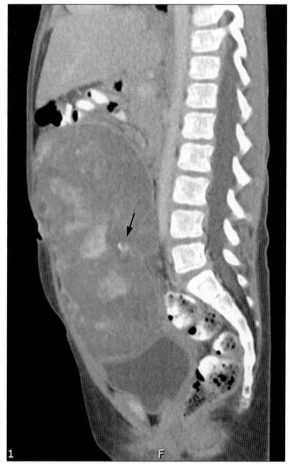

Figure 3. Sagittal reconstructed CT scan shows large size of mass and the heterogeneity, including a focus of calcification (*arrow*). Pathologic analysis revealed the tumor was of mixed germ cell lineage, with a large teratoma component.

Case 118

DEMOGRAPHICS/CLINICAL HISTORY

The patient is a 9-month-old male infant with an incidental finding on ultrasound performed for evaluation of possible splenomegaly.

FINDINGS

Longitudinal ultrasound of the left abdomen (Fig. 1) shows a round, hypoechoic structure that is medial to the spleen and superior to the upper pole of the left kidney. A transverse ultrasound image (Fig. 2) through the mass shows its relationship posterior to the tail of the pancreas and medial to the upper pole of the left kidney. The corresponding axial contrast-enhanced computed tomography (CT) image (Fig. 3) shows the mass as a well-defined, homogeneous structure within the left adrenal gland. Pathologic examination of the surgical specimen confirmed the tumor to be an adrenocortical tumor (i.e., adenoma).

DISCUSSION

Definition/Background
Adrenocortical tumors are rare in children, but are often symptomatic.

Characteristic Clinical Features
Children with adrenocortical tumors often present with virilization or Cushing syndrome. Almost half of patients have hypertension at presentation.

Characteristic Radiologic Findings
Adrenocortical tumors (i.e., adenomas and carcinomas) appear as soft tissue masses within the adrenal gland. Adrenocortical tumors typically are well defined and may contain calcifications, central necrosis, or hemorrhage. The inferior vena cava can be compressed by large tumors, and invasion can occur in cases of adrenocortical carcinoma. Adrenocortical carcinoma can metastasize, and bone scintigraphy and chest CT should be performed for metastatic evaluation.

Differential Diagnosis
- Neuroblastoma (pediatric)

Discussion
Endocrine abnormalities, a thin tumor capsule, and a stellate central zone of necrosis suggest an adrenocortical tumor, rather than a neuroblastoma. Adrenal tumors are typically resected, and pathologic examination of the surgical specimen can differentiate the tumors.

Diagnosis
Adrenocortical tumor

Suggested Readings

Ciftci AO, Senocak ME, Tanyel FC, Büyükpamukçu N: Adrenocortical tumors in children. J Pediatr Surg 36:549-554, 2001.
Ribeiro J, Ribeiro RC, Fletcher BD: Imaging findings in pediatric adrenocortical carcinoma. Pediatr Radiol 30:45-51, 2000.

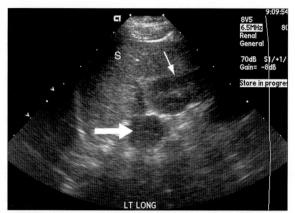

Figure 1. Longitudinal ultrasound of left abdomen shows round, hypoechoic structure (*large arrow*) medial to the spleen (S) and superior to the upper pole of the left kidney (*small arrow*).

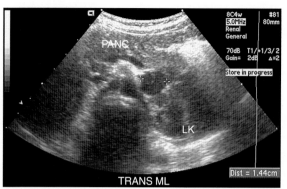

Figure 2. Transverse ultrasound image through mass (*measured*) shows its relationship posterior to tail of the pancreas (PANC) and medial to upper pole of the left kidney (LK).

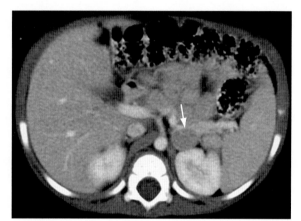

Figure 3. Corresponding axial, contrast-enhanced CT image shows mass (*arrow*) as a well-defined, homogeneous structure within left adrenal gland.

Case 119

DEMOGRAPHICS/CLINICAL HISTORY

The patient is a 16-year-old boy with an enlarging buttock mass.

FINDINGS

Magnetic resonance imaging (MRI) of the pelvis shows a large mass that is isointense to muscle on T1-weighted MRI (Fig. 1), is bright on T2-weighted MRI (Fig. 2), and enhances heterogeneously after administration of contrast agent (Fig. 3). There is diffuse, bony metastatic disease, seen as low signal intensity areas within the bone on T1-weighted MRI (see Fig. 1). Computed tomography (CT) of the chest shows lung metastases (Fig. 4).

DISCUSSION

Definition/Background
Rhabdomyosarcoma is the most common neoplasm of the lower genitourinary tract in children. It arises in the prostate in more than half of cases.

Characteristic Clinical Features
Symptoms include hematuria, urinary frequency, and urinary retention. This patient presented with a palpable buttock mass.

Characteristic Radiologic Findings
CT and MRI are most helpful for evaluating the extent of the disease. T1-weighted MRI is best for evaluating the extent of fat invasion and enlarged lymph nodes. T2-weighted MRI helps to evaluate whether the tumor has spread to other organs or structures.

Differential Diagnosis
- Leiomyosarcoma
- Inflammatory pseudotumor—plasma cell granuloma
- Lymphoma
- Rhabdoid tumor

Discussion
Leiomyosarcoma is a rare malignant neoplasm that may arise from the bladder. Inflammatory pseudotumor is a rare benign tumor of the bladder in children that may simulate rhabdomyosarcoma. Rhabdoid tumor of the lower urinary tract is another rare malignant neoplasm.

Diagnosis
Prostatic rhabdomyosarcoma

Suggested Readings
Agrons GA, Wagner BJ, Lonergan GJ, et al: From the archives of the AFIP. Genitourinary rhabdomyosarcoma in children: Radiologic-pathologic correlation. RadioGraphics 17:919-937, 1997.

Baker ME, Silverman PM, Korobkin M: Computed tomography of prostatic and bladder rhabdomyosarcomas. J Comput Assist Tomogr 9:780-783, 1985.

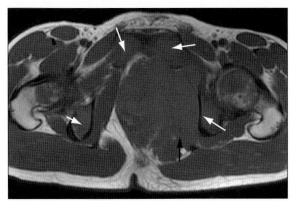

Figure 1. Axial T1-weighted MR image through pelvis shows large soft tissue mass at the level of the pelvic floor that is displacing the rectum and invading the ischiorectal fat (*black arrow*). There is also abnormal bone marrow signal within the pubic bones and ischium bilaterally consistent with metastatic involvement (*white arrows*).

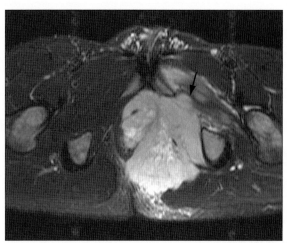

Figure 2. Axial T2-weighted MR image with fat suppression through pelvis shows that mass is invading the adjacent muscles in the left hemipelvis (*arrow*).

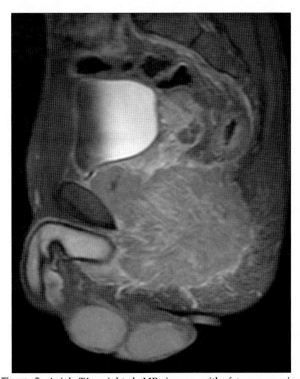

Figure 3. Axial T1-weighted MR image with fat suppression through pelvis after administration of intravenous gadolinium shows heterogeneous enhancement of mass.

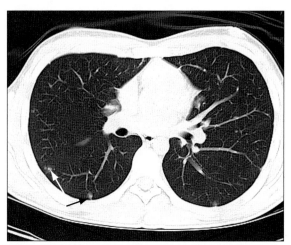

Figure 4. Axial noncontrast CT scan through lungs shows several pulmonary nodules (*arrows*) consistent with metastases.

Case 120

DEMOGRAPHICS/CLINICAL HISTORY

The patient is a 7-month-old infant with prominence of the perirectal and perisacral soft tissues.

FINDINGS

A large presacral mass with cystic and solid components is seen on sagittal T2-weighted (Fig. 1) and T1-weighted (Fig. 2) magnetic resonance imaging (MRI). Postcontrast sagittal MRI (Fig. 3) shows enhancement of the solid components and septa.

DISCUSSION

Definition/Background

Sacrococcygeal teratomas contain elements from all three germ cell layers and are categorized by the amount of external and internal components. Most sacrococcygeal teratomas are diagnosed in utero or in the neonatal period because of a protuberant external component, and benign pathology is typical for external tumors that are diagnosed early.

Characteristic Clinical Features

Because sacrococcygeal teratomas are often diagnosed prenatally, the clinical diagnosis is usually made by visual confirmation of a sacral soft tissue mass at delivery. The internal presacral teratomas typically manifest later in infancy with symptoms from the mass effect of the tumor (e.g., constipation, bladder symptoms, venous or lymphatic obstruction of the legs, lower extremity paralysis).

Characteristic Radiologic Findings

Predominantly external sacrococcygeal teratomas are mostly cystic. Two thirds of teratomas show calcifications on imaging, and fatty components may be seen radiographically. Malignant teratomas are more likely to have solid, enhancing components.

Less Common Radiologic Manifestations

Less commonly, teratomas can extend into the spinal canal. When a presacral mass (e.g., teratoma, sacral meningocele) is seen in conjunction with an anorectal malformation and a sacral bony defect, such as a sickle-shaped sacrum, these findings are referred to as the Currarino triad.

Differential Diagnosis

- Neuroblastoma

Discussion

The presence of fat, a predominantly exophytic and cystic lesion, and minimally enhancing components in a newborn suggest a sacrococcygeal teratoma. Neuroblastoma is predominantly solid, has an internal location, and has a tendency to invade the spinal canal.

Diagnosis

Sacrococcygeal teratoma

Suggested Readings

Isaacs H: Perinatal (fetal and neonatal) germ cell tumors. J Pediatr Surg 39:1003-1013, 2004.

Keslar PJ, Buck JL, Suarez ES: Germ cell tumors of the sacrococcygeal region: Radiologic-pathologic correlation. RadioGraphics 14:607-620, 1994.

Sebire NJ, Fowler D, Ramsay AD: Sacrococcygeal tumors in infancy and childhood: A retrospective histopathological review of 85 cases. Fetal Pediatr Pathol 23:295-303, 2004.

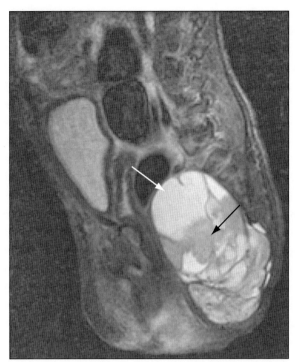

Figure 1. Parasagittal T2-weighted MR image shows large presacral mass with cystic (*white arrow*) and solid (*black arrow*) components.

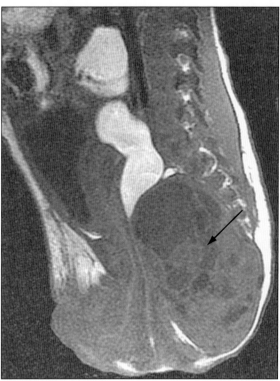

Figure 2. T1-weighted sagittal MR image shows isointense solid portions (*arrow*) and septa.

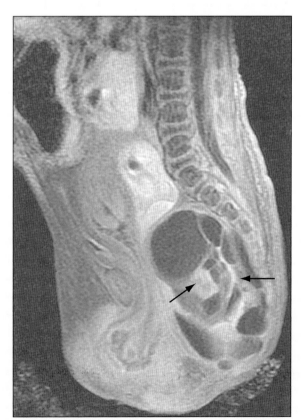

Figure 3. Postcontrast T1-weighted, fat-saturated, sagittal MR image shows enhancement of solid components and septa (*arrows*). There is no intraspinal involvement.

Case 121

DEMOGRAPHICS/CLINICAL HISTORY

The patient is a 14-year-old girl with right lower quadrant pain of acute onset.

FINDINGS

Ultrasound examination of the pelvis (Fig. 1) shows a markedly enlarged, hypoechoic right ovary that is positioned directly posterior to the uterus and contains many small follicles. Doppler ultrasound fails to show any convincing flow within the ovary (Fig. 2). A computed tomography (CT) scan performed immediately after the ultrasound (Fig. 3) shows an enlarged, hypoattenuating, heterogeneous right ovary positioned in the midline and posterior to the uterus.

DISCUSSION

Definition/Background
Ovarian torsion often occurs in peripubertal girls, although any age group may be affected.

Characteristic Clinical Features
Patients present with sudden onset of lower abdominal or pelvic pain.

Characteristic Radiologic Findings
The ovary may have myriad different imaging findings on ultrasound, depending on the presence of an underlying mass or cyst and the amount of hemorrhage.

Classic findings include an enlarged, hypoechoic ovary with many peripheral follicles. Although Doppler ultrasound usually reveals the lack of blood flow to the ovary, ovarian torsion may exist even when there is blood flow to the ovary because of the dual blood supply to the organ.

Less Common Radiologic Manifestations
In other cases, the ovary may contain a large cyst or cystic mass, and it may be difficult to ascertain the presence of blood flow within the cyst.

Differential Diagnosis
- Hemorrhagic ovarian cyst
- Polycystic ovarian syndrome

Discussion
Hemorrhagic ovarian cysts most frequently occur in peripubertal or pubertal girls and tend to resolve over the course of a menstrual cycle.

Diagnosis
Ovarian torsion

Suggested Readings

Servaes S, Zurakowski D, Laufer MR, et al: Sonographic findings of ovarian torsion in children. Pediatr Radiol 37:441-446, 2007.
Stark JE, Siegel MJ: Ovarian torsion in prepubertal and pubertal girls: Sonographic findings. AJR Am J Roentgenol 163:1479-1482, 1994.

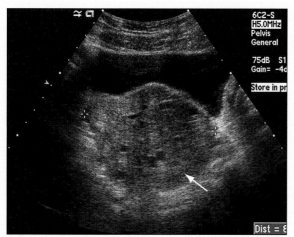

Figure 1. Transverse ultrasound of the pelvis shows enlarged, hypoechoic ovary with many small follicles posterior to the uterus in the region of the cul-de-sac (*arrow*).

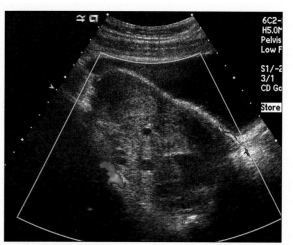

Figure 2. Sagittal ultrasound of the pelvis with color Doppler shows absence of flow to ovary.

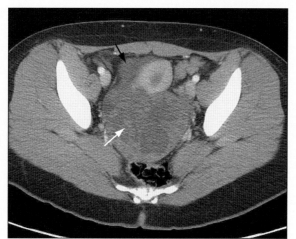

Figure 3. Axial contrast-enhanced CT through pelvis shows large, heterogeneous, hypoattenuating ovary in cul-de-sac (*white arrow*). A small amount of free fluid is present (*black arrow*).

Case 122

DEMOGRAPHICS/CLINICAL HISTORY

The patient is a 16-year-old boy with left scrotal pain for 16 hours.

FINDINGS

Transverse ultrasound shows asymmetric echotextures of the right and left testicles (Fig. 1), with heterogeneity and enlargement of the left testicle. Color Doppler ultrasound of the testicles (Fig. 2) shows normal color flow signal in the right testicle, with no discernible flow in the partially imaged left testicle. Color Doppler ultrasound of the left testicle (Fig. 3) shows no color flow within the testicle and mild color flow around the testicle.

DISCUSSION

Definition/Background

Testicular torsion is a true genitourinary emergency, and rapid diagnosis and treatment are tantamount to salvaging the threatened testicle.

Characteristic Clinical Features

Pain and swelling are the typical presenting features.

Characteristic Radiologic Findings

Ultrasonography is the first-line radiographic study for evaluation of testicular torsion. In the acute presentation, the only finding may be the lack of intratesticular vascular flow. Over time, the avascular testis enlarges and becomes more heterogeneous in echotexture. The scrotal wall becomes edematous and inflamed, causing soft tissue thickening and increased paratesticular flow. If ultrasound cannot be obtained or is equivocal, a nuclear medicine study with technetium 99m (^{99m}Tc) pertechnetate can be performed to show lack of flow into the affected testicle.

Less Common Radiologic Manifestations

Rarely, the twisted vascular pedicle to the testicle can be seen.

Differential Diagnosis

- Testicular hemorrhage
- Testicular mass
- Orchitis

Discussion

A patient with hemorrhage usually has a history of trauma, and flow can be seen in the unaffected testicular tissue. A testicular mass may have a similar gray-scale appearance, but normal to increased intratesticular flow should be seen. Similarly, orchitis may have an echogenic, enlarged appearance with scrotal swelling, but significantly increased flow to the testicle should be seen.

Diagnosis

Testicular torsion

Suggested Reading

Aso C, Enríquez G, Fité M, et al: Gray-scale and color Doppler sonography of scrotal disorders in children: An update. RadioGraphics 25:1197-1214, 2005.

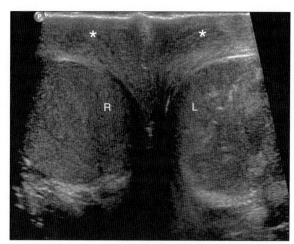

Figure 1. Transverse ultrasound of the testicles shows asymmetric echotextures of right (R) and left (L) testicles, with heterogeneity and enlargement of the left testicle. Mild scrotal edema is seen (*asterisks*).

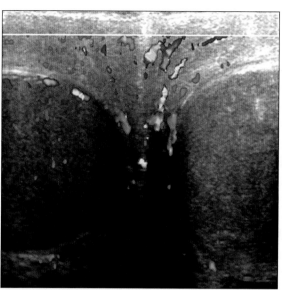

Figure 2. Color Doppler ultrasound of the testicles shows normal color flow signal in right testicle, with no discernible flow in partially imaged left testicle.

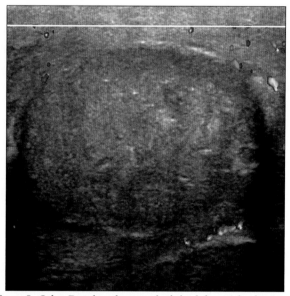

Figure 3. Color Doppler ultrasound of the left testicle shows no color flow within testicle and mild color flow around testicle.

Case 123

DEMOGRAPHICS/CLINICAL HISTORY

The patient is a 19-year-old man with scrotal pain.

FINDINGS

Ultrasound evaluation of the scrotum (Figs. 1 and 2) shows numerous, nonshadowing, punctate echogenic foci scattered throughout both testes.

DISCUSSION

Definition/Background

Testicular microlithiasis has been found in less than 1% of patients referred for scrotal ultrasound imaging, although this figure may be higher given the increased detection of microlithiasis with improving ultrasound imaging technology. Some studies have shown an increased risk of malignancy in patients with testicular microlithiasis compared with patients without this finding.

Characteristic Clinical Features

Most patients who are referred for ultrasound present either with scrotal pain or with a palpable lump, symptoms that are most likely unrelated to the presence of microlithiasis.

Characteristic Radiologic Findings

Imaging shows multiple tiny, nonshadowing echogenic foci scattered throughout the testes.

Diagnosis

Testicular microlithiasis

Suggested Readings

Cast JE, Nelson WM, Early AS, et al: Testicular microlithiasis: Prevalence and tumor risk in a population referred for scrotal sonography. AJR Am J Roentgenol 175:1703-1706, 2000.

Middleton WD, Teefey SA, Santillan CS: Testicular microlithiasis: Prospective analysis of prevalence and associated tumor. Radiology 224:425-428, 2002.

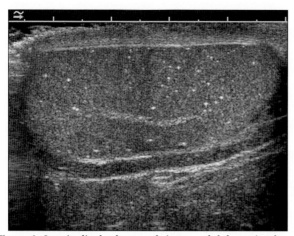

Figure 1. Longitudinal ultrasound image of left testis shows that the testis maintains a normal contour with no focal mass. There are innumerable, punctate, nonshadowing echogenic foci throughout parenchyma.

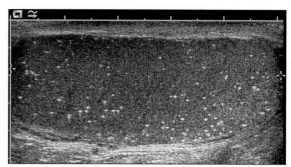

Figure 2. Longitudinal ultrasound image of right testis shows similar findings, with multiple, nonshadowing echogenic foci scattered throughout parenchyma.

Case 124

DEMOGRAPHICS/CLINICAL HISTORY

The patient is a 12-year-old boy with a painless left testicular lump.

FINDINGS

Transverse ultrasound of the left testicle (Fig. 1) shows a well-circumscribed mass within the testicle that has alternating layers of hypoechogenicity and hyperechogenicity. Color Doppler ultrasound (Fig. 2) does not show any internal vascularity within the mass. Histopathology confirmed the mass to be an epidermoid cyst of the testicle.

DISCUSSION

Definition/Background

Epidermoid cyst of the testis is a benign mass within the testicle that contains only ectodermal components.

Characteristic Clinical Features

A painless scrotal mass is the most common presentation.

Characteristic Radiologic Findings

Characteristic ultrasound findings include a well-circumscribed, lamellated or onion-skin appearance, with alternating hypoechogenic and hyperechogenic rings. Similarly, a target pattern or "bull's eye" is often seen because of calcification or keratin in the center. On color Doppler, the epidermoid is avascular.

Differential Diagnosis

- Other testicular masses, such as germ cell tumors

Discussion

Other testicular tumors often have internal vascularity, separating them from benign epidermoid cysts. The lamellated appearance also suggests an epidermoid cyst.

Diagnosis

Epidermoid cyst of the testis

Suggested Reading

Fujino J, Yamamoto H, Kisaki Y, et al: Epidermoid cyst: Rare testicular tumor in children. Pediatr Radiol 34:172-174, 2004.

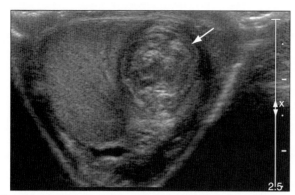

Figure 1. Transverse ultrasound of left testicle shows well-circumscribed mass (*arrow*) within testicle that has alternating layers of hypoechogenicity and hyperechogenicity.

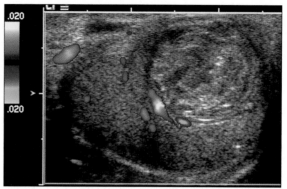

Figure 2. Color Doppler ultrasound does not show any internal vascularity within mass.

Case 125

DEMOGRAPHICS/CLINICAL HISTORY

The patient is a teenage boy with a varicocele suspected during clinical examination.

FINDINGS

Transverse ultrasound of the left scrotum (Fig. 1) shows tortuous, hypoechoic, tubular structures adjacent to the left testicle. A longitudinal view of the left scrotum (Fig. 2) shows a prominent tortuous, tubular structure. A longitudinal view with color Doppler ultrasound (Fig. 3) confirms the tubular structure to be a vessel. Doppler interrogation (Fig. 4) shows a venous waveform that augments with a Valsalva maneuver.

DISCUSSION

Definition/Background

Varicoceles are dilated veins in the pampiniform plexus of the spermatic cord; they are more common on the left side.

Characteristic Clinical Features

Varicoceles are often palpable as cordlike structures within the scrotum.

Characteristic Radiologic Findings

Ultrasound shows tortuous, dilated veins within the scrotum that augment with a Valsalva maneuver. The ipsilateral testicle can be smaller in volume than the contralateral side. Varicoceles are more common on the left side.

Diagnosis

Varicocele

Suggested Reading

Aso C, Enríquez G, Fité M, et al: Gray-scale and color Doppler sonography of scrotal disorders in children: An update. RadioGraphics 25:1197-1214, 2005.

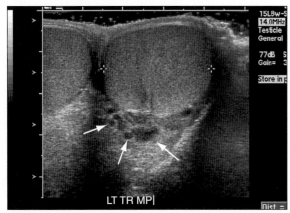

Figure 1. Transverse ultrasound of left scrotum shows tortuous, hypoechoic, tubular structures (*arrows*) adjacent to left testicle.

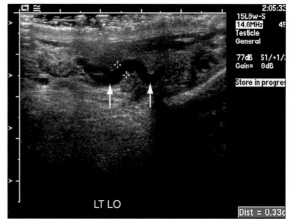

Figure 2. Longitudinal view of left scrotum shows prominent tortuous, tubular structure (*arrows*).

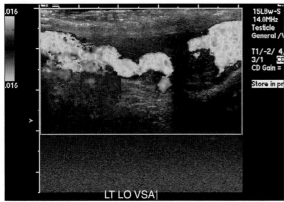

Figure 3. Longitudinal view with color Doppler ultrasound confirms tubular structure to be a vessel.

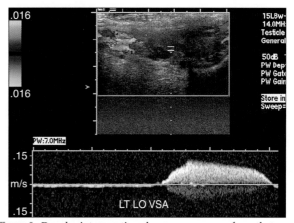

Figure 4. Doppler interrogation shows venous waveform that augments with a Valsalva maneuver.

Case 126

DEMOGRAPHICS/CLINICAL HISTORY

The patient is a 16-year-old boy with scrotal pain.

FINDINGS

Longitudinal ultrasound of the left scrotum (Fig. 1) shows hypoechoic areas adjacent to the left testicle. Color Doppler (Fig. 2) shows normal flow within the testicle and lack of flow in the hypoechoic areas.

DISCUSSION

Definition/Background

Hydroceles are caused by abnormal or lack of closure of the processus vaginalis, with fluid communicating into the scrotum (i.e., funicular hydrocele) or trapped within the inguinal canal (i.e., encysted hydrocele).

Characteristic Clinical Features

Fullness of the scrotum with transillumination suggests a hydrocele.

Characteristic Radiologic Findings

Ultrasonography shows an avascular, hypoechoic collection within the scrotum and inguinal canal. The collection is typically anechoic, but it occasionally contains mobile, tiny, echogenic foci. In an encysted hydrocele, the collection is contained within the inguinal canal, without communication to the peritoneum or tunica vaginalis. Hydroceles can be reactive, resulting from infectious, inflammatory, or neoplastic causes, and findings of these conditions may also be present.

Diagnosis

Hydrocele

Suggested Reading

Bhosale PR, Patnana M, Viswanathan C, Szklaruk J: The inguinal canal: Anatomy and imaging features of common and uncommon masses. RadioGraphics 28:819-835, 2008.

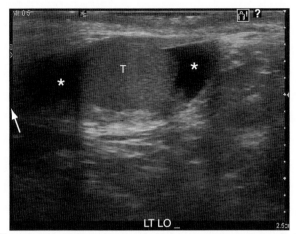

Figure 1. Longitudinal ultrasound of left scrotum shows hypoechoic areas (*asterisks*) adjacent to left testicle (T).

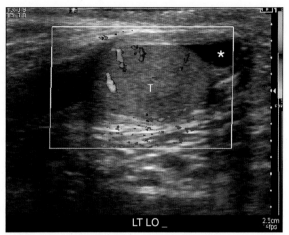

Figure 2. Color Doppler shows normal flow within testicle (T) and lack of flow in hypoechoic areas (*asterisk*).

Case 127

DEMOGRAPHICS/CLINICAL HISTORY

The patient is an 18-year-old male after cardiac surgery with an incidentally identified solitary kidney.

FINDINGS

Four transverse images from ultrasound of the pelvis (Fig. 1) show a cystic structure just right of midline, just superior to the prostate, and posterior to the bladder. Ultrasound of the abdomen (Fig. 2) confirmed absence of the ipsilateral right kidney and an enlarged left kidney. In a different patient, four axial T2-weighted images from magnetic resonance imaging (MRI) of the pelvis (Fig. 3) show a cystic structure just left of midline, just superior to the prostate, and posterior to the bladder. Coronal T2-weighted MRI of the abdomen (Fig. 4) shows absence of the ipsilateral left kidney.

DISCUSSION

Definition/Background
Seminal vesicle cysts are associated with renal anomalies, particularly renal agenesis.

Characteristic Clinical Features
The cysts often are found incidentally. If the cyst is large enough, the patient can experience bladder irritation or obstruction or present with a pelvic mass.

Characteristic Radiologic Findings
Imaging shows a cystic structure extending from the prostate superiorly. Ipsilateral renal agenesis often is observed. Seminal vesicle cysts can be associated with autosomal dominant polycystic kidney disease.

Differential Diagnosis
- True prostate gland cysts
- Ejaculatory duct cysts
- Müllerian duct cysts
- Prostatic utricle
- Hydronephrotic pelvic kidneys
- Bladder diverticula

Discussion
The diagnosis of seminal vesicle cysts is suggested by associated renal anomalies such as renal agenesis and careful imaging.

Diagnosis
Seminal vesicle cyst

Suggested Readings
Arora SS, Breiman RS, Webb EM, et al: CT and MRI of congenital anomalies of the seminal vesicles. AJR Am J Roentgenol 189:130-135, 2007.

Livingston L, Larsen CR: Seminal vesicle cyst with ipsilateral renal agenesis. AJR Am J Roentgenol 175:177-180, 2000.

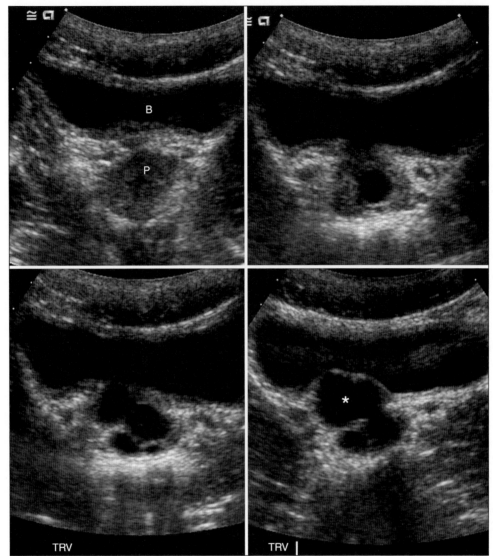

Figure 1. Four transverse images from ultrasound of the pelvis show cystic structure (*asterisk*) just right of midline, just superior to prostate (P), and posterior to bladder (B).

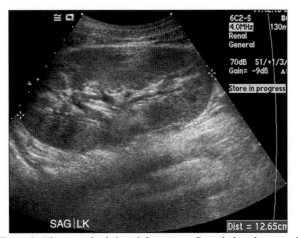

Figure 2. Ultrasound of the abdomen confirmed the absence of ipsilateral right kidney and showed enlarged left kidney.

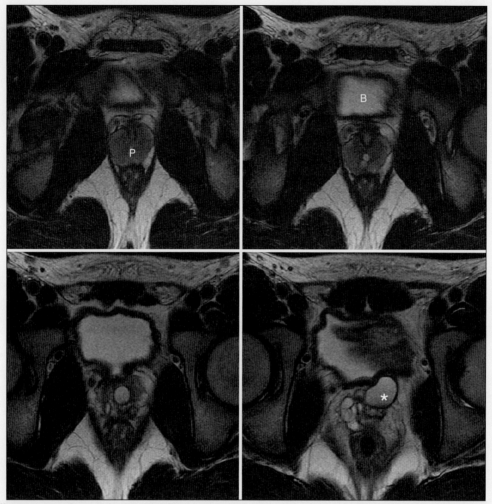

Figure 3. In a different patient, four axial T2-weighted images from MRI of the pelvis show cystic structure (*asterisk*) just left of midline, just superior to prostate (P), and posterior to bladder (B).

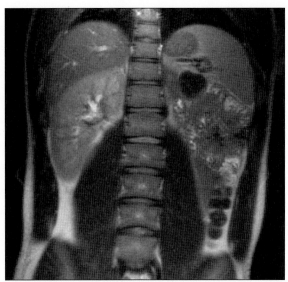

Figure 4. In the same patient shown in Fig. 3, coronal T2-weighted MR image of the abdomen shows absence of ipsilateral left kidney.

Case 128

DEMOGRAPHICS/CLINICAL HISTORY

The patient is a 4-year-old girl with a high fever and a history of recurrent urinary tract infections.

FINDINGS

Ultrasound evaluation of the kidneys reveals that the left kidney is significantly larger than the right kidney (10.3 vs. 7.6 cm). The left kidney is diffusely enlarged, with loss of normal corticomedullary differentiation (Fig. 1). Power Doppler reveals decreased vascularity to the lower pole of the left kidney (Fig. 2). The right kidney is normal (Fig. 3).

DISCUSSION

Definition/Background

Acute pyelonephritis is more common in girls than boys. It is difficult to diagnose in very young children, who are unable to verbalize symptoms.

Characteristic Clinical Features

In a child without other symptoms, a fever of unknown origin may suggest a concomitant cold or flu. The diagnosis is made on the basis of abnormal bacterial growth in a urine specimen.

Characteristic Radiologic Findings

Ultrasound findings in the setting of acute pyelonephritis include diffuse or local parenchymal swelling, poor corticomedullary differentiation, and decreased perfusion on color Doppler ultrasound.

Less Common Radiologic Manifestations

Imaging may show thickening of the urothelium.

Differential Diagnosis

- Xanthogranulomatous pyelonephritis
- Wilms tumor
- Renal lymphoma

Discussion

Xanthogranulomatous pyelonephritis is a rare, chronic infection that occurs most commonly in older women. Typical findings include an enlarged kidney with internal fluid and debris, and a large calculus in the collecting system. Focal forms of acute pyelonephritis may simulate a renal malignancy, such as Wilms tumor or renal lymphoma.

Diagnosis

Acute pyelonephritis

Suggested Readings

Craig WD, Wagner BJ, Travis MD: Pyelonephritis: Radiologic-pathologic review. RadioGraphics 28:255-277, 2008.

Lavocat MP, Granjon D, Allard D, et al: Imaging of pyelonephritis. Pediatr Radiol 27:159-165, 1997.

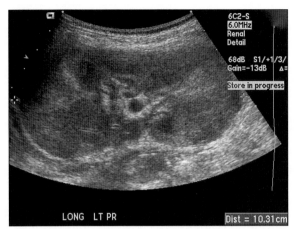

Figure 1. Gray-scale ultrasound shows diffuse enlargement of left kidney, which measures 10.3 cm, and loss of corticomedullary differentiation.

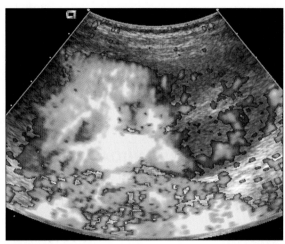

Figure 2. Power Doppler interrogation shows decreased perfusion to lower pole of left kidney.

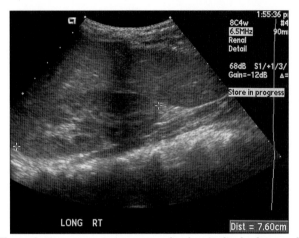

Figure 3. For comparison, gray-scale, longitudinal ultrasound shows normal-appearing right kidney, which measures 7.6 cm.

Case 129

DEMOGRAPHICS/CLINICAL HISTORY

The patient is a 9-month-old girl with fever after pyeloplasty for ureteropelvic junction obstruction.

FINDINGS

Longitudinal ultrasound of the left kidney (Fig. 1) shows a severely dilated renal collecting system with internal debris. A slightly oblique view (Fig. 2) shows the internal debris within the renal pelvis and an echogenic masslike collection of debris within a dilated lower pole calyx. Color Doppler imaging (Fig. 3) does not show any vascularity within the echogenic masslike debris in the lower pole calyx. A transverse view through the left lower pole (Fig. 4) shows layering of the debris and a fluid-debris level.

DISCUSSION

Definition/Background

The collection of infected urine within the collecting system is known as pyonephrosis.

Characteristic Clinical Features

Typical clinical findings are fever and pain.

Characteristic Radiologic Findings

Ultrasound is the recommended initial imaging modality. Low-level echoes are seen within a dilated collecting system dependently. The cause of the obstruction, such as an obstructing calculus, can often be visualized. A fluid-debris level sometimes can be seen.

Differential Diagnosis

- Artifact

Discussion

Low-level echoes should be reproducible because ultrasound artifacts of anechoic collections sometimes can be mistaken for debris.

Diagnosis

Pyonephrosis

Suggested Reading

Baumgarten DA, Baumgartner BR: Imaging and radiologic management of upper urinary tract infections. Urol Clin North Am 24:545-569, 1997.

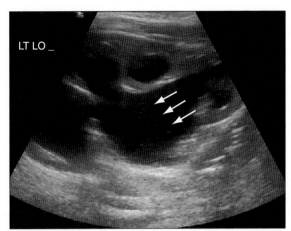

Figure 1. Longitudinal ultrasound of left kidney shows severely dilated renal collecting system with internal debris (*arrows*).

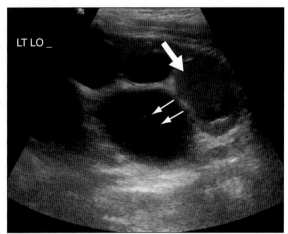

Figure 2. Slightly oblique view shows internal debris within renal pelvis (*small arrows*) and an echogenic masslike collection of debris within dilated lower pole calyx (*large arrow*).

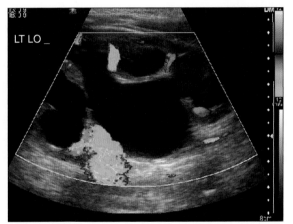

Figure 3. Color Doppler imaging does not show any vascularity within echogenic masslike debris in lower pole calyx.

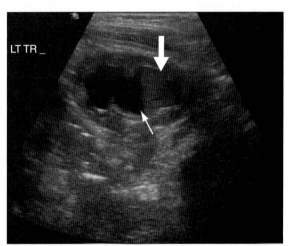

Figure 4. Transverse view through left lower pole shows layering of debris (*large arrow*) with fluid-debris level (*small arrow*).

Case 130

DEMOGRAPHICS/CLINICAL HISTORY

The patient is a 2-year-old child with urinary tract infections.

FINDINGS

Oblique image from a voiding cystourethrogram (VCUG) (Fig. 1) shows right-sided vesicoureteral reflux into a ureter ectopically inserted into the bladder neck. An image of the right renal bed from the VCUG (Fig. 2) shows reflux into a dysmorphic upper pole of a duplicated collecting system.

DISCUSSION

Definition/Background

An ectopic ureter can exist as the malpositioning of a single system ureter or one ureter of a duplicated collecting system.

Characteristic Clinical Features

Children with ectopic ureters may present with febrile urinary tract infections. In girls with ectopic ureters that insert below the bladder neck or into the vagina, the presenting history may be continuous wetness.

Characteristic Radiologic Findings

On VCUG, vesicoureteral reflux is usually seen into ectopically positioned ureters. When part of a duplicated collecting system, ectopic ureters are usually part of the upper pole moiety and typically insert inferomedially to the normal ureteral insertion site (Weigert-Meyer rule). In girls, if the ectopic ureter inserts into the vagina, intravenous urography or magnetic resonance urography often shows contrast agent excreted into the vagina.

Diagnosis

Ectopic ureter

Suggested Readings

Avni FE, Nicaise N, Hall M, et al: The role of MR imaging for the assessment of complicated duplex kidneys in children: Preliminary report. Pediatr Radiol 31:215-223, 2001.

Roy Choudhury S, Chadha R, Bagga D, et al: Spectrum of ectopic ureters in children. Pediatr Surg Int 24:819-823, 2008.

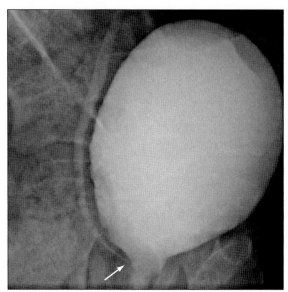

Figure 1. Oblique VCUG shows right-sided vesicoureteral reflux into ureter ectopically inserted into bladder neck (*arrow*).

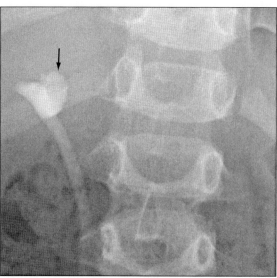

Figure 2. VCUG of right renal bed shows reflux into dysmorphic upper pole of duplicated collecting system (*arrow*).

Case 131

DEMOGRAPHICS/CLINICAL HISTORY

The patient is a newborn with prenatally diagnosed hydronephrosis.

FINDINGS

Transverse ultrasound of the bladder (Fig. 1) shows a thin-walled, cystic structure within the bladder, representing a ureterocele. Posterior to the bladder, a redundant, dilated ureter is identified. A left sagittal ultrasound of the bladder (Fig. 2) shows the ureterocele and the tortuous dilated ureter. Filling image from a voiding cystourethrogram (VCUG) (Fig. 3) shows the ureterocele as a filling defect. Voiding image from VCUG (Fig. 4) shows eversion and prolapse of the ureterocele and vesicoureteral reflux. This ureter was part of an upper pole moiety of a duplicated left collecting system.

DISCUSSION

Definition/Background

A ureterocele is a saccular dilation of the distal ureter into the bladder. The ureterocele often is associated with a duplicated collecting system.

Characteristic Clinical Features

Febrile urinary tract infections typically lead to discovery of a ureterocele.

Characteristic Radiologic Findings

Ultrasound shows a thin-walled, simple cystic structure within the bladder that is off midline. Ureteroceles often are seen with duplicated collecting systems, typically associated with the upper pole moiety. VCUG typically shows the ureterocele during early filling or at the completion of the study, when the small amount of contrast outlines the ureterocele. If the ureterocele everts or prolapses, contrast agent can be seen refluxing into the distal ureter.

Diagnosis

Ureterocel

Suggested Reading

Berrocal T, López-Pereira P, Arjonilla A, Gutiérrez J: Anomalies of the distal ureter, bladder, and urethra in children: Embryologic, radiologic, and pathologic features. RadioGraphics 22:1139-1164, 2002.

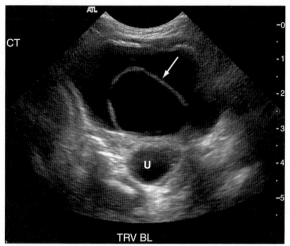

Figure 1. Transverse ultrasound of bladder shows thin-walled, cystic structure (*arrow*) within bladder, representing a ureterocele. Posterior to bladder, redundant dilated ureter is identified (U).

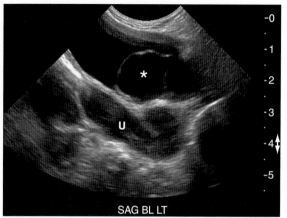

Figure 2. Left sagittal ultrasound of bladder shows ureterocele (*asterisk*) and tortuous dilated ureter (U).

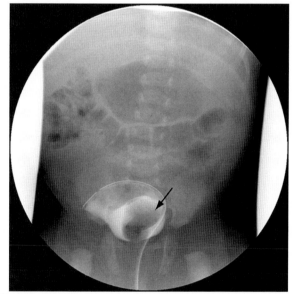

Figure 3. Filling image from VCUG shows ureterocele as filling defect (*arrow*).

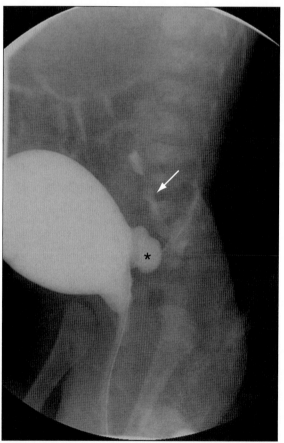

Figure 4. Voiding image from VCUG shows eversion or prolapse of ureterocele (*asterisk*) and vesicoureteral reflux (*arrow*). Ureter was part of upper pole moiety of duplicated left collecting system.

Case 132

DEMOGRAPHICS/CLINICAL HISTORY

The patient is a 6-year-old child with urinary tract infections.

FINDINGS

Oblique image from a voiding cystourethrogram (VCUG) during filling of the bladder does not show an abnormality at the right ureterovesicular junction (Fig. 1). During voiding, bilateral Hutch diverticula are seen, with vesicoureteral reflux into the left ureter (Fig. 2).

DISCUSSION

Definition/Background

Hutch diverticula are bladder diverticula that occur at or adjacent to ureterovesicular junctions.

Characteristic Clinical Features

Hutch diverticula are usually discovered on VCUG performed for urinary tract infections.

Characteristic Radiologic Findings

An outpouching from the bladder typically is seen at the expected site of the ureterovesicular junction. The diverticulum sometimes is seen only during voiding. The diverticulum can enlarge and incorporate the ureteral insertion, causing vesicoureteral reflux.

Diagnosis

Hutch diverticulum

Suggested Reading

Boechat MI, Lebowitz RL: Diverticula of the bladder in children. Pediatr Radiol 7:22, 1978.

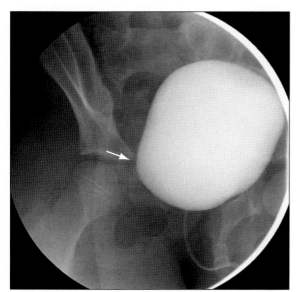

Figure 1. Oblique VCUG image during filling of bladder does not show abnormality at right ureterovesicular junction (*arrow*).

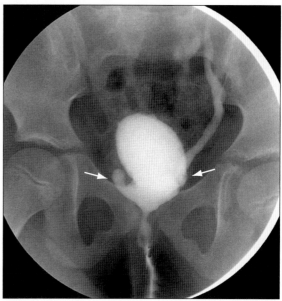

Figure 2. VCUG image during voiding shows bilateral Hutch diverticula (*arrow*) (better on the right), with vesicoureteral reflux into left ureter.

Case 133

DEMOGRAPHICS/CLINICAL HISTORY

The patient is a 2-week-old infant with a two-vessel cord seen on prenatal ultrasound.

FINDINGS

Longitudinal ultrasound view of the left kidney shows moderate to severe hydronephrosis (Fig. 1). Early filling image from a voiding cystourethrogram (VCUG) (Fig. 2) shows elevation of the bladder base above the pubis and bladder diverticula. Another VCUG (Fig. 3) shows marked trabeculation of the bladder, bladder diverticula, dilation of the posterior urethra, and posterior urethral valve (PUV) with a normal-caliber anterior urethra.

DISCUSSION

Definition/Background

PUVs are the most common congenital urethral abnormalities in boys.

Characteristic Clinical Features

A slow, nonforceful urinary stream or dribbling can be seen clinically in boys with PUVs.

Characteristic Radiologic Findings

Diagnosis is made by VCUG, with several classic findings. Elevation of the bladder base from the typical location just above the pubis results from muscular hypertrophy of the bladder. Bladder diverticula and trabeculation are also seen. On voiding images, the posterior urethra is dilated with a typical "valve" or acute narrowing at the junction of the posterior and anterior urethra. The anterior urethra is normal or underdistended because of obstruction by the valve. Because many boys have coexisting vesicoureteral reflux, this is a commonly seen finding on VCUG. Ultrasound can detect bladder hypertrophy and diverticula and hydronephrosis in boys with coexisting reflux. Transperineal ultrasound can better illustrate a dilated posterior urethra.

Less Common Radiologic Manifestations

In patients with coexisting reflux, the pressure from the urinary obstruction because of PUVs can decompress into the renal collecting system. This occasionally causes caliceal rupture and a urinoma.

Differential Diagnosis

- Prune-belly syndrome

Discussion

Prune-belly syndrome has many radiographic findings; one is an enlarged posterior urethra with funneling, which can simulate PUV. The other findings of prune-belly syndrome, particularly the common megalourethra appearance of the anterior urethra and the lack of a distinct PUV, allow distinction from PUV.

Diagnosis

Posterior urethral valves

Suggested Readings

Eklöf O, Ringertz H: Pre- and postoperative urographic findings in posterior urethral valves. Pediatr Radiol 4:43-46, 1975.

Hendren WH: Posterior urethral valves in boys: A broad clinical spectrum. J Urol 106:298-307, 1971.

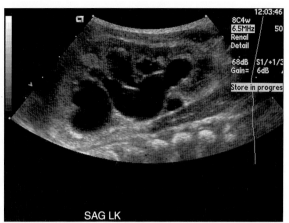

Figure 1. Longitudinal ultrasound view of left kidney shows moderate to severe hydronephrosis.

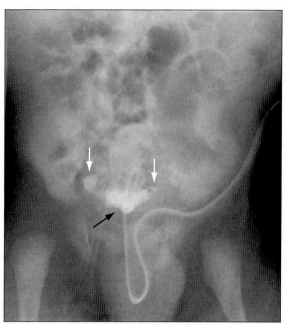

Figure 2. Early filling image from VCUG shows elevation of bladder base (*black arrow*) above pubis and bladder diverticula (*white arrows*). The bladder catheter is seen in place.

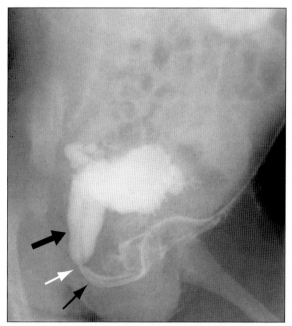

Figure 3. VCUG shows marked trabeculation of bladder, bladder diverticula, dilation of posterior urethra (*large black arrow*), and PUV (*white arrow*) with a normal-caliber anterior urethra (*small black arrow*). The catheter is still in place.

Case 134

DEMOGRAPHICS/CLINICAL HISTORY

The patient is a newborn with prenatal hydronephrosis.

FINDINGS

Transverse ultrasound through the level of the bladder (Fig. 1) shows prominent distal ureters posterior to the bladder. Voiding cystourethrogram (VCUG) (Fig. 2) shows bilateral vesicoureteral reflux into the renal collecting systems, causing blunting of the calices bilaterally. The renal axis of both kidneys is normal, with the upper pole calices closer to the midline. Oblique VCUG (Fig. 3) shows a normal left ureteral insertion site. VCUG in another patient (Fig. 4) shows reflux into a collecting system that has an abnormal axis; this "drooping lily" configuration suggests a duplicated collecting system.

DISCUSSION

Definition/Background

Vesicoureteral reflux is a common condition in young children that often is caused by an abnormality in the angle of ureteral insertion into the bladder. Reflux grades 1 to 5 vary in severity from minimal to severe. Mild cases are commonly outgrown as the child's bladder grows and the insertion angle corrects.

Characteristic Clinical Features

Patients with reflux typically present with febrile urinary tract infections.

Characteristic Radiologic Findings

Ultrasound can show various amounts of renal collecting system and ureteral dilation, including no discernible dilation. VCUG is typically performed for the initial evaluation, allowing resolution of the collecting systems and insertion sites. The grading system is defined as follows: *1,* reflux into the ureter alone; *2,* reflux into the ureter and renal collecting system; *3,* reflux causing mild blunting of the calices; *4,* reflux causing moderate blunting and a tortuous dilated ureter; *5,* reflux causing severe blunting, dilation, and an extremely tortuous dilated ureter. Nuclear medicine scintigraphy can be used to identify reflux, but the resolution is not as good for detecting ureteral abnormalities.

Less Common Radiologic Manifestations

Intrarenal reflux can be seen from the calices into the distal collecting ducts; it may not be related to the grade of reflux.

Diagnosis

Vesicoureteral reflux

Suggested Reading

Lebowitz RL: The detection of vesicoureteral reflux in the child. Invest Radiol 21:519-531, 1986.

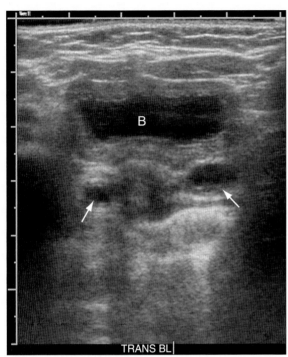

Figure 1. Transverse ultrasound through the level of bladder shows prominent distal ureters (*arrows*) posterior to bladder (B). Fullness of the renal collecting systems was also seen (not shown).

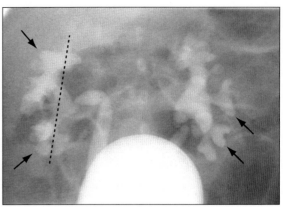

Figure 2. VCUG shows bilateral vesicoureteral reflux into renal collecting systems, causing blunting of calices (*arrows*) bilaterally. Renal axis (*dashed line*) of both kidneys is normal, with upper pole calices closer to midline.

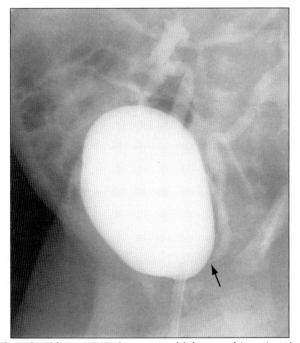

Figure 3. Oblique VCUG shows normal left ureteral insertion site (*arrow*). Right ureteral insertion was also normal.

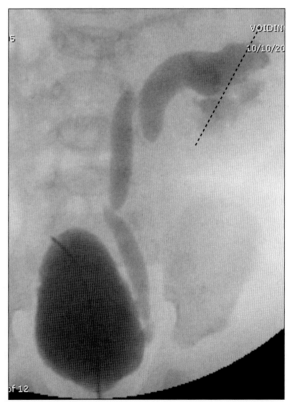

Figure 4. In another patient, VCUG shows reflux into collecting system that has abnormal axis (*dashed line*). This "drooping lily" configuration suggests a duplicated collecting system.

Case 135

DEMOGRAPHICS/CLINICAL HISTORY

The patient is a newborn with a history of prenatal hydronephrosis.

FINDINGS

Transverse color Doppler ultrasound (Fig. 1) of the bladder shows a round, hypoechoic structure posterior to the bladder and right of midline, which does not show vascular flow within it. Longitudinal ultrasound (Fig. 2) of the bladder elongates the hypoechoic structure posterior to the bladder and shows distal tapering at its union with the bladder, representing moderate hydroureter. A longitudinal view of the right kidney (Fig. 3) shows mild dilation of the renal pelvis with mild extension into the caliceal system. Results of a voiding cystourethrogram (VCUG) for the same patient were normal, and there was no evidence of reflux.

DISCUSSION

Definition/Background

Megaureter can be primary or secondary. Obstructing primary megaureter results from an aperistaltic segment of the distal ureter at the ureterovesicular junction, causing dilation of the ureter and obstruction and often causing secondary hydronephrosis.

Characteristic Clinical Features

The clinical presentation of primary megaureter includes prenatal hydronephrosis and infection.

Characteristic Radiologic Findings

Dilation of the ureter of more than 7 mm is typical, with tapering of the distal segment of the ureter at the ureterovesicular junction. Ipsilateral secondary hydronephrosis is often seen.

Differential Diagnosis

- Vesicoureteral reflux

Discussion

Vesicoureteral reflux can have findings similar to hydroureteronephrosis, and VCUG is necessary to evaluate for reflux in these patients. Posterior urethral valves with vesicoureteral reflux can also have this appearance, but bladder wall thickening on ultrasound and posterior urethral valves on VCUG indicate the correct diagnosis.

Diagnosis

Primary megaureter

Suggested Reading

Berrocal T, López-Pereira P, Arjonilla A, Gutiérrez J: Anomalies of the distal ureter, bladder, and urethra in children: Embryologic, radiologic, and pathologic features. RadioGraphics 22:1139-1164, 2002.

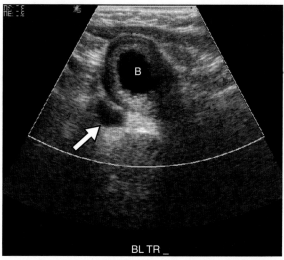

Figure 1. Transverse color Doppler ultrasound of bladder (B) shows round, hypoechoic structure posterior to bladder and right of midline (*arrow*), which does not show vascular flow within it.

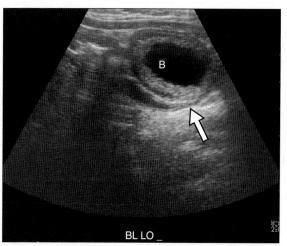

Figure 2. Longitudinal ultrasound of bladder (B) elongates hypoechoic structure posterior to bladder and shows distal tapering at its union with bladder (*arrow*), representing moderate hydroureter.

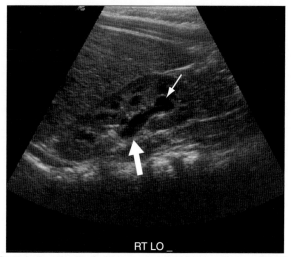

Figure 3. Longitudinal ultrasound of right kidney shows mild dilation of renal pelvis (*large arrow*) with mild extension into caliceal system (*small arrow*).

Case 136

DEMOGRAPHICS/CLINICAL HISTORY

The patient is a 20-year-old female with abdominal pain.

FINDINGS

An axial image from a contrast-enhanced computed tomography (CT) scan (Fig. 1) shows a density along the posterior aspect of the bladder. On a CT image slightly superior (Fig. 2), the density is seen causing obstruction of the left ureter. A coronal reconstruction image of the abdomen (Fig. 3) shows hydronephrosis and delayed excretion of contrast agent in the left kidney. A coronal reconstruction image distally (Fig. 4) shows the obstructing stone at the ureterovesical junction (UVJ) and the dilated distal ureter.

DISCUSSION

Definition/Background

UVJ obstruction can occur because of an obstructing stone or mass. Primary megaureter (see Case 138) can have features similar to UVJ obstruction.

Characteristic Clinical Features

Pain and hematuria are common presentations.

Characteristic Radiologic Findings

Ultrasound is an excellent imaging modality if UVJ obstruction is suspected. Obstruction at the UVJ causes dilation of the ureter and renal collecting system and delays in excretion (visualized during contrast-enhanced CT or nuclear medicine imaging). Chronic obstruction causes renal cortical thinning. Close attention should be focused at the UVJ to determine the etiology of the obstruction.

Differential Diagnosis

■ Primary megaureter

Discussion

Primary megaureter has a distally tapering ureter at the UVJ, as opposed to a mass or stone causing the obstruction.

Diagnosis

Ureterovesical junction obstruction

Suggested Reading

Preston A, Lebowitz RL: What's new in pediatric uroradiology. Urol Radiol 11:217-220, 1989.

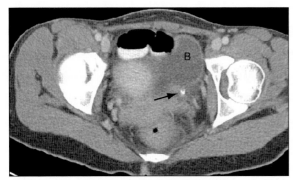

Figure 1. Axial image from contrast-enhanced CT scan shows density (*arrow*) along posterior aspect of bladder (B).

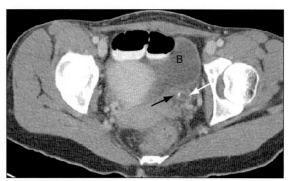

Figure 2. Slightly superiorly, density (*black arrow*) is seen causing obstruction of left ureter (*white arrow*). B, bladder.

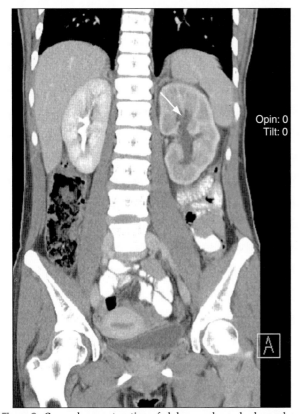

Figure 3. Coronal reconstruction of abdomen shows hydronephrosis and delayed excretion of contrast agent in left kidney (*arrow*).

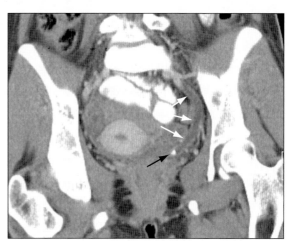

Figure 4. Coronal reconstruction distally shows obstructing stone at UVJ (*black arrow*) and dilated distal ureter (*white arrows*).

Case 137

DEMOGRAPHICS/CLINICAL HISTORY

The patient is a 1-year-old child with hematuria after a fall.

FINDINGS

Longitudinal ultrasound of the left kidney (Fig. 1) shows a very dilated renal pelvis with thinning of the renal cortex. Longitudinal ultrasound of the right kidney (Fig. 2) shows a normal-appearing organ. There is a size discrepancy between the left and right kidneys. Transverse ultrasound of the bladder (Fig. 3) shows a normal-appearing bladder, without a dilated distal left ureter.

DISCUSSION

Definition/Background

Ureteropelvic junction (UPJ) obstruction often is caused by congenital narrowing of the junction between the renal pelvis and proximal ureter. Another possible cause is a vessel crossing the proximal ureter, which produces mass effect and proximal obstruction.

Characteristic Clinical Features

Patients with UPJ obstruction may present with pain, a palpable mass, and hematuria. Prenatal ultrasound has identified patients before they have symptoms.

Characteristic Radiologic Findings

Dilation of the renal pelvis and absence of ureteral dilation are the hallmarks of UPJ obstruction. The bladder appears normal.

Less Common Radiologic Manifestations

Computed tomography (CT) angiography or magnetic resonance angiography (MRA) may be necessary to diagnose a crossing vessel that causes the obstruction.

Differential Diagnosis

- Multicystic dysplastic kidney

Discussion

A multicystic dysplastic kidney has several cysts of different sizes and no definite renal pelvis.

Diagnosis

Ureteropelvic junction obstruction

Suggested Readings

Fernbach SK: The dilated urinary tract in children. Urol Radiol 14: 34-42, 1992.

Rooks VJ, Lebowitz RL: Extrinsic ureteropelvic junction obstruction from a crossing renal vessel: Demography and imaging. Pediatr Radiol 31:120-124, 2001.

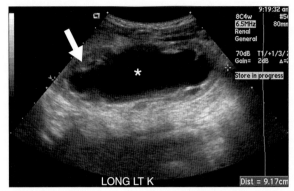

Figure 1. Longitudinal ultrasound of left kidney shows very dilated renal pelvis (*asterisk*) with thinning of renal cortex (*arrow*).

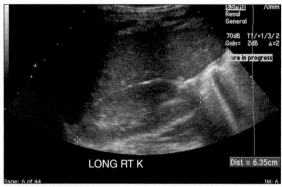

Figure 2. Longitudinal ultrasound of right kidney shows normal-appearing right kidney. Notice the size discrepancy between the left and right kidneys.

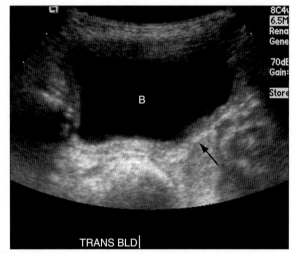

Figure 3. Transverse ultrasound of bladder shows normal-appearing bladder (B), without dilated distal left ureter (*arrow*).

Case 138

DEMOGRAPHICS/CLINICAL HISTORY

The patient is a 2-month-old girl with VACTERL association and cloacal malformation, and currently a diverting ileostomy.

FINDINGS

Images acquired as part of a cloacal contrast study (Figs. 1 and 2) show that contrast medium administered via a catheter placed in the common orifice at the perineum opacifies the rectum, bladder, and vagina. All three structures drain into a long common channel, which exits onto the perineum.

DISCUSSION

Definition/Background
Cloacal malformation is seen exclusively in phenotypic females.

Characteristic Clinical Features
Patients with cloacal malformation have an imperforate anus and a single perineal opening. Vesicoureteral reflux, such as is seen in this patient, is common in cloacal malformation.

Characteristic Radiologic Findings
Contrast studies performed via a catheter placed within the common perineal opening reveal that the bladder, rectum, and vagina all end in the same common channel exiting onto the perineum.

Differential Diagnosis
- Imperforate anus
- Mixed gonadal dysgenesis

Discussion
Imperforate anus is the most common abnormality of the hindgut. Lesions are classified as either high or low (based on whether the blind end of the rectum is above or below the levator muscles), and there is often a fistulous connection between the rectum and the perineum or urethra. Mixed gonadal dysgenesis is a condition of asymmetric gonadal development, which leads to an unassigned sex differentiation.

Diagnosis
Cloacal malformation

Suggested Readings
Hendren WH: Cloacal malformations: Experience with 105 cases. J Pediatr Surg 27:890, 1992.

Jaramillo D, Lebowitz RL, Hendron WH: The cloacal malformation: Radiologic findings and imaging recommendations. Radiology 177:441, 1990.

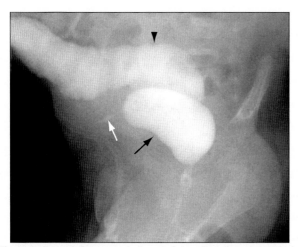

Figure 1. Lateral fluoroscopic image from cloacal contrast study with catheter placed in common orifice at the perineum. Contrast medium administered through this catheter opacifies the dilated vagina (*black arrow*), with a small trickle of contrast medium noted in the cervix (*white arrow*). There also is contrast medium within the rectum (*arrowhead*).

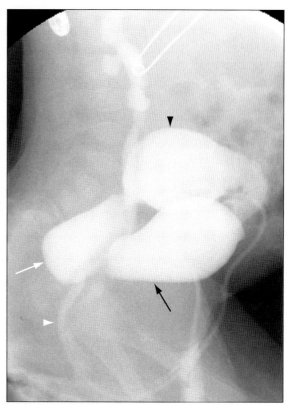

Figure 2. Later fluoroscopic image obtained as part of cloacal contrast study after replacement of catheter more anteriorly in common channel (*white arrowhead*) shows contrast medium within vagina (*white arrow*) and colon (*black arrowhead*). Now there also is contrast medium within the bladder (*black arrow*). Unilateral vesicoureteral reflux is noted.

Case 139

DEMOGRAPHICS/CLINICAL HISTORY

The patient is a newborn girl with no visible vaginal opening.

FINDINGS

A lateral voiding cystourethrogram (VCUG) (Fig. 1) shows contrast agent filling the vagina and the bladder. The distal vagina is attached to the posterior urethra. The flattened contour superiorly is caused by the impression of the cervix. Later in the VCUG study (Fig. 2), contrast agent is seen filling the uterine cavity.

DISCUSSION

Definition/Background
Urogenital sinus anomaly is a rare condition, in which the distal vagina inserts into the urethra.

Characteristic Clinical Features
Because of the common channel, there is no normal vaginal opening.

Characteristic Radiologic Findings
On VCUG, the vagina typically is seen communicating with the urethra between the proximal and distal portions. Contrast agent may enter the uterine cavity. Ultrasound may show fluid within a distended vagina.

Differential Diagnosis
- Congenital adrenal hyperplasia

Discussion
Physical findings of virilization and enlarged adrenal glands can be seen in congenital adrenal hyperplasia; laboratory values should be analyzed to exclude this entity.

Diagnosis
Urogenital sinus anomaly

Suggested Reading
Subramanian S, Sharma R, Gamanagatti S, et al: Antenatal MR diagnosis of urinary hydrometrocolpos due to urogenital sinus. Pediatr Radiol 36:1086-1089, 2006.

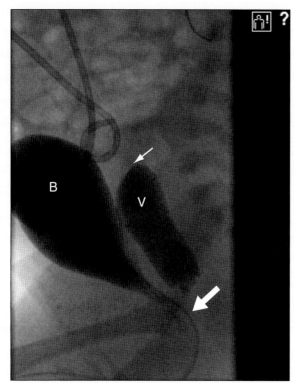

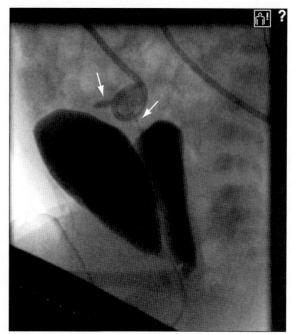

Figure 2. Later in VCUG study, contrast agent is seen filling uterine cavity (*arrows*).

Figure 1. Lateral VCUG shows contrast agent filling vagina (V) and bladder (B). Distal vagina is attached to posterior urethra (*large arrow*). The flattened contour superiorly (*small arrow*) is the impression of the cervix. A pigtail catheter had been placed in a fluid collection of hydrometrocolpos.

Case 140

DEMOGRAPHICS/CLINICAL HISTORY

The patient is a newborn boy with a known diagnosis of bladder exstrophy based on prenatal imaging.

FINDINGS

An anteroposterior radiograph of the abdomen (Fig. 1) reveals diastasis of the symphysis pubis. The patient also has a large scrotal hernia. Magnetic resonance imaging (MRI) of the pelvis (Figs. 2 and 3) better delineates the pelvic anatomy and shows the small, decompressed, exstrophied bladder, which has a nodular contour on this examination.

DISCUSSION

Definition/Background
Bladder exstrophy is a rare disorder in which the entire anterior wall of the bladder, overlying skin, and rectus muscles (inferiorly) are absent. Boys are affected three times as often as girls.

Characteristic Clinical Features
On physical examination, there is an outpouching below the umbilicus. It may be associated with imperforate anus and epispadias.

Characteristic Radiologic Findings
Radiographs show symphyseal diastasis. Cross-sectional computed tomography (CT) or MRI often identifies multiple abnormalities of the pelvic floor musculature.

Differential Diagnosis
- Cloacal exstrophy

Discussion
Compared with bladder exstrophy, cloacal exstrophy is a more complex disorder, in which two hemibladders are separated by bowel mucosa, and the terminal ileum prolapses through the exposed cecum.

Diagnosis
Bladder exstrophy

Suggested Readings
Gargollo PC, Borer JG, Retik AB, et al: Magnetic resonance imaging of pelvic musculoskeletal and genitourinary anatomy in patients before and after complete primary repair of bladder exstrophy. J Urol 174(Pt 2):1559-1566, 2005.

Halachmi S, Farhat W, Konen O, et al: Pelvic floor magnetic resonance imaging after neonatal single stage reconstruction in male patients with classic bladder exstrophy. J Urol 170(Pt 2):1505-1509, 2003.

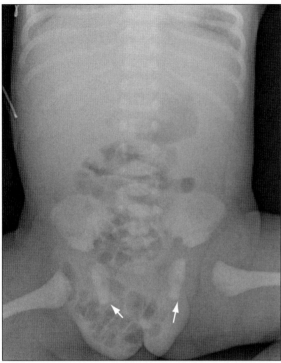

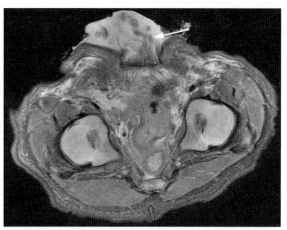

Figure 2. Axial proton density MRI of pelvis better delineates pelvic anatomy and shows small, decompressed, exstrophied bladder (*arrow*), which has a nodular contour likely because of the presence of bladder polyps.

Figure 1. Anteroposterior radiograph of abdomen reveals diastasis of symphysis pubis (*arrows*). The patient also has a large scrotal hernia.

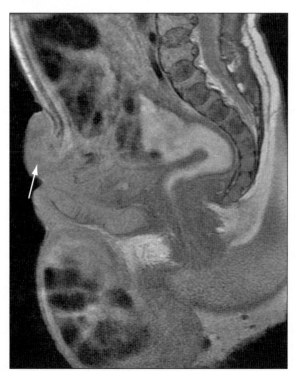

Figure 3. Sagittal proton density MRI of pelvis shows small, decompressed, exstrophied bladder (*arrow*), which has a nodular contour.

Case 141

DEMOGRAPHICS/CLINICAL HISTORY

The patient is a newborn boy with lax abdominal wall musculature and an empty scrotum.

FINDINGS

An anteroposterior radiograph of the abdomen (Fig. 1) reveals a protuberant abdomen resulting from a lack of abdominal wall musculature. A voiding cystourethrogram (VCUG) (Fig. 2) reveals a large-capacity bladder with multiple diverticula and sacculations, vesicoureteral reflux, and a characteristic tubular shape of the bladder base. Ultrasound evaluation of the urinary tract (Fig. 3) shows marked left-sided hydronephrosis and hydroureter.

DISCUSSION

Definition/Background
Prune-belly syndrome occurs in boys with an incidence of 1 in 29,000 to 40,000 births.

Characteristic Clinical Features
Patients with prune-belly syndrome have an absence of the abdominal wall musculature, cryptorchidism, and urinary tract abnormalities.

Characteristic Radiologic Findings
Renal ultrasound shows large bladder capacity and dilation of bilateral collecting systems (the lower ureters appear more dilated than the proximal ureters). In contrast to the posterior urethral valves seen on VCUG, the dilated posterior urethra has a cone-shaped configuration.

Less Common Radiologic Manifestations
Imaging may show a patent urachus.

Differential Diagnosis
- Posterior urethral valve

Discussion
A posterior urethral valve is a congenital, obstructing membrane located within the posterior male urethra. It is thought to result from abnormal embryologic development of the fetal posterior urethra, and the obstruction increases voiding pressures and can alter normal development of the fetal bladder and kidneys. Patients may have a history of oligohydramnios, bilateral hydronephrosis, and incomplete emptying of a thick-walled bladder. Severely affected newborns may have respiratory difficulties because of pulmonary hypoplasia, ascites, and a palpable abdominal mass involving the bladder or ureter. The abnormal valves produce a characteristic "sail-in-the-wind" or "windsock" appearance on VCUG.

Diagnosis
Prune-belly syndrome

Suggested Readings
Das Narla L, Doherty RD, Hingsbergen EA, et al. Pediatric case of the day. Prune-belly syndrome (Eagle-Barrett syndrome, triad syndrome). RadioGraphics 18:1318-1322, 1998.

Jennings RW: Prune belly syndrome. Semin Pediatr Surg 9:115-120, 2000.

Manivel JC, Pettinato G, Reinberg Y, et al: Prune belly syndrome: Clinicopathologic study of 29 cases. Pediatr Pathol 9:711-791, 1989.

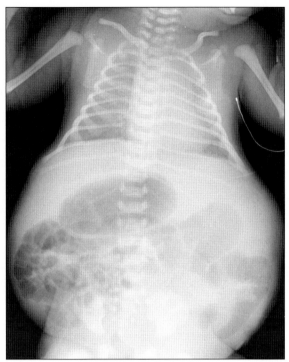

Figure 1. Anteroposterior radiograph of abdomen shows protuberant belly caused by underdeveloped abdominal wall musculature.

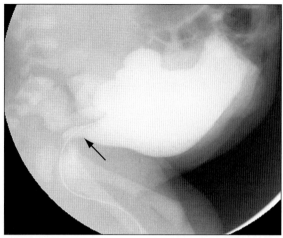

Figure 2. Lateral fluoroscopic spot image from VCUG reveals enlarged, trabeculated bladder; vesicoureteral reflux; and a tubular configuration of the bladder base (*arrow*).

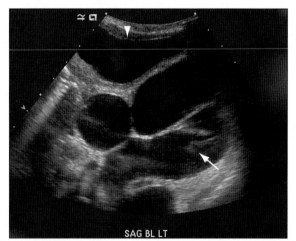

Figure 3. Sagittal ultrasound at level of bladder (*arrowhead*) shows marked dilation and tortuosity of left ureter all the way down to bladder (*arrow*).

Case 142

DEMOGRAPHICS/CLINICAL HISTORY

The patient is a newborn girl with dysmorphic features and respiratory distress.

FINDINGS

An anteroposterior radiograph of the arm reveals hypoplasia of the radius (Fig. 1). An esophagogram shows an abnormal fistula between the trachea and the esophagus (Fig. 2). Renal ultrasound shows a left pelvic kidney (Fig. 3). A radiograph of the thoracic spine in a different patient with VACTERL association reveals multiple vertebral segmentation anomalies (Fig. 4).

DISCUSSION

Definition/Background

VACTERL association refers to a disorder that consists of vertebral anomalies, anorectal malformations, cardiac malformations, tracheoesophageal fistulas, renal anomalies, and limb anomalies. It is thought to result from mesodermal defects occurring in the fifth week of gestation.

Characteristic Clinical Features

Patients with VACTERL association have many defects in various organ systems. At least three of the defects must be present for the diagnosis.

Characteristic Radiologic Findings

Radiologic findings may include hemivertebrae, extra ribs (i.e., 13 pairs), radial hypoplasia, proximal femoral deficiency, fibular hemimelia, renal agenesis, horseshoe kidney, pelvic kidney, anal atresia, tetralogy of Fallot, ventricular septal defect, and tracheoesophageal fistula.

Diagnosis

VACTERL association

Suggested Readings

Harris RD, Nyberg DA, Mack LA, et al: Anorectal atresia: Prenatal sonographic diagnosis. AJR Am J Roentgenol 149:395-400, 1987.

Kuo MF, Tsai Y, Hsu WM, et al: Tethered spinal cord and VACTERL association. J Neurosurg 106(Suppl):201-204, 2007.

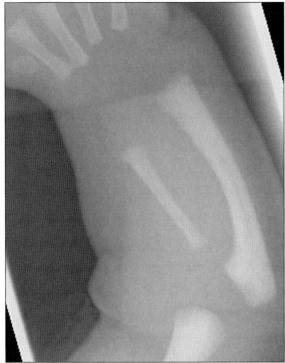

Figure 1. Anteroposterior radiograph of arm reveals hypoplasia of radius.

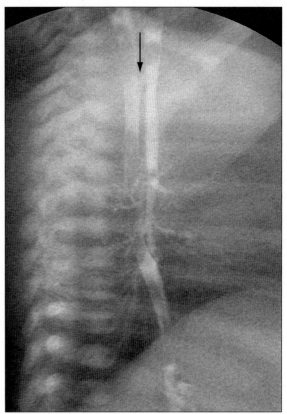

Figure 2. Esophagogram shows abnormal fistula between trachea and esophagus (*arrow*).

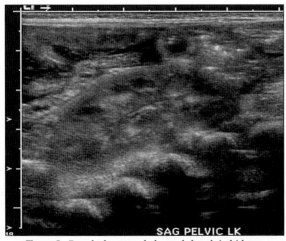

Figure 3. Renal ultrasound shows left pelvic kidney.

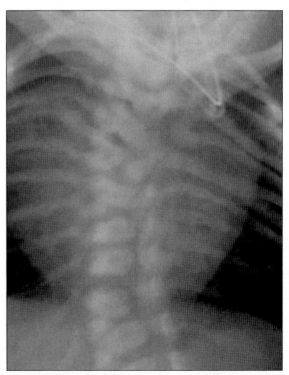

Figure 4. Radiograph of thoracic spine in a different patient reveals multiple vertebral segmentation anomalies.

Case 143

DEMOGRAPHICS/CLINICAL HISTORY

The patient is a 7-day-old girl with an abdominal mass and decreased urine output.

FINDINGS

A plain radiograph of the abdomen shows a markedly distended abdomen with a paucity of bowel gas (Fig. 1). The thorax is small relative to the abdomen. Ultrasound of the abdomen and pelvis (Figs. 2 and 3) reveals bilateral, enlarged, echogenic kidneys. Multiple, small, rounded and tubular-shaped cystic lesions are present throughout both kidneys (see Fig. 3).

DISCUSSION

Definition/Background

The disease affects between 1 in 6000 and 1 in 55,000 live births and is more common in girls.

Characteristic Clinical Features

Patients may have Potter facies: low-set, flattened ears; short, snubbed nose; deep eye creases; and micrognathia.

Characteristic Radiologic Findings

Ultrasound reveals hyperechoic enlarged kidneys with loss of corticomedullary differentiation. Individual cysts are often difficult to appreciate in light of their small size and innumerability.

Differential Diagnosis

- Meckel-Gruber syndrome
- Adult polycystic kidney disease

Discussion

Meckel-Gruber syndrome is an autosomal dominant condition characterized by occipital encephalocele, polycystic kidneys, and polydactyly. Adult polycystic kidney disease is autosomal dominant and is characterized by multiple macrocysts in bilateral kidneys and progressive renal failure.

Diagnosis

Autosomal recessive polycystic kidney disease (prenatal/neonatal)

Suggested Reading

Lonergan GJ, Rice RR, Suarez ES: Autosomal recessive polycystic kidney disease: Radiologic-pathologic correlation. RadioGraphics 20:837-855, 2000.

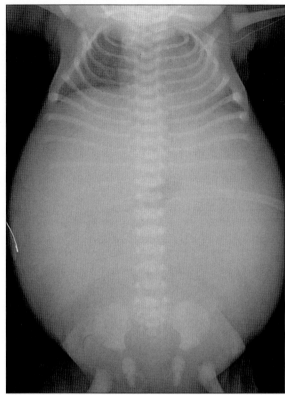

Figure 1. Plain radiograph of abdomen shows markedly distended abdomen with paucity of bowel gas. The thorax is small relative to the abdomen.

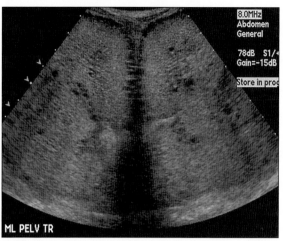

Figure 2. Transverse ultrasound image through lower abdomen/pelvis reveals bilateral, enlarged, echogenic kidneys that fill the entire abdomen. Multiple, small, rounded and tubular-shaped cystic lesions are present throughout both kidneys.

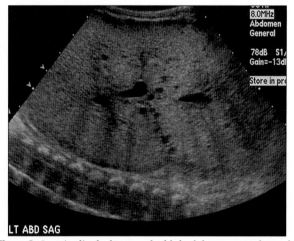

Figure 3. Longitudinal ultrasound of left abdomen reveals markedly enlarged left kidney with multiple, small, rounded and tubular-shaped cystic lesions.

Case 144

DEMOGRAPHICS/CLINICAL HISTORY

The patient is a newborn with an enlarged abdomen.

FINDINGS

Ultrasound of the left abdomen in the longitudinal plane (Fig. 1) shows an enlarged echogenic left kidney with multiple tiny cysts, most within the periphery of the renal cortex. Corticomedullary differentiation is absent. A transverse view of the left upper pole (Fig. 2) shows the tiny peripheral cysts. Findings were symmetric.

DISCUSSION

Definition/Background

Autosomal recessive polycystic kidney disease (ARPCKD) can have a spectrum of severity, and it can manifest from the neonatal period into adolescence.

Characteristic Clinical Features

In severe cases, findings may be suggested on prenatal imaging or at birth by nephromegaly palpated on examination or by respiratory distress from lung hypoplasia. The newborn may present clinically with renal insufficiency and decreased urine output.

Characteristic Radiologic Findings

Ultrasound findings include hyperechoic, enlarged kidneys and loss of corticomedullary differentiation with variable visualization of tiny cysts (1 to 2 mm), representing dilated renal tubules. The cysts are typically found at the peripheries of the renal cortex, and they can be visualized on ultrasound as a hypoechoic rim around the kidney. Findings are typically symmetric. Variable degrees of renal insufficiency and ultrasound findings are seen, correlating with the severity of disease involvement in each patient. Although not usually performed in current practice, intravenous urography (IVU) shows contrast agent within the enlarged kidneys in a radiating, striated pattern. Magnetic resonance imaging (MRI) can show findings similar to those of ultrasound (e.g., nephromegaly, tiny cysts that often are subcapsular). The kidneys are hyperintense on T2-weighted MRI, and the enhancement pattern is similar to the findings on IVU. Along with renal findings, these patients can have hepatic fibrosis, and radiographs can be obtained to look for fibrosis. The severity of hepatic fibrosis is often inversely proportional to renal involvement in patients with ARPCKD.

Less Common Radiologic Manifestations

In the most severe cases, patients can present with Potter syndrome, including lung hypoplasia, oligohydramnios, and Potter facies (i.e., low-set ears, flattened nose, and micrognathia).

Differential Diagnosis

- Autosomal dominant polycystic kidney disease

Discussion

Autosomal dominant polycystic kidney disease manifests later in childhood with larger cysts compared with ARPCKD.

Diagnosis

Autosomal recessive polycystic kidney disease (ARPCKD)

Suggested Reading

Lonergan GJ, Rice RR, Suarez ES: Autosomal recessive polycystic kidney disease: Radiologic-pathologic correlation. RadioGraphics 20:837-855, 2000.

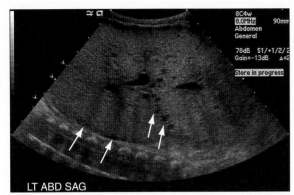

Figure 1. Ultrasound of left abdomen in longitudinal plane shows enlarged, echogenic left kidney with multiple tiny cysts (*arrows*), most within the periphery of the renal cortex. Corticomedullary differentiation is absent.

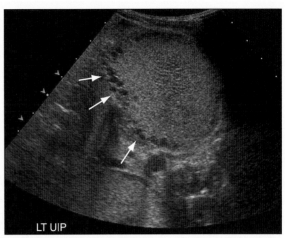

Figure 2. Transverse view of left upper pole shows tiny peripheral cysts (*arrows*).

Case 145

DEMOGRAPHICS/CLINICAL HISTORY

The patient is an 18-year-old female with a father and uncle with polycystic kidney disease.

FINDINGS

A longitudinal ultrasound of the right kidney (Fig. 1) shows several cysts approximately 1 to 2 cm in diameter throughout the renal parenchyma. Longitudinal ultrasound of the left kidney (Fig. 2) shows similar findings.

DISCUSSION

Definition/Background

Autosomal dominant polycystic kidney disease (ADPCKD) results from mutations in *PKD1* (approximately 85% of cases) and *PKD2* (approximately 15% of cases) genes; patients with the *PKD1* mutation have more severe manifestations.

Characteristic Clinical Features

In pediatric patients, there is usually a clinical history of familial renal disease only.

Characteristic Radiologic Findings

Ultrasound usually is performed as a screening tool and to follow disease progression. Renal parenchymal cysts are usually numerable in pediatric patients and innumerable in more severely affected adult patients.

Differential Diagnosis

- Renal cysts associated with tuberous sclerosis or von Hippel-Lindau disease
- Autosomal recessive polycystic kidney disease (ARPCKD)

Discussion

Tuberous sclerosis and von Hippel-Lindau disease predispose patients to renal cyst formation, but each condition has a spectrum of other clinical and radiographic abnormalities, such as angiomyolipomas (in tuberous sclerosis) and pancreatic cysts (in von Hippel-Lindau disease), which can help distinguish them. ARPCKD typically manifests with enlarged, echogenic kidneys containing tiny cysts (1 to 2 mm), particularly in the subcapsular region.

Diagnosis

Autosomal dominant polycystic kidney disease (ADPCKD)

Suggested Readings

Pei Y: Diagnostic approach in autosomal dominant polycystic kidney disease. Clin J Am Soc Nephrol 1:1108-1114, 2006.

Torres VE, Harris PC, Pirson Y: Autosomal dominant polycystic kidney disease. Lancet 369:1287-1301, 2007.

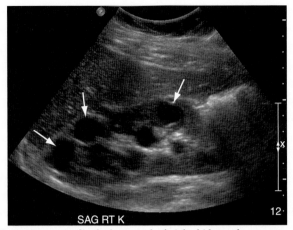

Figure 1. Longitudinal ultrasound of right kidney shows several cysts (*arrows*), approximately 1 to 2 cm in diameter, throughout renal parenchyma.

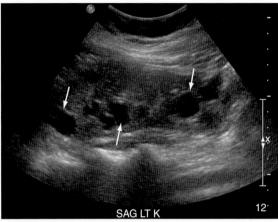

Figure 2. Longitudinal ultrasound of left kidney shows similar findings (*arrows*).

Case 146

DEMOGRAPHICS/CLINICAL HISTORY

The patient is a newborn (37 weeks' gestational age) with respiratory distress and an enlarged abdomen.

FINDINGS

A radiograph of the neonate's chest and abdomen (Fig. 1) shows small lung volumes and a large abdomen with a paucity of bowel gas. Ultrasound of the right abdomen in the longitudinal plane (Fig. 2) shows an enlarged, echogenic left kidney with multiple, peripheral, tiny cysts and a loss of corticomedullary differentiation, which is consistent with autosomal recessive polycystic kidney disease (ARPCKD).

DISCUSSION

Definition/Background

Potter syndrome was originally described as a syndrome because of bilateral renal or ureteral agenesis. The term has since been applied to other causes of in utero severe oligohydramnios, which results in lung hypoplasia and abnormal facies.

Characteristic Clinical Features

Manifestations typically include prenatal oligohydramnios, respiratory distress at birth, and abnormal facies (i.e., low-set ears, flattened nose, and micrognathia).

Characteristic Radiologic Findings

Radiographic findings reflect the underlying entity that causes decreased fetal urine output and severe oligohydramnios. The initial description of Potter syndrome accounted for cases of bilateral renal or ureteral agenesis. Chest radiographs show hypoplastic lungs, and pneumothoraces or pneumomediastinum often is present.

Less Common Radiologic Manifestations

Prune-belly syndrome and severe ARPCKD can cause severe in utero oligohydramnios, resulting in lung hypoplasia and Potter facies.

Diagnosis

Potter syndrome

Suggested Readings

Dhundiraj KM, Madhukar DN, Ambadasrao PG, et al: Potter's syndrome: A report of 5 cases. Indian J Pathol Microbiol 49:254-257, 2006.

Herman TE, Siegel MJ: Special imaging casebook. Oligohydramnios sequence with bilateral renal agenesis (Potter's syndrome). J Perinatol 20:397-398, 2000.

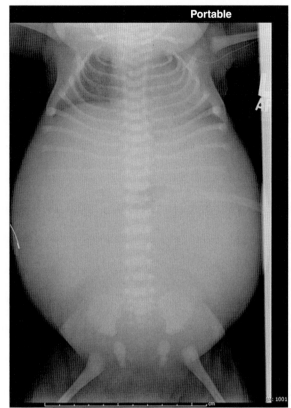

Figure 1. Radiograph of chest and abdomen shows small lung volumes and large abdomen with paucity of bowel gas.

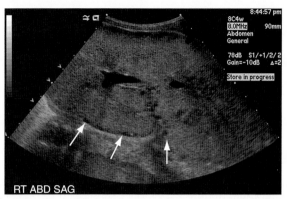

Figure 2. Ultrasound of right abdomen in longitudinal plane shows enlarged, echogenic right kidney with multiple, tiny, peripheral cysts (*arrows*) and an absence of corticomedullary differentiation.

Case 147

DEMOGRAPHICS/CLINICAL HISTORY

The patient is a 10-year-old child with an incidental radiographic finding.

FINDINGS

Axial computed tomography (CT) image with contrast agent (Fig. 1) shows a prominent collecting system in the upper pole of the left kidney at the level of the inferior aspect of the liver. Inferiorly on CT (Fig. 2), dysmorphic-appearing renal parenchyma is seen along the lower aspect of the left kidney, with a separate collecting system. Intravenous urography (IVU) (Fig. 3) during the excretory phase shows two separate collecting systems, with the ureter from the lower collecting system crossing from the left side and inserting into the right side of the bladder.

DISCUSSION

Definition/Background

Crossed fused renal ectopia is abnormal fusion of both kidneys, with the fused renal parenchyma located on one side of the retroperitoneum.

Characteristic Clinical Features

Crossed fused renal ectopia is usually incidentally identified.

Characteristic Radiologic Findings

Radiologic findings include an enlarged unilateral kidney with the apparent absence of the contralateral kidney. Evaluation of the kidney reveals a dysmorphic appearance and the presence of two separate collecting systems. The fused ectopic kidney still has a normal ureterovesicular junction, which is located on the side contralateral to the renal parenchyma.

Less Common Radiologic Manifestations

Crossed fused renal ectopia is considered a predisposing factor for ureteropelvic junction obstruction, stasis and stone formation, and neoplasia of the urinary system.

Differential Diagnosis

- Horseshoe kidney

Discussion

Horseshoe kidney is a fused kidney, but the upper poles of the kidneys are located in relatively normal positions, with midline fusion of the lower poles.

Diagnosis

Crossed fused renal ectopia

Suggested Reading

Boyan N, Kubat H, Uzum A: Crossed renal ectopia with fusion: Report of two patients. Clin Anat 20:699-702, 2007.

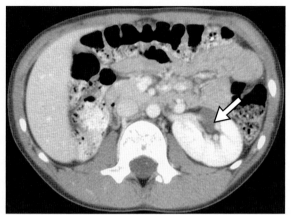

Figure 1. Axial CT image with contrast agent shows prominent collecting system in upper pole of left kidney (*arrow*) at level of inferior aspect of the liver.

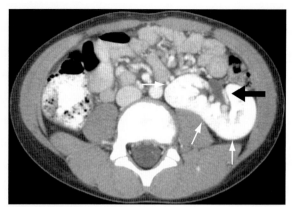

Figure 2. Inferiorly, dysmorphic-appearing renal parenchyma (*white arrows*) is seen along lower aspect of left kidney, with a separate collecting system (*black arrow*).

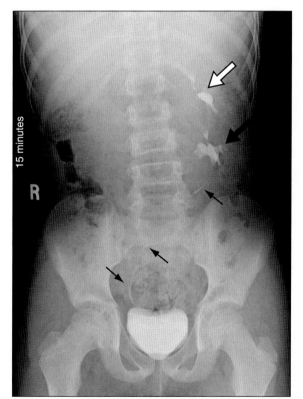

Figure 3. IVU during excretory phase shows two separate collecting systems (*large black and white arrows*) and ureter (*lower small arrows*) from lower collecting system (*upper small arrow*) crossing from left side and inserting into right side of bladder.

Case 148

DEMOGRAPHICS/CLINICAL HISTORY

The patient is a 16-year-old girl with hypertension.

FINDINGS

Longitudinal ultrasound of the left kidney (Fig. 1) shows increased echogenicity within the medullary pyramids. A longitudinal view of the right kidney (Fig. 2) shows similar findings.

DISCUSSION

Definition/Background

Medullary nephrocalcinosis can have many causes, including furosemide treatment, medullary sponge kidney, acute tubular acidosis, and hypercalcemia.

Characteristic Clinical Features

Patients typically present with abnormal renal function.

Characteristic Radiologic Findings

Echogenic renal medullary pyramids are seen on ultrasonography. On noncontrast computed tomography (CT), increased density in the pyramids may suggest the diagnosis.

Differential Diagnosis

- Tamm-Horsfall proteinuria

Discussion

Tamm-Horsfall proteinuria occurs in the neonatal period, whereas medullary nephrocalcinosis occurs at any age, but it is less likely in neonates.

Diagnosis

Medullary nephrocalcinosis

Suggested Reading

Shultz PK, Strife JL, Strife CF, McDaniel JD: Hyperechoic renal medullary pyramids in infants and children. Radiology 181:163-167, 1991.

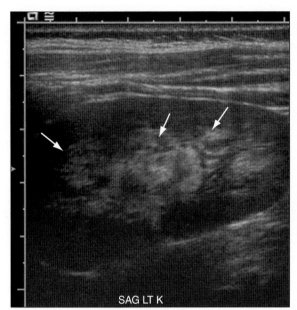

Figure 1. Longitudinal ultrasound of left kidney shows increased echogenicity within medullary pyramids (*arrows*).

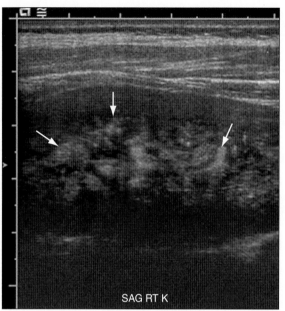

Figure 2. Longitudinal ultrasound of right kidney shows increased echogenicity within medullary pyramids (*arrows*).

Case 149

DEMOGRAPHICS/CLINICAL HISTORY

The patient is a newborn with a prenatal diagnosis of cystic kidney.

FINDINGS

Longitudinal ultrasound of the left kidney (Fig. 1) shows multiple cysts of various sizes, and the spleen is seen superiorly. A longitudinal view of the right kidney (Fig. 2) shows the normal contralateral neonatal kidney. Follow-up longitudinal ultrasound of the left kidney 4 months later (Fig. 3) shows an interval decrease in size of the kidney and multiple cysts, and the spleen is seen superiorly. At the 9-month follow-up, the left kidney was no longer visualized.

DISCUSSION

Definition/Background

Multicystic dysplastic kidney manifests with cystic changes throughout the renal parenchyma. These cysts do not communicate with the collecting system, and over time, the kidney typically regresses.

Characteristic Clinical Features

Multicystic dysplastic kidney is often suggested on prenatal ultrasonography, but may be found incidentally.

Characteristic Radiologic Findings

Multiple cysts of various sizes are seen throughout the affected kidney, and there is no discernible collecting system. On follow-up ultrasound, the cysts and overall kidney size decrease, and the kidney usually completely regresses with time. Nuclear medicine scintigraphy may show a rim of radiotracer uptake, without collection or excretion.

Differential Diagnosis

■ Hydronephrosis

Discussion

If the cysts of a multicystic dysplastic kidney all are similar in size, it can simulate dilated calices, but with careful examination, the cysts can be individually discerned, and they do not communicate with each other.

Diagnosis

Multicystic dysplastic kidney

Suggested Reading

Thomsen HS, Levine E, Meilstrup JW, et al: Renal cystic diseases. Eur Radiol 7:1267-1275, 1997.

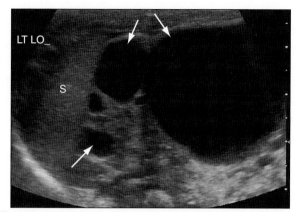

Figure 1. Longitudinal ultrasound of left kidney shows multiple cysts of various sizes (*arrows*). The spleen (S) is seen superiorly.

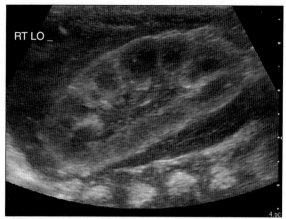

Figure 2. Longitudinal ultrasound of right kidney shows normal contralateral kidney.

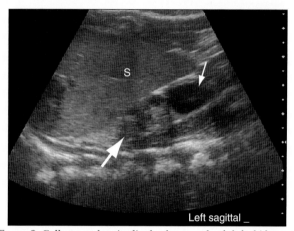

Figure 3. Follow-up longitudinal ultrasound of left kidney 4 months later shows an interval decrease in size of the kidney and multiple cysts (*arrows*). The spleen (S) is seen superiorly. At 9-month follow-up, the left kidney was no longer visualized.

Case 150

DEMOGRAPHICS/CLINICAL HISTORY

The patient is a 2-day-old boy with a two-vessel umbilical cord detected at birth.

FINDINGS

Longitudinal ultrasound of the right kidney (Fig. 1) shows normal, hypoechoic medullary pyramids. Hyperechogenicity is seen at the tips of the medullary pyramids, and a normal adrenal gland is seen. A transverse view of the right kidney (Fig. 2) shows the medullary pyramid and the hyperechoic tip. Findings were less prominent on the contralateral side. On a transverse view of the bladder (Fig. 3), echogenic debris is seen within the bladder.

DISCUSSION

Definition/Background
Renal medullary hyperechogenicity can be a transient ultrasound finding in normal neonates. A proposed explanation for this finding is the excretion of Tamm-Horsfall proteins, which are commonly found in amniotic fluid and which often form casts in the renal tubules.

Characteristic Clinical Features
Patients may have elevation of neonatal urine protein levels.

Characteristic Radiologic Findings
Characteristic findings are hyperechoic tips of the hypoechoic renal pyramids during the first 2 weeks of life. Follow-up ultrasound in 2 to 3 weeks shows resolution of the hyperechogenicity.

Differential Diagnosis
- Medullary nephrocalcinosis
- Renal tubular acidosis

Discussion
Medullary nephrocalcinosis causes hyperechogenicity within the renal medullary pyramids and can have an appearance similar to that of patients with Tamm-Horsfall proteinuria, but the entire pyramid is often hyperechoic, rather than just the distal tip. Tamm-Horsfall proteinuria is seen in the neonatal period, whereas medullary nephrocalcinosis can occur at any age. Renal tubular acidosis may cause more prominent medullary echogenicity and is accompanied by signs of compromised renal function.

Diagnosis
Tamm-Horsfall proteinuria

Suggested Reading
Howlett DC, Greenwood KL, Jarosz JM, et al: The incidence of transient renal medullary hyperechogenicity in neonatal ultrasound examination. Br J Radiol 70:140-143, 1997.

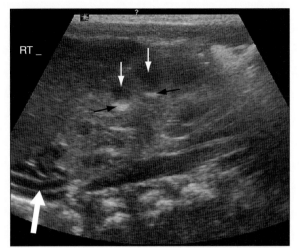

Figure 1. Longitudinal ultrasound of right kidney shows normal, hypoechoic medullary pyramids (*small white arrows*). Hyperechogenicity is seen at tips of medullary pyramids (*black arrows*). Normal adrenal gland (*large white arrow*) can be seen.

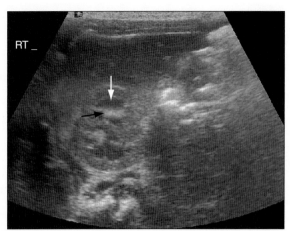

Figure 2. Transverse ultrasound of right kidney shows medullary pyramid (*white arrow*) and hyperechoic tip (*black arrow*). Findings were less prominent on contralateral side.

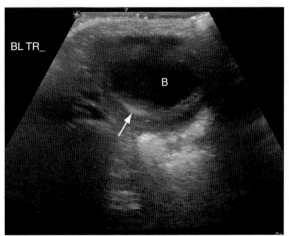

Figure 3. Transverse ultrasound of bladder shows echogenic debris (*arrow*) within bladder (B).

Case 151

DEMOGRAPHICS/CLINICAL HISTORY

The patient is a 5-month-old girl with acute renal failure after cardiac surgery.

FINDINGS

Longitudinal ultrasound of the right kidney (Fig. 1) shows slight increased echogenicity within the renal cortex compared with the liver parenchyma. Medullary hypoechogenicity is predominantly maintained. Free fluid is seen within the abdomen. Doppler interrogation of the main renal artery (Fig. 2) shows a high-resistance arterial waveform with reversal of flow in diastole. A small pleural effusion is suggested.

DISCUSSION

Definition/Background

Acute tubular necrosis (ATN) typically results from hypoxia or ischemia. Although ATN typically is reversible, it may lead to permanent renal damage.

Characteristic Clinical Features

Patients with ATN usually present with decreased urine output to complete anuria.

Characteristic Radiologic Findings

Ultrasonography findings may be variable with increased cortical echogenicity, decreased corticomedullary differentiation, or a normal gray-scale appearance. Doppler imaging shows decreased peripheral flow with increased arterial resistance and decreased diastolic flow. Elevated resistive indices are typically present.

Differential Diagnosis

- Hemolytic uremic syndrome

Discussion

The appearance of hemolytic uremic syndrome can be similar to ATN, but the presentation and cause usually suggest the diagnosis.

Diagnosis

Acute tubular necrosis

Suggested Reading

Khati NJ, Hill MC, Kimmel PL: The role of ultrasound in renal insufficiency: The essentials. Ultrasound 21(4):227-244, 2005.

Platt JF, Rubin JM, Ellis JH: Acute renal failure: Possible role of duplex Doppler US in distinction between acute prerenal failure and acute tubular necrosis. Radiology 179:419-423, 1991.

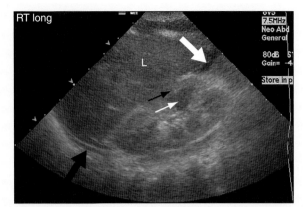

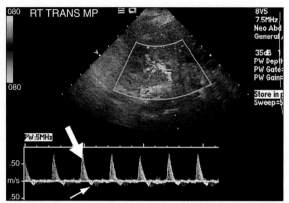

Figure 1. Longitudinal ultrasound of right kidney shows increased echogenicity within renal cortex (*small arrows*) compared with liver (L) parenchyma. Free fluid is seen within abdomen (*large white arrow*). A small pleural effusion is suggested (*large arrow*).

Figure 2. Doppler interrogation of main renal artery shows high-resistance arterial waveform (*large white arrow*) with reversal of flow in diastole (*small white arrow*).

Case 152

DEMOGRAPHICS/CLINICAL HISTORY

The patient is a 3-year-old girl with abdominal pain and acute renal failure.

FINDINGS

Longitudinal ultrasound of the right kidney (Fig. 1) shows increased echogenicity in the renal cortex compared with the liver echotexture, and the hypoechoic medullary pyramids are preserved. Color Doppler interrogation (Fig. 2) reveals an elevated resistive index value.

DISCUSSION

Definition/Background
Hemolytic uremic syndrome is an illness characterized by hemolytic anemia, thrombocytopenia, and acute renal failure. This syndrome is most often seen in children rather than adults. Diarrhea is the typical prodrome and is most commonly caused by *Escherichia coli* O157:H7 infection.

Characteristic Clinical Features
After a prodrome of diarrhea, hemolytic uremic syndrome typically manifests with decreased urine output and other signs of uremia, such as neurologic dysfunction.

Characteristic Radiologic Findings
Ultrasonography is the preferred imaging modality for evaluation. Findings include nephromegaly, increased cortical echogenicity, and increased resistive indices on Doppler interrogation.

Differential Diagnosis
- Acute tubular necrosis

Discussion
Findings for hemolytic uremic syndrome are similar to findings of acute tubular necrosis. The clinical presentation and evidence of hemolytic anemia and thrombocytopenia often lead to the diagnosis.

Diagnosis
Hemolytic uremic syndrome

Suggested Readings
Kenney PJ, Brinsko RE, Patel DV, et al: Sonography of the kidneys in hemolytic uremic syndrome. Invest Radiol 21:547-550, 1986.
Platt JF: Doppler ultrasound of the kidney. Semin Ultrasound CT MR 18:22-32, 1997.

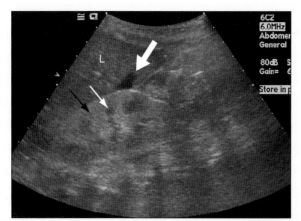

Figure 1. Longitudinal ultrasound of right kidney shows increased echogenicity in renal cortex (*black arrow*) compared with liver (L) echotexture; hypoechoic medullary pyramids (*small white arrow*) are preserved. Free fluid in the abdomen is seen (*large white arrow*).

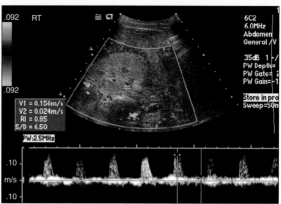

Figure 2. Color Doppler interrogation shows elevated resistive index value.

Case 153

DEMOGRAPHICS/CLINICAL HISTORY

The patient is a newborn with spina bifida.

FINDINGS

Transverse ultrasound of the abdomen (Fig. 1) shows the upper poles of the kidneys on both sides of the retroperitoneum. The aorta is anterior to the vertebral body. More inferiorly, an isthmus of renal parenchyma is contiguous between the inferior poles (Fig. 2). The isthmus is anterior to the aorta, and the vertebral body is well visualized. Axial T2-weighted magnetic resonance imaging (MRI) (Fig. 3), performed for evaluation of the patient's spina bifida, shows the upper poles of the kidneys and the aorta and vertebral body. More inferiorly, the crossing isthmus of renal parenchyma is seen connecting the inferior poles (Fig. 4). The corresponding orientation of the aorta and vertebral body can be seen.

DISCUSSION

Definition/Background

Horseshoe kidneys have an isthmus of tissue that fuses the poles, typically the inferior poles.

Characteristic Clinical Features

Horseshoe kidneys are found more often in patients with trisomy 18, Turner syndrome, and neural tube defects. Patients can present with pain or hematuria after midline trauma.

Characteristic Radiologic Findings

Imaging reveals an isthmus of renal tissue connecting two poles, commonly the inferior poles, anterior to the aorta. Concomitant findings, such as obstruction, stones, or tumor, should be evaluated because there is increased incidence of these conditions with horseshoe kidneys.

Differential Diagnosis

- Crossed fused renal ectopia

Discussion

In cases of crossed fused renal ectopia, all of the renal parenchyma is typically on one side of the patient, whereas in patients with a horseshoe kidney, portions of the kidney lie on both sides of midline.

Diagnosis

Horseshoe kidney

Suggested Reading

Cohen HL, Kravets F, Zucconi W, et al: Congenital abnormalities of the genitourinary system. Semin Roentgenol 39:282-303, 2004.

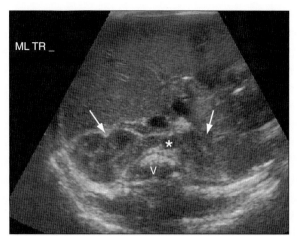

Figure 1. Transverse ultrasound of abdomen shows upper poles of kidneys (*arrows*) on both sides of the retroperitoneum. The aorta (*asterisk*) is anterior to the vertebral body (V).

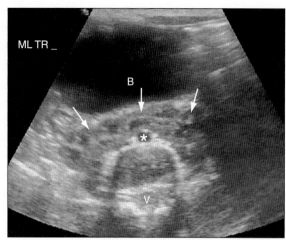

Figure 2. More inferiorly than the position in Fig. 1, isthmus of renal parenchyma is contiguous between inferior poles (*arrows*). The isthmus is anterior to the aorta (*asterisk*). The vertebral body is well visualized (V). B, bladder.

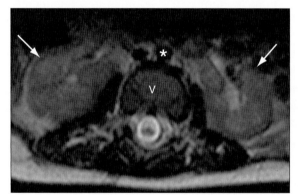

Figure 3. Axial T2-weighted MR image shows upper poles of kidneys (*arrows*), aorta (*asterisk*), and vertebral body (V).

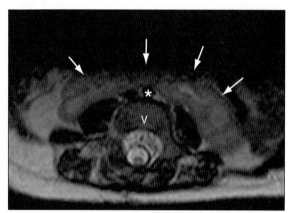

Figure 4. More inferiorly, crossing isthmus of renal parenchyma is seen on MRI connecting inferior poles (*arrows*). The corresponding orientation of aorta (*asterisk*) and vertebral body (V) can be seen. Kidneys were incidentally imaged on spine MRI.

Case 154

DEMOGRAPHICS/CLINICAL HISTORY

The patient is a 14-year-old girl with abdominal pain.

FINDINGS

Longitudinal ultrasound of the right renal fossa (Fig. 1) shows a normal-appearing right kidney inferior to the liver. Longitudinal ultrasound of the left renal fossa (Fig. 2) shows the normal spleen and absence of the left kidney. On ultrasound of the pelvis (not shown), hematometrocolpos was seen with no evidence of a pelvic kidney. Coronal T2-weighted magnetic resonance imaging (MRI) (Fig. 3) shows the normal right kidney, absence of the left kidney, and a distended vagina.

DISCUSSION

Definition/Background

Renal agenesis is typically unilateral and can be associated with syndromes and other genitourinary anomalies.

Characteristic Clinical Features

Because of the increase in prenatal ultrasound, renal agenesis often is detected in the fetus. It can be found postnatally during the work-up for other genitourinary or syndromic problems, such as a urinary tract infection, mullerian duct anomaly, or VACTERL (vertebral anomalies, anorectal malformations, cardiac malformations, tracheoesophageal fistulas, renal anomalies, and limb anomalies) association. Bilateral renal agenesis is not typically compatible with life. Patients can have Potter facies and clubfeet from oligohydramnios.

Characteristic Radiologic Findings

Imaging reveals the absence of the kidney and ureter. The contralateral kidney shows compensatory enlargement. Other genitourinary abnormalities can be seen, such as an ipsilateral seminal vesicle cyst in boys or mullerian duct anomalies in girls. Many patients have abnormalities of the contralateral kidney, such as ureteropelvic junction obstruction or vesicoureteral reflux.

Less Common Radiologic Manifestations

Other radiologic findings can be seen if renal agenesis is associated with syndromes such as VACTERL association, branchio-oto-renal syndrome, and Kallmann syndrome.

Differential Diagnosis

- Pelvic kidney
- Crossed fused renal ectopia

Discussion

Absence of the kidney from the renal fossa can indicate renal agenesis, but a thorough evaluation of the abdomen and pelvis is necessary to look for an ectopic location. The contralateral kidney should be evaluated for any change in morphology that might suggest crossed fused renal ectopia.

Diagnosis

Renal agenesis

Suggested Reading

Cohen HL, Kravets F, Zucconi W, et al: Congenital abnormalities of the genitourinary system. Semin Roentgenol 39:282-303, 2004.

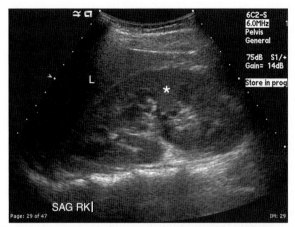

Figure 1. Longitudinal ultrasound of right renal fossa shows normal-appearing right kidney (*asterisk*) inferior to liver (L).

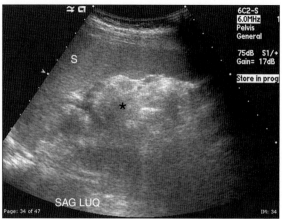

Figure 2. Longitudinal ultrasound of left renal fossa shows normal spleen (S) and absence of left kidney (*asterisk*).

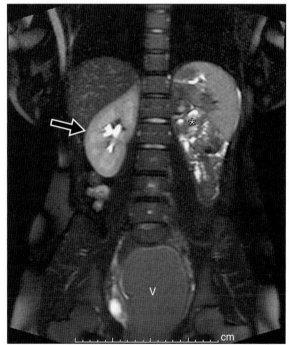

Figure 3. Coronal T2-weighted MR image shows normal right kidney (*arrow*), absence of left kidney (*asterisk*), and distended vagina (V).

Case 155

DEMOGRAPHICS/CLINICAL HISTORY

The patient is an 18-year-old woman with right adnexal tenderness and abnormal pelvic examination.

FINDINGS

Ultrasound evaluation of the pelvis shows a hypoechoic collection in the right adnexa (Fig. 1). The lesion is intimately associated with the right ovary (Fig. 2). An axial image from a contrast-enhanced computed tomography (CT) scan of the pelvis shows an irregular, rim-enhancing fluid collection in the right adnexa with surrounding inflammatory change in the mesentery with thickening of adjacent bowel loops, including the sigmoid colon (Fig. 3).

DISCUSSION

Definition/Background

Tubo-ovarian abscess is a complication of pelvic inflammatory disease, which is an infection of the gynecologic tract caused by sexually transmitted diseases.

Characteristic Clinical Features

Women often present with adnexal or lower abdominal pain, often associated with fever and elevated white blood cell count.

Characteristic Radiologic Findings

A tubo-ovarian abscess is best appreciated on cross section imaging modalities, such as ultrasound or CT. Ultrasound reveals a hypoechoic fluid collection intimately associated with the adnexa. On CT, the abscess appears as a ring-enhancing fluid collection.

Differential Diagnosis

- Hemorrhagic ovarian cyst
- Perforated appendix with abscess

Discussion

A hemorrhagic ovarian cyst may have various imaging appearances, although it often manifests on ultrasound as a hypoechoic collection in the ovary with multiple thin septations in a lacelike reticular pattern. A perforated appendix may subsequently lead to abdominal or pelvic abscess formation. If an abscess develops in the right adnexa, this may be nearly indistinguishable from a tubo-ovarian abscess.

Diagnosis

Tubo-ovarian abscess

Suggested Readings

Bulas DI, Ahlstrom PA, Sivit CJ, et al: Pelvic inflammatory disease in the adolescent: Comparison of transabdominal and transvaginal sonographic evaluation. Radiology 183:435, 1992.

Ellis JH, Francis IR, Rhodes M, et al: CT findings in tuboovarian abscess. J Comput Assist Tomogr 15:589, 1991.

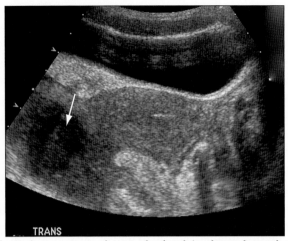

Figure 1. Transverse ultrasound of pelvis shows hypoechoic collection in right adnexa adjacent to uterus (*arrow*).

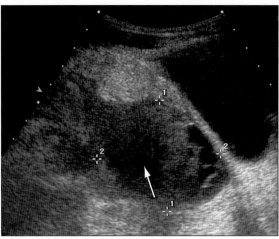

Figure 2. Longitudinal ultrasound in region of right adnexa shows hypoechoic collection in right adnexa (*arrow*) intimately related to right ovary, which contains several follicles.

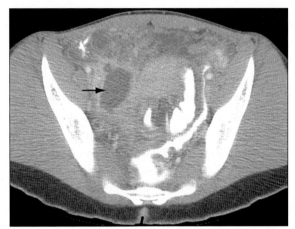

Figure 3. Axial image from contrast-enhanced CT scan of pelvis shows irregular, rim-enhancing fluid collection in right adnexa (*arrow*) with surrounding inflammatory change in mesentery with thickening of adjacent bowel loops, including sigmoid colon.

Case 156

DEMOGRAPHICS/CLINICAL HISTORY

The patient is a 15-year-old girl with pelvic pain.

FINDINGS

Transverse ultrasound of the pelvis (Fig. 1) shows the uterus posterior to the bladder. The uterus has two distinct hyperechoic endometrial stripes, suggesting a uterine anomaly. Axial T2-weighted magnetic resonance imaging (MRI) (Fig. 2) shows the two distinct uterine cavities and a left ovarian hemorrhagic cyst and free fluid. An axial T2-weighted MR image slightly more cephalad (Fig. 3) shows separation of the uterine horns superiorly, which assists in distinguishing this bicornuate uterus from a septate uterus.

DISCUSSION

Definition/Background

Bicornuate uterus is within the spectrum of müllerian duct anomalies and is caused by incomplete fusion of the two uterine horns.

Characteristic Clinical Features

Müllerian duct anomalies can manifest because of fertility problems or can be found incidentally during imaging for other reasons. If there is agenesis of a portion of the vagina or an imperforate hymen, pain from hydrometrocolpos can be the presenting symptom.

Characteristic Radiologic Findings

Bicornuate uterus has two distinct uterine cavities and endometria. There is some fusion of the lower uterine segment and some degree of nonfusion of the upper uterus; this gives the bicornuate uterus the appearance of a fundal cleft (> 1 cm indentation in the contour of the uterine fundus), considered to be the feature that distinguishes it from a septate uterus. A bicornuate uterus can have complete separation to the internal (i.e., bicornuate unicollis) or external (i.e., bicornuate bicollis) os.

Differential Diagnosis

- Septate uterus
- Uterus didelphys

Discussion

Differentiation from a septate uterus is usually made by the presence of a cleft greater than 1 cm along the fundal surface of the uterus in a bicornuate uterus. The septate uterus can have a fibrous or muscular separation of the uterus, but it has a normal fundal contour. Differentiation from a didelphys typically is made by the lack of fusion of the lower uterine segment. The didelphys usually has complete separation of the uterine horns without a fibrous or muscular common lower uterine segment.

Diagnosis

Bicornuate uterus

Suggested Reading

Troiano RN, McCarthy SM: Mullerian duct anomalies: Imaging and clinical issues. Radiology 233:19-34, 2004.

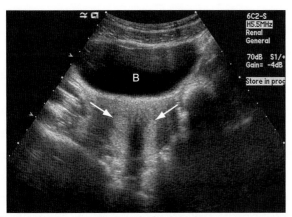

Figure 1. Transverse ultrasound of pelvis shows uterus posterior to bladder (B). Uterus has two distinct hyperechoic endometrial stripes (*arrows*), suggesting a uterine anomaly.

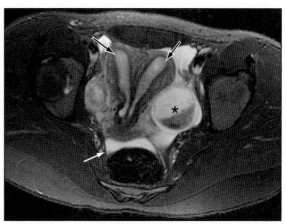

Figure 2. Axial T2-weighted MR image shows two distinct uterine cavities (*black arrows*), left ovarian hemorrhagic cyst (*asterisk*), and free fluid (*white arrow*).

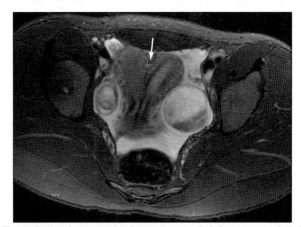

Figure 3. Axial T2-weighted MR image slightly more cephalad shows separation of uterine horns superiorly (*arrow*), resulting in a fundal cleft.

Case 157

DEMOGRAPHICS/CLINICAL HISTORY

The patient is a newborn girl with a palpable pelvic mass.

FINDINGS

A portable radiograph of the abdomen (Fig. 1) shows a rounded soft tissue density in the lower abdomen or pelvis. A composite, longitudinal ultrasound examination (Fig. 2) through the abdomen and pelvis shows a large cystic mass with debris, corresponding to a dilated, fluid-filled and debris-filled vagina and uterus. The bladder is decompressed and seen anteriorly. A transverse ultrasound (Fig. 3) through the pelvis shows the fluid-debris level in the dilated, obstructed vagina and the decompressed bladder anteriorly.

DISCUSSION

Definition/Background

Hydrometrocolpos refers to a collection of fluid, debris, or blood within a distended vagina and uterus. It is caused by vaginal obstruction.

Characteristic Clinical Features

Patients have a palpable pelvic mass and pelvic pain.

Characteristic Radiologic Findings

Ultrasonography is usually the first radiologic study performed. A thin-walled, fluid-filled structure is seen in the midline, posterior to the bladder and often with debris layering dependently. When T2-weighted magnetic resonance imaging (MRI) is used to evaluate the pelvic structures, similar findings are seen, with low signal intensity representing blood products and high signal intensity representing fluid within the distended uterus and vagina.

Differential Diagnosis
- Ovarian dermoid cyst
- Hemorrhagic cyst

Discussion

Dermoids and hemorrhagic cysts may have cystic components with fluid-debris levels, but they often are more complicated than hydrometrocolpos, and they are less likely to be midline. The presence of two normal-appearing ovaries also leads away from ovarian pathology.

Diagnosis

Hydrometrocolpos

Suggested Readings

El-Messidi A, Fleming NA: Congenital imperforate hymen and its life-threatening consequences in the neonatal period. J Pediatr Adolesc Gynecol 19:99-103, 2006.

Messina M, Severi FM, Bocchi C, et al: Voluminous perinatal pelvic mass: A case of congenital hydrometrocolpos. J Matern Fetal Neonatal Med 15:135-137, 2004.

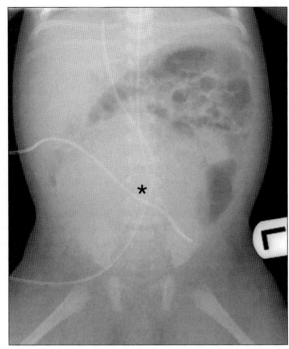

Figure 1. Portable radiograph of abdomen shows rounded soft tissue density in lower abdomen or pelvis (*asterisk*).

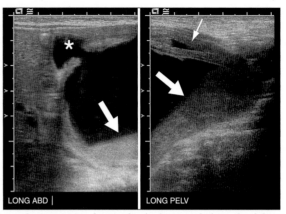

Figure 2. Composite, longitudinal ultrasound through abdomen and pelvis shows large cystic mass with debris (*large arrows*), corresponding to a dilated fluid-filled and debris-filled vagina and uterus (*asterisk*). The bladder is decompressed and seen anteriorly (*small arrow*).

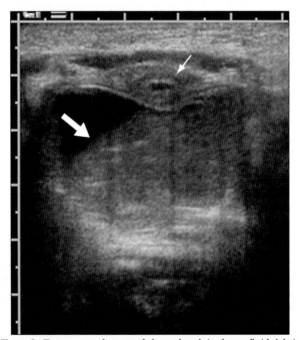

Figure 3. Transverse ultrasound through pelvis shows fluid-debris level in dilated, obstructed vagina (*large arrow*) and decompressed bladder anteriorly (*small arrow*).

Case 158

DEMOGRAPHICS/CLINICAL HISTORY

The patient is a 12-year-old girl with a suprapubic mass and imperforate hymen.

FINDINGS

Ultrasound of the pelvis (Figs. 1 and 2) shows a lobular mass in the pelvis, posterior to the bladder, in the midline in the expected location of the vagina. The uterus is seen separate from this mass and superiorly (Fig. 3). The mass is uniformly hypoechoic with low-level echoes within the mass. Color Doppler revealed no blood flow within the mass.

DISCUSSION

Definition/Background
Girls often present at the time of menarche.

Characteristic Clinical Features
Patients most often present with symptoms of cyclic abdominal or pelvic pain. A mass also may be palpable. Physical examination often reveals a bulging hymen.

Characteristic Radiologic Findings
Ultrasound evaluation of the pelvis shows a round, hypoechoic mass posterior to the bladder, which represents a blood-distended vagina. When the uterus is similarly involved (hematometrocolpos), the mass extends superiorly, and only a thin rind of normal uterine tissue is appreciated. In hematocolpos, the uterus appears normal, and a normal cervix is outlined by blood in the vagina.

Differential Diagnosis
- Hemorrhagic ovarian cyst

Discussion
Although hemorrhagic ovarian cyst may have similar imaging features, the midline location of this mass should readily distinguish these two entities, as should the identification of two normal ovaries.

Diagnosis
Hematocolpos

Suggested Readings
Blask AR, Sanders RC, Gearhart JP: Obstructed ureterovaginal anomalies: Demonstration with sonography, part I: Neonates and infants. Radiology 179:79, 1991.
Blask AR, Sanders RC, Rock JA: Obstructed ureterovaginal anomalies: Demonstration with sonography, part II: Teenagers. Radiology 179:84, 1991.

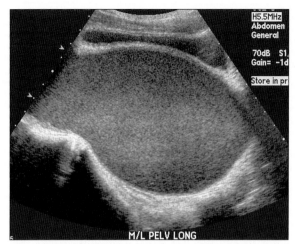

Figure 1. Longitudinal ultrasound of pelvis shows lobular mass in pelvis, posterior to bladder, in midline in expected location of vagina. Mass is uniformly hypoechoic with low-level echoes within mass.

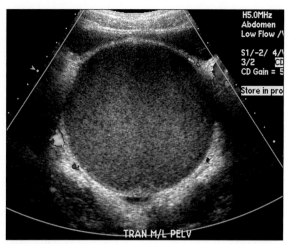

Figure 2. Color Doppler reveals no blood flow within mass.

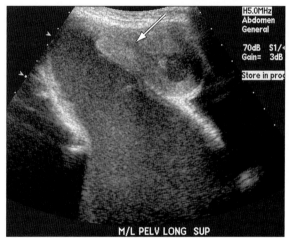

Figure 3. Longitudinal ultrasound of pelvis more superiorly than Fig. 1 shows lobular mass in pelvis, posterior to bladder, in midline in expected location of vagina. The uterus is seen separate from this mass and superiorly (*arrow*).

Case 159

DEMOGRAPHICS/CLINICAL HISTORY

The patient is a newborn with rugose labioscrotal folds; a small, male-configuration phallus; and a small peno-scrotal perineal opening with a blind-ending dimple at the tip of the phallus.

FINDINGS

Ultrasound of the right labioscrotal region (Fig. 1) shows a normal configuration testicle, which is mobile into the right inguinal canal. A less mobile mass is palpable on the left in an inguinal position. Ultrasound of the left inguinal region (Fig. 2) shows alternating hypoechoic and hyperechoic bands that correspond to a neonatal uterus. A lateral view of the patient's genitogram (Fig. 3) shows contrast agent within the bladder, vagina, and uterine cavity. The distal junction of the vaginal opening into the urethra is suggested. A frontal view of the genitogram (Fig. 4) shows the uterine cavity herniated into the left inguinal canal. The imaging findings are most in keeping with the diagnosis of hernia uteri inguinale (i.e., persistent müllerian duct syndrome), a rare form of male pseudohermaphroditism.

DISCUSSION

Definition/Background
The term *ambiguous genitalia* encompasses a spectrum of urogenital and hormonal abnormalities.

Characteristic Clinical Features
Ambiguous genitalia can have various clinical features, with an overlying concern about the uncertainty of the patient's phenotypic (and subsequently genetic) gender.

Characteristic Radiologic Findings
Radiologic findings depend on the underlying cause of the ambiguous genitalia. Ultrasound is performed to look for gonads (i.e., ovaries or testicles) and the presence or absence of a uterus. A voiding cystourethrogram (VCUG) (i.e., genitogram) is performed to look for the location of the distal vaginal insertion (when not on the perineum) or the presence of a utricle (in boys with hypospadias).

Differential Diagnosis
- Congenital adrenal hyperplasia
- Hypospadias

Discussion
Ambiguous genitalia can have many underlying causes. Two of the most common are congenital adrenal hyperplasia and hypospadias. Full clinical, radiologic, and genetic analyses are needed to differentiate the causes of ambiguous genitalia.

Diagnosis
Ambiguous genitalia

Suggested Readings
Low Y, Hutson JM: Murdoch Children's Research Institute Sex Study Group: Rules for clinical diagnosis in babies with ambiguous genitalia. J Paediatr Child Health 39:406-413, 2003.
Sultan C, Paris F, Jeandel C, et al: Ambiguous genitalia in the newborn. Semin Reprod Med 20:181-188, 2002.

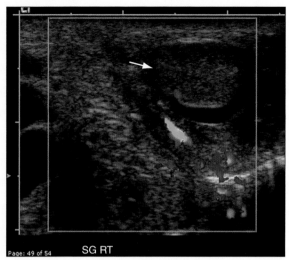

Figure 1. Ultrasound of right labioscrotal region shows normal-configuration testicle (*arrow*), which is mobile into the right inguinal canal.

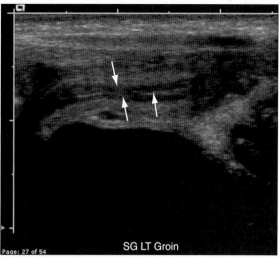

Figure 2. Ultrasound of left inguinal region shows alternating hypoechoic and hyperechoic bands (*arrows*) that correspond to a neonatal uterus.

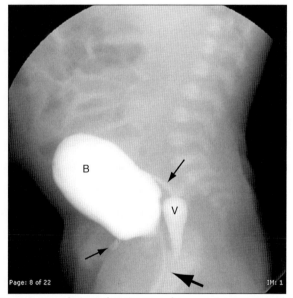

Figure 3. Lateral view of genitogram shows contrast agent within bladder (B), vagina (V), and uterine cavity (*small arrows*). Distal junction of vaginal opening into urethra is suggested (*large arrow*).

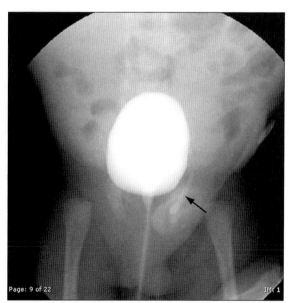

Figure 4. Frontal view of genitogram shows uterine cavity (*arrow*) herniated into left inguinal canal.

Case 160

DEMOGRAPHICS/CLINICAL HISTORY

The patient is an 11-year-old child with spina bifida and ventriculoperitoneal shunt being evaluated for shunt malfunction.

FINDINGS

A pelvic radiograph (Fig. 1) shows rounded densities in the left pelvis. Spinal fusion defects in the lumbosacral spine and a portion of the patient's ventriculoperitoneal shunt are seen. Transverse ultrasound of the bladder (Fig. 2) shows an echogenic focus within the dependent portion of the bladder and posterior shadowing. Color Doppler imaging (Fig. 3) shows a twinkle artifact that is posterior to the echogenic focus. When the patient was positioned obliquely, the echogenic focus and its shadow move dependently (Fig. 4).

DISCUSSION

Definition/Background

Bladder calculi typically are found in patients with chronic infections, neurogenic bladder, or other cause of urinary stasis.

Characteristic Clinical Features

Patients may present with hematuria and other signs of bladder irritation.

Characteristic Radiologic Findings

Ultrasound typically reveals a clinically significant bladder stone. A mobile, echogenic focus can be seen with posterior shadowing. Color Doppler often shows a sparkle artifact resulting from calcification. Computed tomography (CT) shows a calcific density within the dependent portion of the bladder. Magnetic resonance imaging (MRI) shows a rounded, T2-weighted hypointensity layering dependently.

Differential Diagnosis

- Bladder mass
- Cystitis

Discussion

A key to the ultrasound diagnosis of a bladder calculus is the finding of mobility of the echogenic calculus. If any irregularities of the bladder (e.g., mass, cystitis) are seen, additional imaging or follow-up is necessary.

Diagnosis

Bladder calculus

Suggested Reading

Dyer RB, Chen MY, Zagoria RJ: Abnormal calcifications in the urinary tract. RadioGraphics 18:1405-1424, 1998.

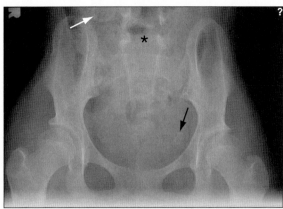

Figure 1. Pelvic radiograph shows rounded densities in left pelvis (*black arrow*). Spinal fusion defects are seen in lumbosacral spine (*asterisk*), and a portion of the patient's ventriculoperitoneal shunt (*white arrow*) can be seen.

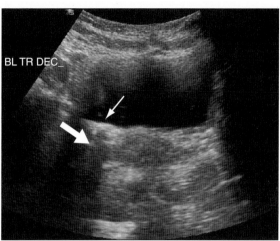

Figure 2. Transverse ultrasound of bladder shows echogenic focus within dependent portion of bladder (*small arrow*) with posterior shadowing (*large arrow*).

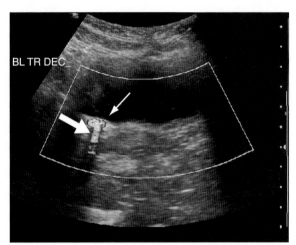

Figure 3. Color Doppler imaging shows twinkle artifact (*large arrow*) that is posterior to echogenic focus (*small arrow*).

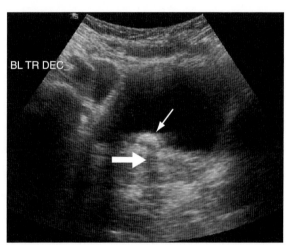

Figure 4. When patient was positioned obliquely, echogenic focus (*small arrow*) and its shadow (*large arrow*) move dependently.

Case 161

DEMOGRAPHICS/CLINICAL HISTORY

The patient is a 14-year-old boy with cerebral palsy and scoliosis, undergoing radiography.

FINDINGS

A frontal radiograph of the chest and abdomen for scoliosis evaluation (Fig. 1) shows a density projecting over the left renal collecting system. An enlarged view of the left renal fossa (Fig. 2) shows that the density corresponds to a calcified cast of the renal collecting system, and the renal calices can be seen. A lateral view (Fig. 3) shows a corresponding density. An enlarged lateral view (Fig. 4) shows the renal calices and casting of the renal collecting system.

DISCUSSION

Definition/Background

Staghorn calculi are branched renal stones that can cause obstruction and eventually lead to stasis, sepsis, and renal failure.

Characteristic Clinical Features

Patients can present with pain from obstruction. If the calculus is infected, the patient also can have fever.

Characteristic Radiologic Findings

A calcified branching stone is visualized on imaging studies. Stones can be partial (involving at least two calices) or complete (involving virtually the entire collecting system). Secondary obstruction and infection can be seen within the involved kidney.

Diagnosis

Staghorn calculus

Suggested Reading

Preminger GM, Assimos DG, Lingeman JE, et al: AUA Nephrolithiasis Guideline Panel: AUA guideline on management of staghorn calculi: Diagnosis and treatment recommendations. J Urol 173: 1991-2000, 2005.

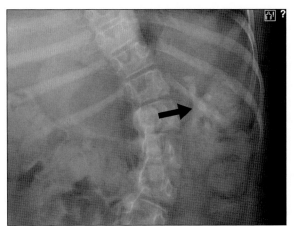

Figure 1. Frontal radiograph of chest and abdomen for scoliosis evaluation shows density projecting over left renal collecting system (*arrow*).

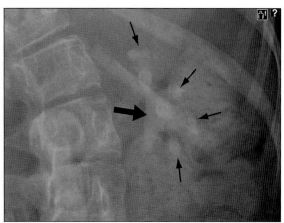

Figure 2. Enlarged view of left renal fossa shows density (*large arrow*) corresponding to calcified cast of renal collecting system, with visualization of the renal calices (*small arrows*).

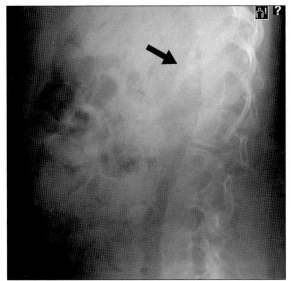

Figure 3. Lateral view shows corresponding density (*arrow*).

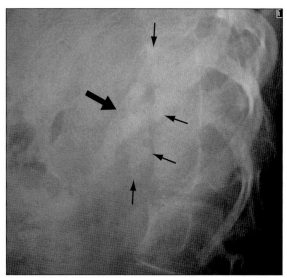

Figure 4. Enlarged lateral view shows renal calices (*small arrows*) and casting of renal collecting system (*large arrow*).

Case 162

DEMOGRAPHICS/CLINICAL HISTORY

The patient is a newborn with prenatal imaging showing an adrenal mass.

FINDINGS

Prenatal ultrasound (Fig. 1) shows a heterogeneous mass (calipers) superior to the right fetal kidney and inferior to the fetal liver. Fetal ribs are also seen. Longitudinal postnatal ultrasound (Fig. 2) shows the heterogeneous mass within the right adrenal gland, superior to the right kidney and inferior to the liver. Transverse postnatal color Doppler (Fig. 3) shows no evidence for vascularity in the mass within the right adrenal gland. Follow-up longitudinal ultrasound (Fig. 4) shows interval increased echogenicity and interval decrease in size of the mass within the adrenal gland.

DISCUSSION

Definition/Background
Adrenal hemorrhage is often unilateral; is typically right-sided; and is usually a benign, self-limited process.

Characteristic Clinical Features
Adrenal hemorrhage is typically incidentally found, particularly in neonates or trauma patients.

Characteristic Radiologic Findings
Ultrasonography is the preferred imaging modality for neonatal hemorrhage. Acute hemorrhage can manifest as a heterogeneous adrenal mass. Over the following weeks, involution of the hemorrhage is seen, often with cystic components, eventually resorbing and possibly calcifying. No vascularity should be seen within the mass.

Differential Diagnosis
■ Neuroblastoma

Discussion
Early-stage neuroblastoma can have a similar heterogeneous appearance; however, neuroblastoma shows vascularity and does not typically show significant improvement within a few weeks.

Diagnosis
Adrenal hemorrhage

Suggested Readings
Paterson A: Adrenal pathology in childhood: A spectrum of disease. Eur Radiol 12:2491-2508, 2002.
Westra SJ, Zaninovic AC, Hall TR, et al: Imaging of the adrenal gland in children. RadioGraphics 14:1323-1340, 1994.

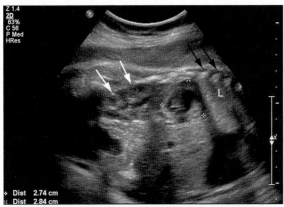

Figure 1. Prenatal ultrasound shows heterogeneous mass (*calipers*) superior to right fetal kidney (*white arrows*) and inferior to the fetal liver (L). Fetal ribs are also seen (*black arrows*).

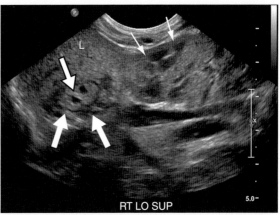

Figure 2. Longitudinal postnatal ultrasound shows heterogeneous mass (*white-filled arrow*) within right adrenal gland (*large white arrows*), superior to the right kidney (*small white arrows*) and inferior to the liver (L).

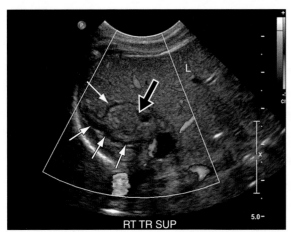

Figure 3. Transverse postnatal color Doppler shows no evidence for vascularity in mass (*black-filled arrow*) within right adrenal gland (*small arrows*). The liver (L) is seen adjacent.

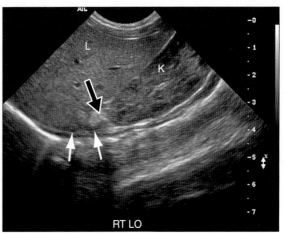

Figure 4. Follow-up longitudinal ultrasound shows interval increased echogenicity and interval decrease in size of mass (*black-filled arrow*) within adrenal gland (*white arrows*). Liver (L) and kidney (K) are also well visualized.

Case 163

DEMOGRAPHICS/CLINICAL HISTORY

The patient is a 4-year-old girl with a past history of pyloric atresia, now with bilateral hydronephrosis and bilateral nephrostomy tubes in place.

FINDINGS

An anteroposterior fluoroscopic spot image from a voiding cystourethrogram (VCUG) (Fig. 1) shows multiple smooth filling defects at the base of the bladder and right-sided vesicoureteral reflux. A transverse ultrasound image at the level of the bladder (Fig. 2) shows prominent, irregular bladder wall thickening, most severe along the posterior wall of the bladder base. In a different patient, a lateral oblique fluoroscopic spot image from a barium swallow (Fig. 3) shows a high-grade proximal esophageal stricture.

DISCUSSION

Definition/Background
Epidermolysis bullosa (EB) refers to several disorders that are characterized by extreme fragility of the skin related to defects in the basement membrane.

Characteristic Clinical Features
Patients with junctional EB may also have congenital pyloric atresia, pseudosyndactyly of the hands and feet, oral ulcers, esophageal strictures, and bladder outlet obstruction.

Characteristic Radiologic Findings
Barium esophagogram in patients with EB may show an esophageal stricture that may cause severe obstructive symptoms. In a newborn with EB and pyloric atresia, an upper gastrointestinal (GI) examination reveals a distended stomach, and no contrast agent passes through the pyloric channel into the duodenum.

Less Common Radiologic Manifestations
Cystograms in patients with bladder involvement may show a small-capacity bladder with filling defects within the bladder secondary to blistering in the bladder wall.

Differential Diagnosis
- Peptic esophageal stricture
- Caustic ingestion
- Infectious esophagitis

Discussion
Peptic esophageal strictures are often in the distal esophagus and are related to gastroesophageal reflux. Caustic ingestion, typically with alkali agents, causes diffuse mucosal irregularity within the midesophagus and distal esophagus with areas of esophageal stricturing. Infectious esophagitis is most often secondary to fungal or viral causes and occurs in immunocompromised children.

Diagnosis
Epidermolysis bullosa

Suggested Readings
Freeman EB, Koglmeier J, Martinez AE, et al: Gastrointestinal complications of epidermolysis bullosa in children. Br J Dermatol 158:1308-1314, 2008.
Horn HM, Tidman MJ: The clinical spectrum of dystrophic epidermolysis bullosa. Br J Dermatol 146:267-274, 2002.

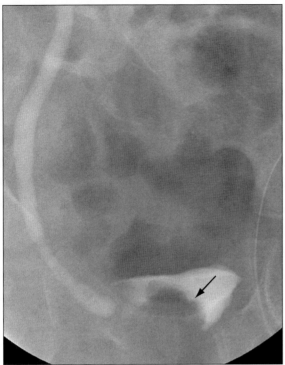

Figure 1. Anteroposterior fluoroscopic spot image from VCUG shows multiple smooth filling defects at base of bladder (*arrow*) and right-sided vesicoureteral reflux.

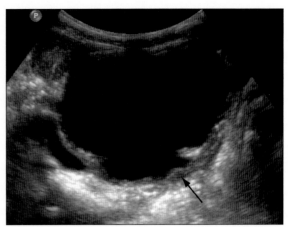

Figure 2. Transverse ultrasound image at level of bladder shows irregular blistering of bladder wall, most severe along posterior wall of bladder base (*arrow*).

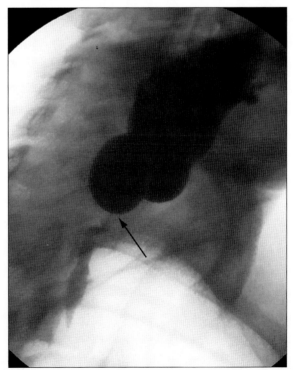

Figure 3. Lateral oblique fluoroscopic spot image from a barium swallow in a 22-year-old man with EB shows high-grade proximal esophageal stricture (*arrow*).

Case 164

DEMOGRAPHICS/CLINICAL HISTORY

The patient is a newborn boy with protuberant abdomen, no urine output, respiratory distress, and unable to pass bladder catheter.

FINDINGS

A plain radiograph of the abdomen obtained shortly after birth shows a protuberant abdomen with centralization of bowel loops secondary to a large amount of ascites (Fig. 1). The lungs are hypoplastic. Ultrasound of the abdomen shows a large amount of intra-abdominal ascites (Fig. 2). The kidneys are dysplastic with loss of normal corticomedullary differentiation and bilateral hydroureteronephrosis (Fig. 3). The urinary bladder was also markedly distended.

DISCUSSION

Definition/Background

Urinary ascites may occur secondary to rupture of a loculated urinoma into the peritoneal space, transudation of urine from a dilated collecting system or urinoma into the peritoneum, or direct bladder rupture. Urinary ascites is present in approximately 25% of fetuses with urethral obstruction.

Characteristic Clinical Features

Patients present at birth with a distended abdomen, which may make delivery difficult. Given the association of oligohydramnios with urinary ascites (because of urinary output obstruction), patients have hypoplastic lungs and respiratory compromise, which is often the cause of death. Patients also present with characteristic flattened facial features (i.e., Potter facies).

Characteristic Radiologic Findings

Infants with urinary ascites have a distended abdomen in plain radiographs, and the presence of ascites can be deduced by the centralization of air-filled bowel loops. The lungs appear hypoplastic.

Less Common Radiologic Manifestations

Ultrasound confirms the presence of intra-abdominal ascites. Ultrasound can also assess the abnormal urinary system and reveal hydroureteronephrosis and bladder distention secondary to urethral obstruction.

Differential Diagnosis

- Meconium peritonitis
- Biliary ascites
- Chylous ascites

Discussion

Meconium peritonitis is a sequela of in utero bowel rupture with escape of meconium into the peritoneal cavity. In addition to ascites, which may or may not be present, intra-abdominal calcifications are often detected on radiographs and ultrasound. Biliary ascites is rare, and neonates usually present with jaundice, distended abdomen, and feeding intolerance. Chylous ascites is also rare in infants and manifests with abdominal distention and poor feeding. Aspiration of ascites reveals high triglycerides. Many patients respond to nonoperative treatment.

Diagnosis

Urinary ascites

Suggested Readings

Chen C, Shih SL, Liu FF, et al: In utero bladder perforation, urinary ascites, and bilateral contained urinomas secondary to posterior urethral valves: clinical and imaging findings. Pediatr Radiol 27:3-5, 1997.

Herman TE, Siegel MJ: Special imaging casebook: Oligohydramnios sequence with bilateral renal agenesis (Potter's syndrome). J Perinatol 20:397-398, 2000.

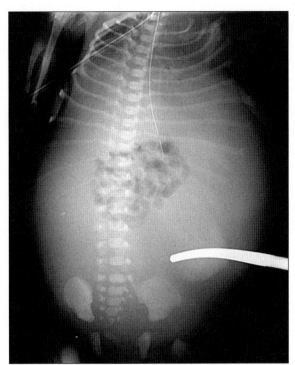

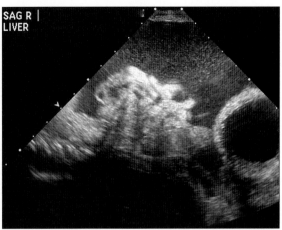

Figure 2. Sagittal image in right lower quadrant from ultrasound of abdomen shows large amount of intra-abdominal ascites.

Figure 1. Plain radiograph of abdomen performed shortly after birth shows protuberant abdomen with centralization of bowel loops secondary to large amount of ascites. Lungs are hypoplastic.

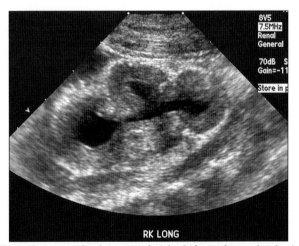

Figure 3. Longitudinal image of right kidney shows dysplastic parenchyma with loss of normal corticomedullary differentiation and increased cortical echogenicity with associated hydroureteronephrosis.

Case 165

DEMOGRAPHICS/CLINICAL HISTORY

The patient is a newborn with prenatal diagnosis of urinoma, contralateral hydroureteronephrosis, and posterior urethral valves.

FINDINGS

Longitudinal ultrasound of the right kidney (Fig. 1) shows pockets of fluid around the kidney. Transverse ultrasound (Fig. 2) shows multiple septations and a large amount of fluid surrounding the kidney. Drainage of the fluid confirmed that this septated fluid collection was a urinoma.

DISCUSSION

Definition/Background
Urinomas are collections of urine that are formed from rupture of the collecting system.

Characteristic Clinical Features
Clinical features may be secondary to underlying cause of urinoma formation, such as poor urinary stream in boys with posterior urethral valves. A palpable mass may be felt on physical examination.

Characteristic Radiologic Findings
A perinephric fluid collection is seen, often with septations or debris.

Differential Diagnosis
- Cystic abdominal/retroperitoneal masses
- Ascites

Discussion
Urinomas are intimately associated with the kidney in the retroperitoneal space, whereas cystic abdominal masses and ascites are intraperitoneal. Cystic retroperitoneal masses may be difficult to distinguish if intimately associated with the kidney, but delayed postcontrast imaging shows urinary excretion of contrast agent into a urinoma.

Diagnosis
Urinoma

Suggested Readings
Titton RL, Gervais DA, Hahn PF, et al: Urine leaks and urinomas: Diagnosis and imaging-guided intervention. RadioGraphics 23:1133-1147, 2003.

Yang DM, Jung DH, Kim H, et al: Retroperitoneal cystic masses: CT, clinical, and pathologic findings and literature review. RadioGraphics 24:1353-1365, 2004.

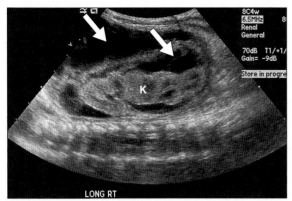

Figure 1. Longitudinal ultrasound of right kidney (K) shows pockets of fluid (*arrows*) around kidney.

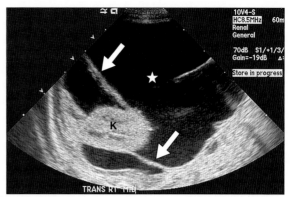

Figure 2. Transverse ultrasound shows multiple septations (*arrows*) and large amount of fluid (*star*) surrounding kidney (K).

Case 166

DEMOGRAPHICS/CLINICAL HISTORY

The patient is an 11-month-old girl with inverted umbilicus with discharge.

FINDINGS

A longitudinal ultrasound scan along the midline lower abdomen (Fig. 1) shows a round hypoechoic collection with internal echoes and a thick isoechoic rim connected to the umbilicus and just superior to the bladder. Using a high-frequency linear transducer in the longitudinal plane (Fig. 2), the tract from the umbilicus to the collection is better visualized. Using the high-frequency transducer in the transverse plane (Fig. 3), the internal echoes, debris, and thick rim of the collection are better visualized. A transverse view of the bladder (Fig. 4) shows the fibrous connection of the urachal remnant to the bladder.

DISCUSSION

Definition/Background
The urachus is a primitive communication from the bladder to the umbilicus. If incomplete resorption occurs during fetal development, urachal remnants can be seen.

Characteristic Clinical Features
Patients usually present with leakage of urine from the umbilicus or infection of a urachal cyst.

Characteristic Radiologic Findings
Ultrasound may show a cystic mass in the midline lower abdomen/upper pelvis. Debris or peripheral vascularity or both can be seen, particularly if complicated by infection. If computed tomography (CT) or magnetic resonance imaging (MRI) is performed, often the urachal fistula or fibrous remnant can also be shown extending from the bladder or urachal cyst to the umbilicus.

Differential Diagnosis
- Other pelvic cystic masses (e.g., ovarian cysts, duplication cysts, mesenteric cysts)
- Other causes of fistulous formation (e.g., Crohn disease)

Discussion
In evaluating cystic masses, the presence of the ovaries should be confirmed, and the relationship with the cystic mass to the bladder and its position in the midline should be evaluated. Typically, patients with Crohn disease have other radiographic manifestations before cutaneous fistula formation.

Diagnosis
Infected urachal cyst

Suggested Reading
Berrocal T, López-Pereira P, Arjonilla A, et al: Anomalies of the distal ureter, bladder, and urethra in children: Embryologic, radiologic, and pathologic features. RadioGraphics 22:1139, 2002.

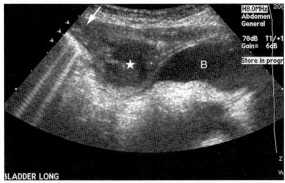

Figure 1. Longitudinal ultrasound along midline lower abdomen shows round hypoechoic collection (*star*) with internal echoes and thick isoechoic rim connected to umbilicus (*arrow*) and just superior to bladder (B).

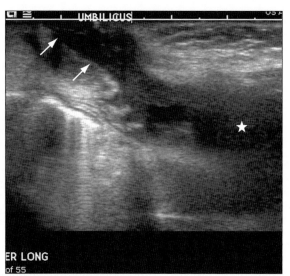

Figure 2. Using high-frequency linear transducer in longitudinal plane, tract from umbilicus (*arrows*) to collection (*star*) is better visualized.

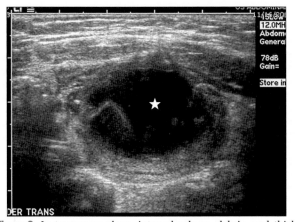

Figure 3. In transverse plane, internal echoes, debris, and thick rim of collection (*star*) are better visualized.

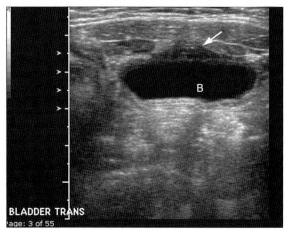

Figure 4. Transverse view of bladder shows fibrous connection (*arrow*) of urachal remnant to bladder (B).

Case 167

DEMOGRAPHICS/CLINICAL HISTORY

The patient is an 11-year-old girl 24 hours after a motor vehicle accident.

FINDINGS

Coronal reconstructed contrast-enhanced computed tomography (CT) (Fig. 1) shows linear low attenuation in the lower pole of the right kidney, representing a renal laceration. A more posterior coronal view (Fig. 2) shows stranding along the retroperitoneum. Axial contrast-enhanced CT (Fig. 3) shows multiple linear hypointensities in the lower pole of the right kidney and a surrounding perirenal fluid collection. A more inferior view (Fig. 4) shows fluid tracking down the retroperitoneum. No contrast extravasation was observed into the perirenal fluid collection or along the retroperitoneum.

DISCUSSION

Definition/Background
Trauma to the kidneys can injure the vascular or collecting systems.

Characteristic Clinical Features
Patients may present with hematuria and costophrenic angle tenderness.

Characteristic Radiologic Findings
Radiologic findings depend on the severity of injury. Injury to the renal parenchyma can cause perinephric fluid collections. These collections can contain blood or urine or both. Intravenous contrast agent can help identify collecting system injury during excretory phase imaging. Subcapsular hematomas can cause compression of the renal parenchyma. Renal arteries and veins should be imaged to look for evidence of avulsion or thrombus.

Differential Diagnosis
- Renal mass
- Infection

Discussion
Areas of heterogeneous attenuation in small renal masses can mimic renal injury, but masses typically have a rounded configuration. Linear low attenuation seen in pyelonephritis may look similar to renal laceration, but the history and presence of dense fluid (i.e., blood) suggest the diagnosis of renal injury.

Diagnosis
Renal trauma

Suggested Reading
Vasile M, Bellin MF, Hélénon O, et al: Imaging evaluation of renal trauma. Abdom Imaging 25:424-430, 2000.

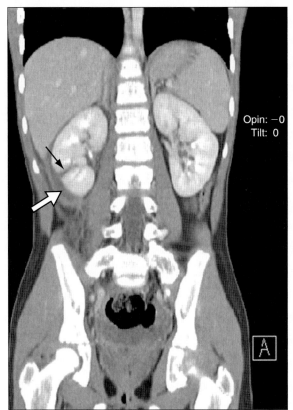

Figure 1. Coronal reconstructed contrast-enhanced CT image shows linear area of low attenuation in lower pole of right kidney (*black arrow*), representing renal laceration. Perirenal hematoma can be seen (*black outlined arrow*).

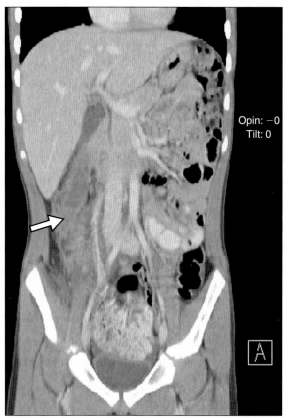

Figure 2. More posterior coronal view shows stranding along retroperitoneum (*arrow*).

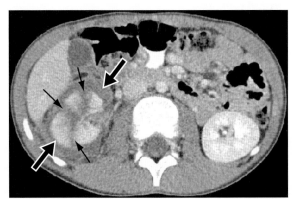

Figure 3. Axial contrast-enhanced CT image shows multiple linear hypointensities in lower pole of right kidney (*small arrows*) and surrounding perirenal fluid collection (*large arrows*).

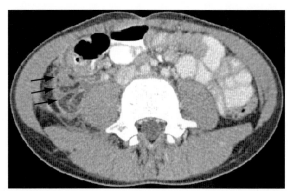

Figure 4. More inferiorly, fluid is seen tracking down the retroperitoneum (*arrows*). No contrast extravasation was seen into the perirenal fluid collection or along the retroperitoneum.

Case 168

DEMOGRAPHICS/CLINICAL HISTORY

The patient is a 6-year-old boy presenting after a fall from a chair.

FINDINGS

Contrast-enhanced axial and coronal reformatted images from a computed tomography (CT) scan of the abdomen and pelvis (Figs. 1 and 2) show a focal defect within the interlobar region of the right kidney that does not enhance, consistent with a renal laceration. The laceration does not extend into the renal pelvis. There is a small amount of perinephric fluid.

DISCUSSION

Definition/Background
Injury to the kidney occurs in 4% to 14% of children presenting with blunt abdominal trauma. Most (64% to 96%) renal injuries are mild (grades 1 or 2 out of 5).

Characteristic Clinical Features
Most patients with significant renal injury present with hematuria, although many present with history of trauma and no other symptoms.

Characteristic Radiologic Findings
On CT, a renal contusion appears as an ill-defined, hypoattenuating lesion in the parenchyma. Grade 2 injuries include lacerations that do not involve the collecting system or the deep renal medulla. Grade 3 injuries are deeper lacerations that may or may not have associated urinary extravasation.

Less Common Radiologic Manifestations
Grade 4 injuries are catastrophic injuries, including lacerations that involve the collecting system at the ureteropelvic junction and major renal pedicle injuries.

Differential Diagnosis
- Renal infarct
- Lobar nephronia

Discussion
Renal infarct manifests as a wedge-shaped perfusion defect in the kidney, usually toward the periphery of the kidney with a preserved enhancing cortical rim. Lobar nephronia is a focal area of infection of the kidney that may manifest as an area of decreased attenuation and enhancement on CT.

Diagnosis
Renal trauma

Suggested Readings
Kawashima A, Sandler CM, Corl FM, et al: Imaging of renal trauma: A comprehensive review. RadioGraphics 21:557-574, 2001.

Mirvis S: Injuries to the urinary system and retroperitoneum. In Mirvis SE, Shanmuganathan K, (eds): Imaging in Trauma and Critical Care, 2nd ed, Philadelphia: Saunders, 2003, pp 483-517.

Morey AF, Bruce JE, McAninch JW: Efficacy of radiographic imaging in pediatric blunt renal trauma. J Urol 156:2014-2018, 1996.

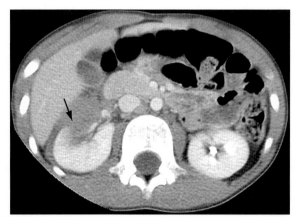

Figure 1. Contrast-enhanced axial image from CT scan of abdomen and pelvis shows focal defect within interlobar region of right kidney that does not enhance, consistent with renal laceration (*arrow*). Laceration does not extend into renal pelvis.

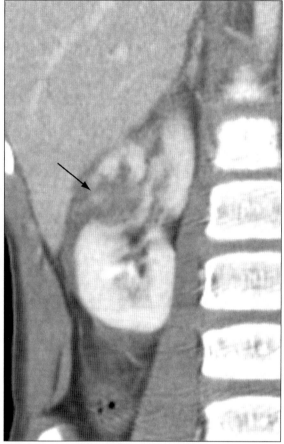

Figure 2. Contrast-enhanced coronal reformatted image from CT scan of abdomen and pelvis shows focal defect within interlobar region of right kidney that does not enhance, consistent with renal laceration (*arrow*). Laceration does not extend into the renal pelvis. There is a small amount of perinephric fluid.

Case 169

DEMOGRAPHICS/CLINICAL HISTORY

The patient is a 3-year-old Haitian boy with hematuria.

FINDINGS

Ultrasound examination of the pelvis (Figs. 1 and 2) shows a moderately full urinary bladder with large, echogenic, shadowing calculi layering along the dependent wall of the bladder. There is also a mild amount of debris in the bladder.

DISCUSSION

Definition/Background

Schistosomiasis is a parasitic disease that most often occurs in parts of South America and Africa, the Caribbean, and the Middle East.

Characteristic Clinical Features

Infection may affect many different organs, including the central nervous system, colon, liver, and spleen. When the bladder is infected, symptoms include cystitis and ureteritis with hematuria, which may progress to bladder cancer.

Characteristic Radiologic Findings

In this case, the patient's prior urinary tract infection led to the formation of bladder calculi, which manifest as echogenic, shadowing structures on ultrasound.

Differential Diagnosis

- Urinary stasis
- Transitional cell carcinoma

Discussion

Patients with urinary stasis, including patients with bladder outlet obstruction or myelodysplasia, develop bladder calculi, which may be indistinguishable from the calculi that develop in patients as a result of schistosomiasis infection. Although bladder wall calcifications may be present in patients with transitional cell carcinoma, this disease is rare in children.

Diagnosis

Schistosomiasis.

Suggested Readings

Abdel-Wahab MF, Ramzy I, Esmat G, et al: Ultrasound for detecting *Schistosoma haematobium* urinary tract complications: Comparison with radiographic procedures. J Urol 148(2 Pt 1):346, 1992.

Dyer RB, Chen MY, Zagoria RJ: Abnormal calcifications in the urinary tract. RadioGraphics 18:1405, 1998.

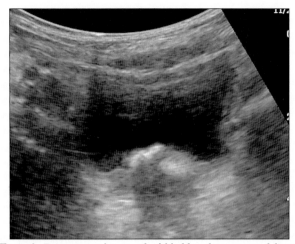

Figure 1. Transverse ultrasound of bladder shows several large, echogenic, shadowing calculi along nondependent bladder wall.

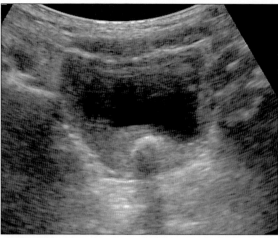

Figure 2. Transverse ultrasound of bladder shows large, dominant calculus layered dependently in bladder, which is surrounded by bladder debris.

Case 170

DEMOGRAPHICS/CLINICAL HISTORY

The patient is a 5-year-old girl with renal failure.

FINDINGS

Longitudinal ultrasound images of the right and left kidneys (Figs. 1 and 2) show increased echogenicity of the renal parenchyma with loss of normal corticomedullary differentiation.

DISCUSSION

Definition/Background

Primary oxalosis (or primary hyperoxaluria) is a rare, heritable, inborn error of metabolism secondary to a deficient liver enzyme, which results in excessive synthesis and urinary excretion of oxalate. Renal stone formation and deposition of calcium oxalate in the kidney and other organs occur.

Characteristic Clinical Features

Patients present with progressive renal dysfunction, which may eventually necessitate renal transplantation.

Characteristic Radiologic Findings

There are two ultrasound patterns in primary hyperoxaluria: cortical nephrocalcinosis (increased cortical echogenicity) and medullary nephrocalcinosis (increased echogenicity in the medullary pyramids).

Differential Diagnosis

- Cortical necrosis
- Alport syndrome
- Hemolytic uremic syndrome

Discussion

Cortical necrosis of the kidney is a cause of renal failure that is secondary to ischemic necrosis of the parenchyma. It is also a cause of cortical nephrocalcinosis. Alport syndrome is an inherited disorder that causes progressive nephritis and sensorineural hearing loss. This syndrome also causes cortical nephrocalcinosis. Hemolytic uremic syndrome is the most common cause of acute renal failure in children. It usually follows an infectious illness, and is characterized by hemolytic anemia, thrombocytopenia, and acute renal failure.

Diagnosis

Oxalosis

Suggested Readings

Akhan O, Oxmen MN, Coskun M, et al: Systemic oxalosis: Pathognomonic renal and specific extrarenal findings on US and CT. Pediatr Radiol 25:15, 1995.

Orazi C, Picca S, Schingo PM, et al: Oxalosis in primary hyperoxaluria in infancy: Report of a case in a 3-month-old baby: Follow-up for 3 years and review of literature. Skeletal Radiol 38:387-391, 2009.

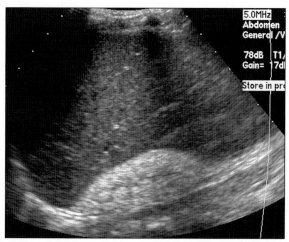

Figure 1. Longitudinal ultrasound image of right kidney shows diffusely and markedly increased echogenicity of renal parenchyma compared with adjacent liver parenchyma.

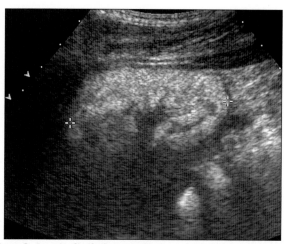

Figure 2. Longitudinal ultrasound image of left kidney shows diffusely increased echogenicity of renal parenchyma with loss of normal corticomedullary differentiation.

Case 171

DEMOGRAPHICS/CLINICAL HISTORY

The patient is a 5-year-old girl who fell off the monkey bars and landed on an outstretched arm.

FINDINGS

Radiograph (Fig. 1) shows a fracture through the proximal shaft of the ulna with an associated radial head dislocation.

DISCUSSION

Characteristic Clinical Features

This injury is treated with closed reduction under conscious sedation and long arm casting.

Characteristic Radiologic Findings

Radiography shows ulnar fracture with associated radial head dislocation.

Diagnosis

Monteggia fracture

Suggested Readings

Kay RM, Skaggs DL: The pediatric Monteggia fracture. Am J Orthop 27:606-609, 1998.

Perron AD, Hersh RE, Brady WJ, et al: Orthopedic pitfalls in the ED: Galeazzi and Monteggia fracture-dislocation. Am J Emerg Med 19:225-228, 2001.

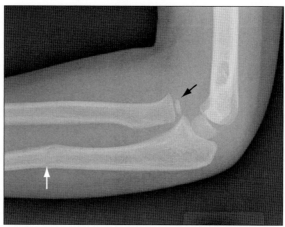

Figure 1. Lateral view of elbow that includes proximal forearm reveals fracture through proximal ulna (*black arrow*) with associated dislocation of radial head (*white arrow*).

Case 172

DEMOGRAPHICS/CLINICAL HISTORY

The patient is a 5-year-old boy who fell off a slide several days ago and injured the left elbow, with persistent pain and swelling.

FINDINGS

Anteroposterior (Fig. 1) and lateral (Fig. 2) views of the elbow show a lucency within the lateral condyle of the distal humerus and an associated joint effusion.

DISCUSSION

Characteristic Clinical Features

Treatment for this fracture depends on the degree of displacement of the fracture fragment.

Characteristic Radiologic Findings

Radiographs show linear lucency within the lateral condyle with an associated joint effusion. In some cases, the fracture line is not appreciated, but the presence of a joint effusion should raise concern for the diagnosis.

Differential Diagnosis

- Supracondylar fracture

Diagnosis

Lateral condylar fracture

Suggested Readings

Chapman VM, Grottkau BE, Albright M, et al: Multidetector computed tomography of pediatric lateral condylar fractures. J Comput Assist Tomogr 29:842-846, 2005.

Song KS, Kang CH, Min BW, et al: Internal oblique radiographs for diagnosis of nondisplaced or minimally displaced lateral condylar fractures of the humerus in children. J Bone Joint Surg Am 89: 58-63, 2007.

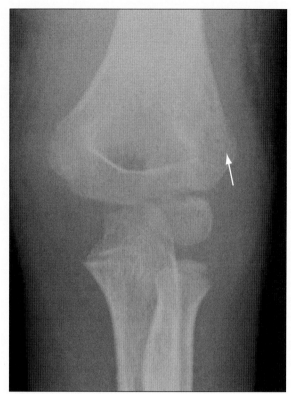

Figure 1. Anteroposterior radiograph of left elbow reveals nondisplaced fracture through lateral condyle (*arrow*) with associated periosteal new bone formation.

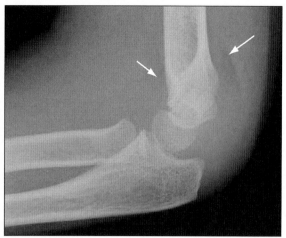

Figure 2. Lateral radiograph of elbow shows large joint effusion with elevation of anterior and posterior fat pads (*arrows*).

Case 173

DEMOGRAPHICS/CLINICAL HISTORY

The patient is a 25-month-old girl favoring the left leg after injury.

FINDINGS

Radiographs of the left lower leg (Figs. 1 and 2) show a nondisplaced spiral fracture involving the distal tibial metadiaphysis. Radiographs performed 2 weeks later (Figs. 3 and 4) reveal periosteal new bone formation indicative of healing.

DISCUSSION

Characteristic Clinical Features

If there is a high suspicion of fracture, but anteroposterior and lateral radiographs are normal, oblique radiographs of the lower leg are recommended.

Characteristic Radiologic Findings

Radiography shows oblique/spiral fracture of the tibia.

Less Common Radiologic Manifestations

Fracture also can involve the cuboid (although not in this case).

Diagnosis

Toddler fracture

Suggested Readings

John SD, Moorthy CS, Swischuk LE: Expanding the concept of the toddler's fracture. RadioGraphics 17:367-376, 1997.

Miller JH, Sanderson RA: Scintigraphy of toddler's fracture. J Nucl Med 29:2001-2003, 1988.

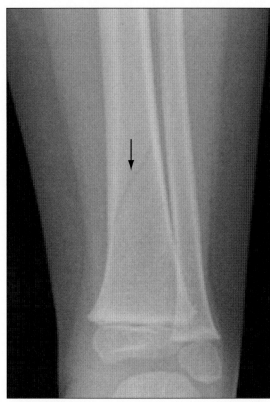

Figure 1. Anteroposterior radiograph of lower leg at time of injury shows spiral fracture of distal tibial diametaphysis (*arrow*).

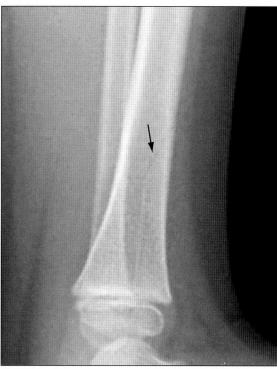

Figure 2. Lateral radiograph of left lower leg also shows spiral fracture of tibia (*arrow*).

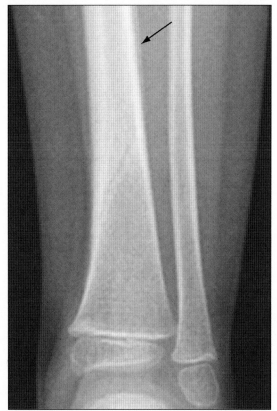

Figure 3. Anteroposterior radiograph of lower leg performed 2 weeks later shows subtle periosteal new bone formation (*arrow*) indicative of healing.

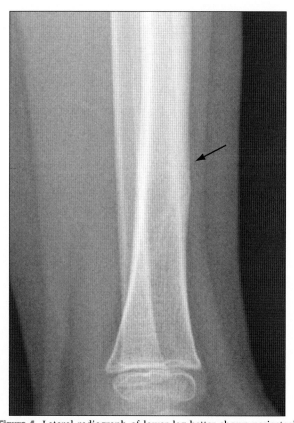

Figure 4. Lateral radiograph of lower leg better shows periosteal new bone formation (*arrow*).

Case 174

DEMOGRAPHICS/CLINICAL HISTORY

The patient is a 12-year-old boy with pain, swelling, and limited range of motion after an arm injury.

FINDINGS

Plain radiographs of the elbow (Figs. 1 and 2) reveal a transversely oriented fracture through the supracondylar aspect of the humerus. There is an associated joint effusion (see Fig. 2).

DISCUSSION

Definition/Background
Supracondylar fractures are the most common fracture to occur at the pediatric elbow.

Characteristic Clinical Features
A common mechanism of injury is a hyperextension injury.

Characteristic Radiologic Findings
A fracture lucency often is identified in the supracondylar humerus, and most often the distal fracture fragment is posteriorly displaced. A line drawn along the anterior humeral cortex should intersect the middle third of the capitellum, but in cases of supracondylar fracture this line passes through the anterior third of the capitellum, or anterior to the capitellum entirely.

Differential Diagnosis
- Lateral condylar fracture

Diagnosis
Supracondylar fracture

Suggested Readings
Hindman BW, Schreiber RR, Wiss DA, et al: Supracondylar fractures of the humerus: Prediction of the cubitus varus deformity with CT. Radiology 168:513-515, 1988.

Skaggs DL, Mirzayan R: The posterior fat pad sign in association with occult fracture of the elbow in children. J Bone Joint Surg Am 81:1429-1433, 1999.

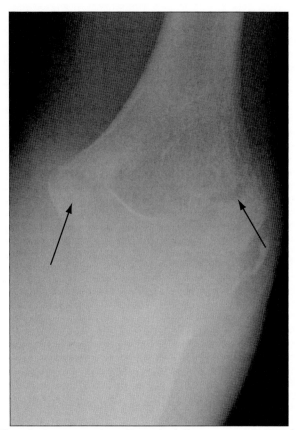

Figure 1. Anteroposterior radiograph of elbow reveals transversely oriented fracture involving supracondylar aspect of humerus (*arrows*).

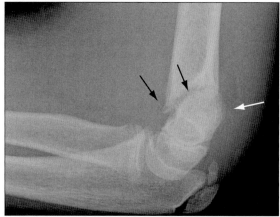

Figure 2. Lateral radiograph of elbow reveals supracondylar fracture (*black arrows*) and associated joint effusion (*white arrow*). There is mild posterior displacement of distal fracture fragment.

Case 175

DEMOGRAPHICS/CLINICAL HISTORY

The patient is a 12-year-old gymnast with right hip pain.

FINDINGS

Anteroposterior (Fig. 1) and frog-leg lateral (Fig. 2) views of the hips and pelvis show avulsion of the right ischial tuberosity at the insertion site of the hamstring tendons. Coronal T2-weighted magnetic resonance imaging (MRI) of the pelvis shows bone marrow edema in the ischium at the site of the avulsion injury (Fig. 3).

DISCUSSION

Definition/Background

Pelvic avulsion injuries are most commonly encountered in adolescent athletes, particularly gymnasts and soccer players.

Characteristic Clinical Features

Avulsion of the ischial tuberosity is related to sudden, excessive lengthening of the hamstring muscles. The epiphyseal plate is weaker than the hypertrophied muscles and is avulsed, which produces pain often described as hip pain.

Characteristic Radiologic Findings

Routine radiographs are the best imaging modality to visualize the avulsed fragment and its donor site.

Less Common Radiologic Manifestations

MRI may be helpful in some cases by showing the degree of surrounding bone marrow edema, the presence and size of hematoma, and the status of the attached tendons.

Differential Diagnosis

- Osteomyelitis

Discussion

The avulsion injury of the ischial tuberosity has a characteristic appearance and is not often mistaken for other entities. During the reparative phase of healing, the proliferative bone response may appear similar, however, to an infectious process (i.e., osteomyelitis) or a malignant neoplasm.

Diagnosis

Avulsion of the ischial tuberosity

Suggested Readings

Fernbach SK, Wilkinson RH: Avulsion injuries of the pelvis and proximal femur. AJR Am J Roentgenol 137:581-584, 1981.

Rossi F, Dragoni S: Acute avulsion fractures of the pelvis in adolescent competitive athletes: Prevalence, location and sports distribution of 203 cases collected. Skeletal Radiol 30:127-131, 2001.

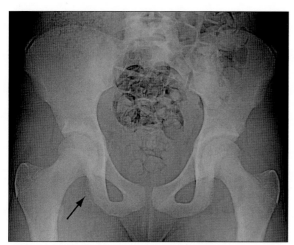

Figure 1. Anteroposterior radiograph of pelvis reveals irregular, avulsed, crescentic bony fragment (*arrow*) and donor site from the right ischial tuberosity.

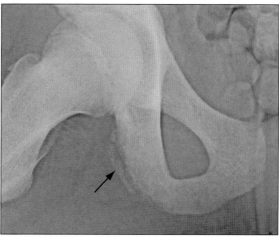

Figure 2. Magnified frog-leg lateral radiograph of pelvis reveals irregular, avulsed, crescentic bony fragment (*arrow*) and donor site from right ischial tuberosity.

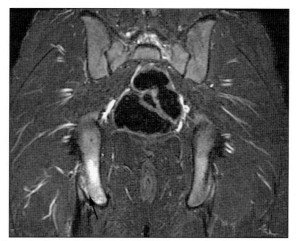

Figure 3. Coronal T2-weighted MR image of pelvis shows bone marrow edema in right ischial tuberosity at site of attachment of hamstring tendons (*arrow*).

Case 176

DEMOGRAPHICS/CLINICAL HISTORY

The patient is an 11-year-old boy with left hip pain.

FINDINGS

Plain radiographs of the hips and pelvis (Figs. 1 and 2) show posteromedial displacement of the left femoral head with respect to the femoral neck. After surgical fixation, there is a new, acute slip on the right (Fig. 3).

DISCUSSION

Definition/Background

Slipped capital femoral epiphysis most commonly occurs in preadolescent children. Obesity is a risk factor.

Characteristic Clinical Features

Patients often present with hip pain, although the pain may radiate to the knee or lower leg.

Characteristic Radiologic Findings

Diagnosis is made on the basis of plain radiographs, which show the characteristic posteromedial displacement of the femoral head and the widening of the physis. These findings are best appreciated on a frog-leg lateral view plain radiograph of the hip.

Differential Diagnosis

- Legg-Calvé-Perthes disease

Diagnosis

Slipped capital femoral epiphysis

Suggested Readings

Katz DA: Slipped capital femoral epiphysis: The importance of early diagnosis. Pediatr Ann 35:102-111, 2006.

Kocher MS, Bishop JA, Weed B, et al: Delay in diagnosis of slipped capital femoral epiphysis. Pediatrics 113:e322-e325, 2004.

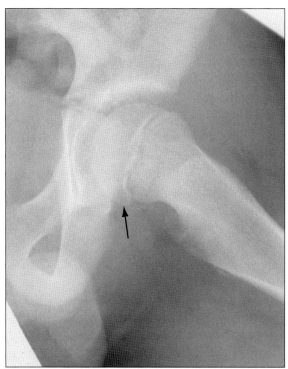

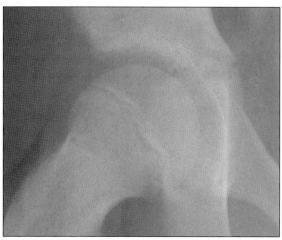

Figure 2. Frog-leg lateral view of right hip reveals no abnormality.

Figure 1. Frog-leg lateral radiograph of left hip shows mild, posteromedial slip of left capital femoral epiphysis (*arrow*).

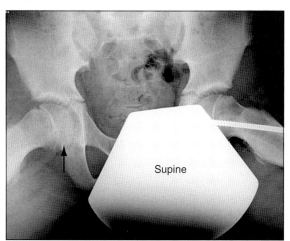

Figure 3. Anteroposterior radiograph of pelvis performed 9 months after surgical pinning of left hip. There is a new slip on the right (*arrow*).

Case 177

DEMOGRAPHICS/CLINICAL HISTORY

The patient is a 15-year-old male baseball pitcher with right-sided shoulder pain.

FINDINGS

An anteroposterior radiograph of the right shoulder shows relative widening of the proximal humeral growth plate (Fig. 1) compared with the normal left shoulder (Fig. 2).

DISCUSSION

Definition/Background

Little League shoulder is most commonly seen in high-performance male pitchers 11 to 14 years old. The syndrome involves chronic stress changes in the proximal humeral physis.

Characteristic Clinical Features

Patients complain of shoulder pain.

Characteristic Radiologic Findings

Radiographs show widening of the proximal humeral physis.

Differential Diagnosis

- Proximal humerus fracture

Diagnosis

Little League shoulder

Suggested Readings

Barnett LS: Little League shoulder syndrome: Proximal humeral epiphysiolysis in adolescent baseball pitchers: A case report. J Bone Joint Surg Am 67:495-496, 1985.

Kocher MS, Waters PM, Micheli LJ: Upper extremity injuries in the paediatric athlete. Sports Med 30:117-135, 2000.

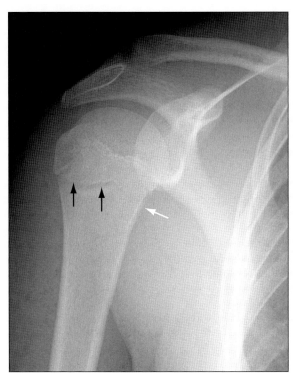

Figure 1. Anteroposterior radiograph of right shoulder shows widening of proximal humeral physis (*black arrows*). Subtle periosteal reaction can be seen along medial cortex of humerus (*white arrow*).

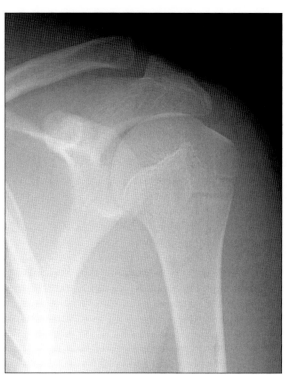

Figure 2. For comparison, anteroposterior radiograph of left shoulder shows that it is normal.

Case 178

DEMOGRAPHICS/CLINICAL HISTORY

The patient is an 11-year-old baseball pitcher with medial elbow pain.

FINDINGS

An anteroposterior radiograph of the elbow (Fig. 1) shows mild widening of the physis separating the medial epicondyle from the distal humerus. Radiographs otherwise were normal. Coronal fluid-sensitive magnetic resonance imaging (MRI) of the elbow (Fig. 2) shows abnormal bone marrow signal within the medial epicondyle and within the adjacent soft tissues. The patient also sustained a partial tear of the ulnar collateral ligament (not shown).

DISCUSSION

Definition/Background

Little League elbow refers to a group of conditions around the elbow joint in young pitchers. The types of injuries that occur are age-dependent, with medial epicondylitis occurring most often in childhood, avulsion fractures of the medial epicondyle occurring more commonly in adolescents, and ulnar collateral ligament tears occurring more commonly in young adults.

Characteristic Clinical Features

Patients experience pain along the medial aspect of the elbow.

Characteristic Radiologic Findings

Plain radiographs either are normal or may show hypertrophy of the medial epicondyle with apophyseal widening. The apophysis of the medial epicondyle may appear irregular and fragmented.

Less Common Radiologic Manifestations

MRI shows thickening and increased signal intensity of the common flexor tendon and surrounding soft tissue edema. Abnormal signal within the medial epicondyle is also often present.

Differential Diagnosis

- Ulnar collateral ligament tear
- Medial epicondylitis

Discussion

Ulnar collateral ligament tears usually occur after acute valgus stress injury to the elbow and typically occur in overhead-throwing athletes. Most tears involve the anterior bundle of the ulnar collateral ligament. Medial epicondylitis refers to an inflammation of the common flexor tendon at its origin from the medial epicondyle of the humerus. It is also mainly seen in athletes—particularly golfers, tennis players, swimmers, and pitchers.

Diagnosis

Little League elbow

Suggested Readings

Cassas KJ, Cassettari-Wayhs A: Childhood and adolescent sports-related overuse injuries. Am Fam Physician 73:1014-1022, 2006.

Kijowski R, De Smet AA: Magnetic resonance imaging findings in patients with medial epicondylitis. Skeletal Radiol 34:196-202, 2005.

Kocher MS, Waters PM, Micheli LJ: Upper extremity injuries in the paediatric athlete. Sports Med 30:117-135, 2000.

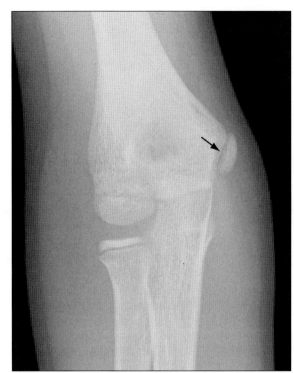

Figure 1. Anteroposterior radiograph of elbow shows mild widening of physis separating medial epicondyle from distal humerus (*arrow*). Radiographs otherwise were normal.

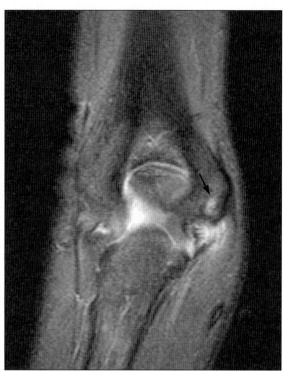

Figure 2. Coronal fluid-sensitive MRI of elbow shows abnormal bone marrow signal within medial epicondyle (*arrow*) and within adjacent soft tissues.

Case 179

DEMOGRAPHICS/CLINICAL HISTORY

The patient is a 9-year-old girl involved in a motor vehicle accident.

FINDINGS

An axial computed tomography (CT) image (Fig. 1) through the thorax shows a complex fracture through a vertebral body. Sagittal reconstruction of the CT scan (Fig. 2) shows the significant loss of vertebral height in two of the fractured and compressed vertebral bodies. Coronal reconstruction of the CT scan (Fig. 3) shows the multilevel fractures and findings of pulmonary hemorrhage.

DISCUSSION

Definition/Background

The burst fracture is the most common thoracic vertebral fracture in children, typically caused by a fall.

Characteristic Clinical Features

Back pain is the typical clinical symptom. If retropulsed fracture fragments are causing spinal cord compression, lower extremity symptoms can be present.

Characteristic Radiologic Findings

Radiographs often underestimate the extensive nature of traumatic fractures. Radiographs may show anterior wedging, kyphosis, disruption of the posterior cortex of the vertebral body, and widening of the interpediculate distance. CT shows the fractures better, and often shows multiple fractures not seen on plain radiographs. If anterior wedging is greater than 25%, posterior ligamentous injury and instability are likely present.

Differential Diagnosis

■ Chance fracture

Discussion

Chance fractures classically occur at the thoracolumbar junction from injuries related to seatbelts in motor vehicle accidents.

Diagnosis

Burst fracture

Suggested Reading

Roche C, Carty H: Spinal trauma in children. Pediatr Radiol 31:677, 2001.

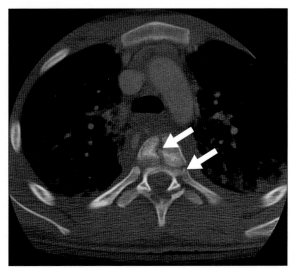

Figure 1. Axial CT image through thorax shows complex fracture through vertebral body (*arrows*).

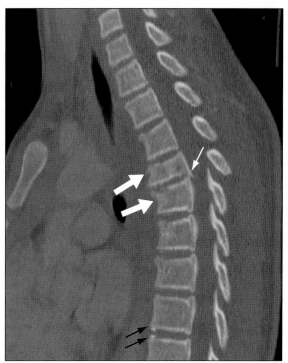

Figure 2. Sagittal reconstruction of CT scan shows significant loss of vertebral height in two fractured and compressed vertebral bodies (*large white arrows*). Retropulsion of portion of fractured vertebral body (*small arrow*) into spinal canal is seen. Normal ring apophyses are seen in lower thoracic spine (*small black arrows*).

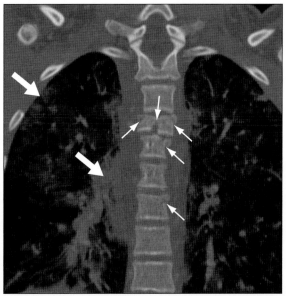

Figure 3. Coronal reconstruction of CT scan shows multilevel fractures (*small arrows*) and findings of pulmonary hemorrhage (*large arrows*).

Case 180

DEMOGRAPHICS/CLINICAL HISTORY

The patient is a 3-month-old boy with vomiting and leg swelling.

FINDINGS

An anteroposterior (AP) radiograph of the right lower leg (Fig. 1) shows a spiral fracture involving the right tibia. An AP radiograph of the chest (Fig. 2) shows multiple healing right-sided rib fractures and an acute left posterior rib fracture. An AP radiograph of the right humerus (Fig. 3) shows a healing classic metaphyseal lesion with exuberant periosteal new bone formation.

DISCUSSION

Definition/Background
Child abuse refers to any form of nonaccidental injury, most often involving the skeletal system in the form of fractures.

Characteristic Clinical Features
Patients usually present with a history of trauma, but the mechanism of trauma is believed to be an inappropriate explanation for the injury sustained. Lower extremity injuries in a child who is not yet walking are suspicious for child abuse.

Characteristic Radiologic Findings
Skeletal survey usually reveals multiple fractures of varying ages. Fractures with high specificity for child abuse include classic metaphyseal lesions, scapular fractures, and posterior rib fractures.

Differential Diagnosis
- Osteogenesis imperfecta (pediatric)
- Accidental trauma

Discussion
Patients with osteogenesis imperfecta have brittle bones and sustain fractures with very little trauma. The bones are often diffusely osteopenic. In some cases, multiple fractures in a patient are a result of accidental trauma, and abuse is not a factor.

Diagnosis
Child abuse

Suggested Readings
Kleinman PK: Problems in the diagnosis of metaphyseal fractures. Pediatr Radiol 38(Suppl 3):S388-S394, 2008.
Nimkin K, Kleinman PK: Imaging of child abuse. Radiol Clin North Am 39:843-864, 2001.

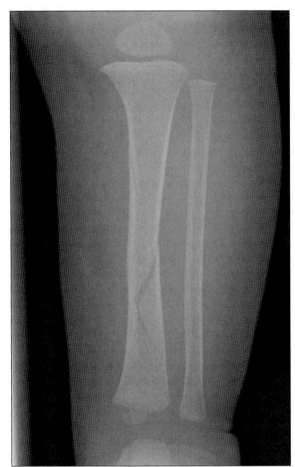

Figure 1. AP radiograph of right lower leg shows spiral fracture involving the right tibia.

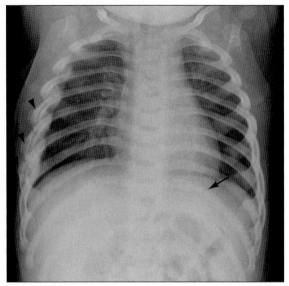

Figure 2. AP radiograph of chest shows multiple healing right-sided rib fractures (*arrowheads*) and acute left posterior rib fracture (*arrow*).

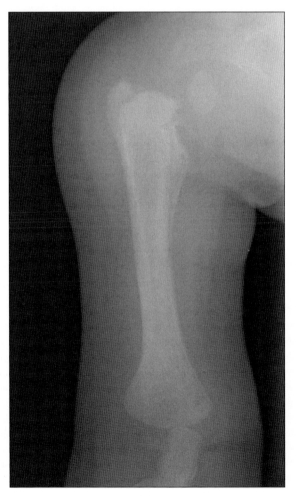

Figure 3. AP radiograph of right humerus shows healing classic metaphyseal lesion with exuberant periosteal new bone formation.

Case 181

DEMOGRAPHICS/CLINICAL HISTORY

The patient is a 3-month-old boy with leg swelling and vomiting, and multiple fractures noted on a prior skeletal survey.

FINDINGS

Bilateral oblique radiographs of the ribs (Figs. 1 and 2) show multiple healing left-sided posterior rib fractures. Incidentally, this patient also had multiple right-sided anterolateral rib fractures.

DISCUSSION

Definition/Background

Posterior rib fractures are highly specific for nonaccidental injury.

Characteristic Clinical Features

Posterior rib fractures may be unsuspected clinically, but are commonly identified in infants who have been the victims of child abuse.

Characteristic Radiologic Findings

Chest radiographs show fractures involving the posterior aspects of the ribs adjacent to the costovertebral junction. Depending on the stage of healing, there are variable amounts of callus formation.

Differential Diagnosis

- Osteogenesis imperfecta (pediatric)
- Cardiopulmonary resuscitation (CPR)

Discussion

Osteogenesis imperfecta is a metabolic disorder that causes brittle bone disease. Patients with this disorder sustain fractures with relatively little trauma. Patients who have been resuscitated with CPR also may sustain rib fractures if chest compressions were performed, although these fractures tend to occur in a different location.

Diagnosis

Nonaccidental trauma—rib fracture

Suggested Readings

Maguire S, Mann M, John N, et al: Does cardiopulmonary resuscitation cause rib fractures in children? A systematic review. Child Abuse Negl 30:739-751, 2006.

Nimkin K, Kleinman PK: Imaging of child abuse. Radiol Clin North Am 39:843-864, 2001.

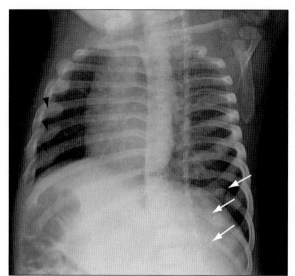

Figure 1. Right lateral oblique radiograph of the ribs shows multiple healing left-sided posterior rib fractures (*arrows*). This patient also had multiple right-sided anterolateral rib fractures (*arrowheads*).

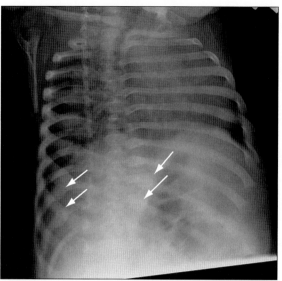

Figure 2. Left lateral oblique radiograph of the ribs better shows multiple healing bilateral posterior rib fractures (*arrows*).

Case 182

DEMOGRAPHICS/CLINICAL HISTORY

The patient is a 10-month-old boy with irritability, and swelling and tenderness of the left forearm.

FINDINGS

An anteroposterior radiograph of the wrist (Fig. 1) shows cupping, fraying, and widening of the distal metaphyses of the radius and ulna. The patient also sustained non-displaced fractures to the distal shafts of the radius and ulna, likely related to the precipitating injury. Over time, the metaphyseal changes normalized as the patient was treated with vitamin D replacement (Figs. 2 and 3).

DISCUSSION

Definition/Background

The patient presented 2 days after his older sister fell onto him. Laboratory analysis reveals critically low calcium of 5.4 mg/dL. The patient breastfeeds four to five times per day.

Characteristic Clinical Features

This infant was exclusively breastfed and was not receiving vitamin D supplementation.

Characteristic Radiologic Findings

Radiography shows metaphyseal cupping and fraying. Osteopenia also is apparent.

Differential Diagnosis

- Scurvy
- Renal osteodystrophy
- Osteogenesis imperfecta

Diagnosis

Rickets

Suggested Reading

Ecklund K, Doria AS, Jaramillo D: Rickets on MR images. Pediatr Radiol 29:673-675, 1999.

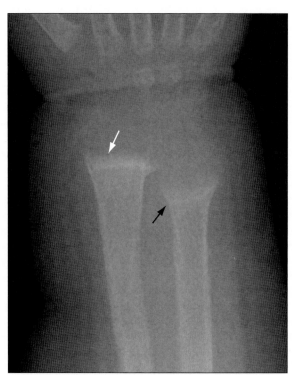

Figure 1. Anteroposterior radiograph of the wrist shows widening (*black arrow*), cupping, and fraying (*white arrow*) of the distal metaphyses of the radius and ulna. There is periosteal new bone formation along the distal radius and ulna with buckle fractures of the distal radius and ulna, likely related to the precipitating injury.

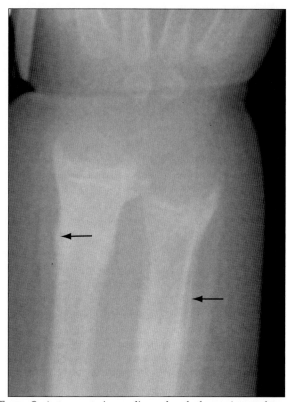

Figure 2. Anteroposterior radiograph of the wrist performed 3 weeks later after the patient was started on calcium replacement and vitamin D supplementation. There is persistent periosteal new bone formation (*arrows*). The zones of provisional calcification appear more dense, and the degree of metaphyseal irregularity has improved.

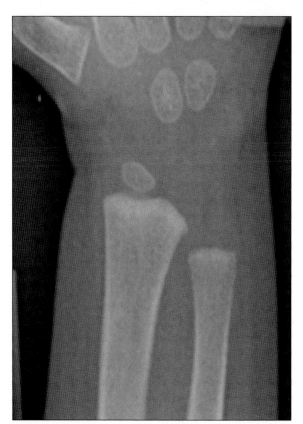

Figure 3. Anteroposterior radiograph of the wrist performed 1 year later. The distal radial and ulnar metaphyses now are normal.

Case 183

DEMOGRAPHICS/CLINICAL HISTORY

The patient is a 1-year-old girl with an abnormal gait.

FINDINGS

A standing anteroposterior radiograph (Fig. 1) of both legs shows bilateral, moderate genu varum deformities and bilateral widening and fraying of the distal femoral and proximal tibial metaphyses. A lateral radiograph (Fig. 2) of the knee better reveals metaphyseal cupping and fraying involving the distal femur and proximal tibia. A lateral radiograph (Fig. 3) of the humerus shows diffuse bony demineralization and a mild bowing deformity of the bone.

DISCUSSION

Definition/Background

This condition is an X-linked hypophosphatemia that causes a phosphate-wasting syndrome resulting from a deficiency in phosphate resorption in the proximal tubules of the kidney.

Characteristic Clinical Features

Patients usually present with short stature and bowing deformities of the legs.

Characteristic Radiologic Findings

Radiographs show abnormal bowing deformities of the extremities and rachitic changes in the femurs, tibias, and distal forearms. The appendicular skeleton appears mildly demineralized.

Less Common Radiologic Manifestations

Imaging may show looser zones or areas of pseudofracture that occur at sites of stress.

Differential Diagnosis

- Vitamin D–deficient rickets
- Renal tubular disease

Discussion

Type 1 vitamin D–deficient rickets is an autosomal recessive disorder that manifests with myopathy, hypocalcemia, moderate hypophosphatemia, secondary hyperparathyroidism, and subnormal concentrations of 1,25-dihydroxyvitamin D. The defect causing this form of rickets is absent or reduced activity of calcidiol 1-monooxygenase. Although skeletal deformities occur in hypophosphatemic rickets, hypocalcemia, myopathy, and tetany do not, and serum parathyroid hormone levels are normal. Hypophosphatemic rickets also can be caused by defects in renal tubular function that may be hereditary (i.e., familial hypophosphatemic rickets) or acquired.

Diagnosis

Hypophosphatemic rickets

Suggested Readings

Novais E, Stevens PM: Hypophosphatemic rickets: The role of hemi-epiphysiodesis. J Pediatr Orthop 26:238-244, 2006.

Shore RM, Langman CB, Poznanski AK: Lumbar and radial bone mineral density in children and adolescents with X-linked hypophosphatemia: Evaluation with dual x-ray absorptiometry. Skeletal Radiol 29:90-93, 2000.

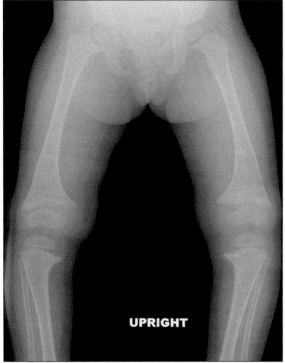

Figure 1. Standing anteroposterior radiograph of both legs shows moderate genu varum deformity bilaterally. There is bilateral widening and fraying of the distal femoral and proximal tibial metaphyses. Mild, convex, lateral bowing deformities of the femur are seen.

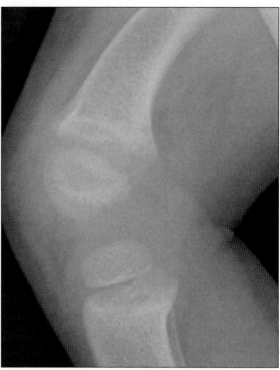

Figure 2. Lateral radiograph of knee better reveals metaphyseal cupping and fraying involving distal femur and proximal tibia.

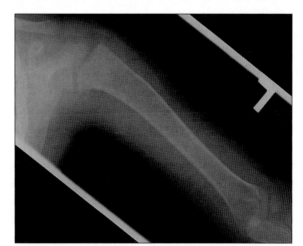

Figure 3. Lateral radiograph of humerus shows diffuse bony demineralization and mild bowing deformity of the bone.

Case 184

DEMOGRAPHICS/CLINICAL HISTORY

The patient is a 9-month-old girl with failure to thrive.

FINDINGS

Anteroposterior and lateral radiographs of the knee (Figs. 1 and 2) show diffuse osteopenia. The distal femoral epiphysis is centrally demineralized with a peripheral mineralized ring (i.e., Wimberger sign).

DISCUSSION

Definition/Background

The condition caused by lack of sufficient ascorbic acid (vitamin C) in the diet is known as scurvy.

Characteristic Clinical Features

Patients are usually older than 6 months. The diagnosis may be suggested on the basis of history and other dietary deficiencies, or children may present with focal bone pain or swelling related to fracture or subperiosteal hemorrhage.

Characteristic Radiologic Findings

Skeletal radiographs show a radiopaque line at the zone of provisional calcification (the white line of Frankel) with an adjacent radiolucent zone. The epiphyses appear demineralized with a peripheral mineralized ring (also called the Wimberger sign).

Less Common Radiologic Manifestations

The bones are brittle, and fractures are common. Subperiosteal hemorrhage is also associated with scurvy.

Differential Diagnosis
- Vitamin D–deficient rickets
- Congenital syphilis
- Osteogenesis imperfecta

Discussion

Rickets is caused by inadequate stores of vitamin D and is characterized by metaphyseal cupping and fraying at the zone of provisional calcification and diffuse osteopenia. Congenital syphilis is characterized by broad bands of metaphyseal radiolucency. Destructive change in the metaphyses of the proximal tibias is referred to as Wimberger sign. Osteogenesis imperfecta is characterized by decreased bone density with or without fractures, all related to a collagen abnormality.

Diagnosis

Scurvy

Suggested Reading

Weinstein M, Babyn P, Zlotkin S: An orange a day keeps the doctor away. Scurvy in the year 2000. Pediatrics 108:E55, 2001

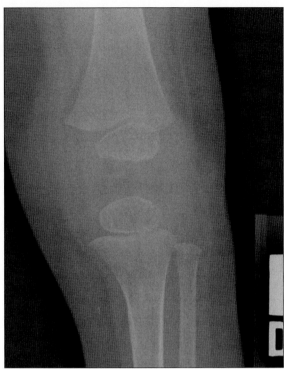

Figure 1. Anteroposterior radiograph of knee shows diffuse osteopenia. Distal femoral epiphysis is centrally demineralized with peripheral mineralized ring (i.e., Wimberger ring).

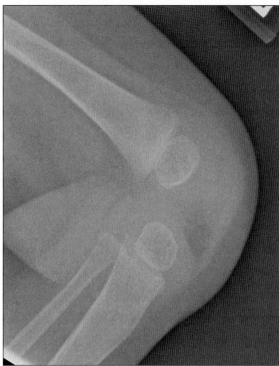

Figure 2. Lateral radiograph of knee shows diffuse osteopenia.

Case 185

DEMOGRAPHICS/CLINICAL HISTORY

The patient is a 2-month-old girl (born at 30 weeks' gestation) with blue sclerae and multiple fractures noticed at the time of birth.

FINDINGS

Plain radiographs of the axial and appendicular skeleton (Figs. 1-3) reveal many osseous fractures in various stages of healing and bowing deformities of the long bones. A lateral radiograph of the thoracic spine shows several compression fractures (Fig. 4).

DISCUSSION

Definition/Background

Osteogenesis imperfecta encompasses a large group of bone dysplasias characterized by a collagen abnormality that makes the bones brittle.

Characteristic Clinical Features

Patients present with many fractures. In severe cases, the diagnosis is made in utero based on ultrasound findings.

Characteristic Radiologic Findings

Radiographs of the bones reveal diffuse osteopenia with many fractures. The vertebral bodies may appear collapsed.

Less Common Radiologic Manifestations

Radiographs of the skull show many wormian bones.

Differential Diagnosis

- Child abuse

Diagnosis

Osteogenesis imperfecta, type III

Suggested Readings

Ablin DS: Osteogenesis imperfecta: A review. Can Assoc Radiol J 49:110-123, 1998.
Zeitlin L, Fassier F, Glorieux FH: Modern approach to children with osteogenesis imperfecta. J Pediatr Orthop B 12:77-87, 2003.

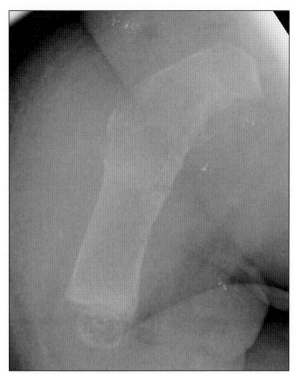

Figure 1. Lateral radiograph of right femur shows bowing deformity of bone with evidence of an old fracture.

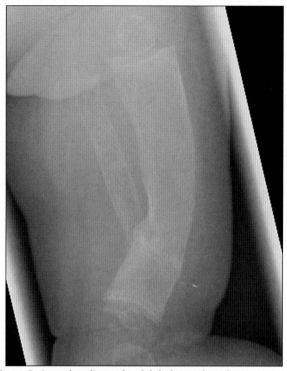

Figure 2. Lateral radiograph of left lower leg shows anterior bowing of tibia with several healing fractures.

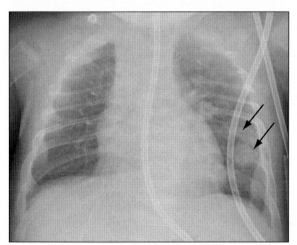

Figure 3. Anteroposterior radiograph of chest reveals several healing left posterior rib fractures (*arrows*).

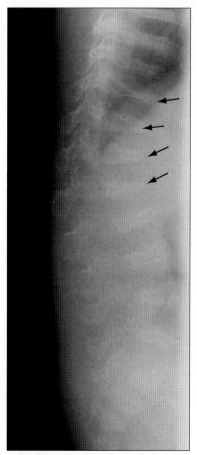

Figure 4. Lateral radiograph of vertebral column shows platyspondylisis at several levels (*arrows*).

Case 186

DEMOGRAPHICS/CLINICAL HISTORY

The patient is a 21-month-old boy with left facial swelling.

FINDINGS

An anteroposterior radiograph of the skull and facial bones shows a lucent lesion at the angle of the left mandible (Fig. 1). An axial image from a contrast-enhanced computed tomography (CT) scan of the face shows an enhancing mass with a soft tissue component causing destruction of the angle of the left mandible (Fig. 2).

DISCUSSION

Definition/Background

Langerhans cell histiocytosis (LCH) is a spectrum of disease that ranges from a localized osseous lesion to a fulminant, disseminated, multiorgan disorder. It is most common in whites, and boys are affected twice as frequently as girls.

Characteristic Clinical Features

Patients usually present with localized pain and swelling referable to a localized osseous lesion. Systemic symptoms may also be present.

Characteristic Radiologic Findings

Radiographic features of LCH lesions in the facial bones consist of a destructive lesion with an associated soft tissue mass. LCH in the long bones consists of an aggressive-appearing, lytic lesion with endosteal scalloping and cortical destruction. In the calvaria, the lesions have a "punched-out" appearance with a thin, sclerotic border.

Less Common Radiologic Manifestations

When LCH affects the vertebral body, a vertebra plana deformity ensues.

Differential Diagnosis

- Ewing sarcoma
- Primary lymphoma of bone
- Leukemia
- Osteomyelitis

Discussion

Ewing sarcoma is a malignancy of bone that often involves the metadiaphyseal region of long bones, although it can involve flat bones as well. Patients usually present with a lytic bone lesion with an associated soft tissue mass. Primary lymphoma of bone is a rare disease in children; it may manifest as a mixed lytic/sclerotic lesion in the metaphyses of long bones. Children with leukemia most often present with no radiographic abnormality, although the bones may appear diffusely osteopenic. More uncommonly, leukemia may manifest with a focal osseous lesion. Osteomyelitis is an infection of bone that may mimic an aggressive neoplasm. Although early radiographs are normal, radiographs 2 to 3 weeks into the infection show a permeative pattern of bone destruction that may mimic a neoplastic process.

Diagnosis

Langerhans cell histiocytosis of the mandible

Suggested Readings

Azouz EM, Saigal G, Rodriguez MM, et al: Langerhans' cell histiocytosis: Pathology, imaging and treatment of skeletal involvement. Pediatr Radiol 35:103-115, 2005.

Hoover KB, Rosenthal DI, Mankin H: Langerhans cell histiocytosis. Skeletal Radiol 36:95-104, 2007.

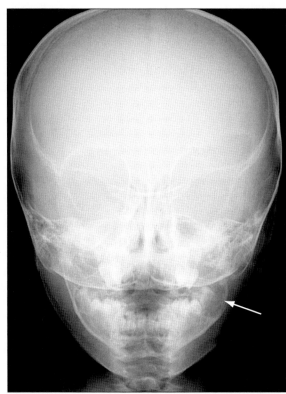

Figure 1. Anteroposterior radiograph of skull and facial bones shows lucent lesion at angle of left mandible (*arrow*).

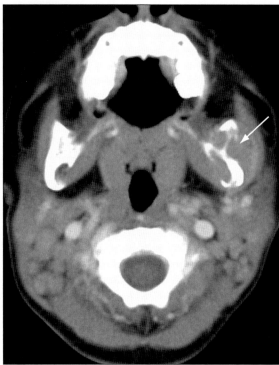

Figure 2. Axial image from contrast-enhanced CT scan of face shows enhancing mass with soft tissue component causing destruction of angle of left mandible (*arrow*).

Case 187

DEMOGRAPHICS/CLINICAL HISTORY

The patient is a 2-year-old boy with a mass adjacent to the right orbit.

FINDINGS

Computed tomography (CT) of the head (Figs. 1 and 2) shows a soft tissue mass centered within the right sphenoid bone with associated osseous destruction. T1-weighted fat-suppressed images obtained after administration of contrast agent from a magnetic resonance imaging (MRI) study through the orbits (Figs. 3 and 4) show heterogeneous enhancement of the mass.

DISCUSSION

Definition/Background
Langerhans cell histiocytosis (LCH) is a spectrum of disease that ranges from a localized osseous lesion to a fulminant, disseminated, multiorgan disorder. LCH is most common in whites, and boys are affected twice as frequently as girls.

Characteristic Clinical Features
Patients usually present with localized pain and swelling referable to a localized osseous lesion. Systemic symptoms also may be present.

Characteristic Radiologic Findings
Radiographic features of LCH lesions in the long bones consist of aggressive-appearing, lytic lesions with endosteal scalloping and cortical destruction. In the calvaria, the lesions have a "punched-out" appearance with a thin, sclerotic border.

Less Common Radiologic Manifestations
When LCH affects the vertebral body, a vertebra plana deformity ensues.

Differential Diagnosis
- Ewing sarcoma
- Primary lymphoma of bone
- Leukemia
- Osteomyelitis

Discussion
Ewing sarcoma is a malignant bone tumor that affects children usually in their teens. It has a predilection for long bones, and radiographic features include a permeative pattern of bone destruction and an associated soft tissue mass, findings that may mimic LCH. Primary lymphoma of bone is rare in children; when it occurs, it most commonly affects the lower extremities. Radiographs may reveal lytic or sclerotic or a mixed pattern of bone destruction, which is similar to that seen in Ewing sarcoma or other malignant bone lesions. Disseminated osseous involvement is a common finding in children with leukemia. More rarely, leukemia may manifest with a focal, destructive, lytic osseous lesion. A chloroma is a localized collection of granulocyte precursors that may involve bone. Osteomyelitis is an infection in bone that is often caused by a bacterial organism. Although the history and symptoms may suggest the correct diagnosis, the imaging features of osteomyelitis often mimic aggressive bone tumors.

Diagnosis
Langerhans cell histiocytosis

Suggested Readings
Azouz EM, Saigal G, Rodriguez MM, et al: Langerhans' cell histiocytosis: Pathology, imaging and treatment of skeletal involvement. Pediatr Radiol 35:103, 2005.

Hoover KB, Rosenthal DI, Mankin H: Langerhans cell histiocytosis. Skeletal Radiol 36:95, 2007.

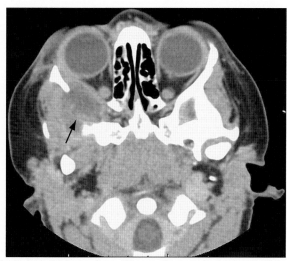

Figure 1. Axial image from CT scan through the brain reveals soft tissue mass centered within right sphenoid bone with destruction of underlying bone (*arrow*). The mass extends into retro-orbital fat with mild anterior displacement of globe.

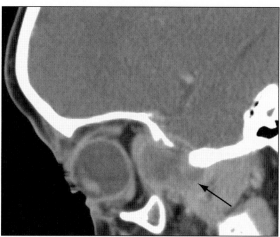

Figure 2. Sagittal reformatted image of right orbit from CT scan through the brain shows soft tissue mass with lytic destruction of sphenoid bone posterior to orbit (*arrow*).

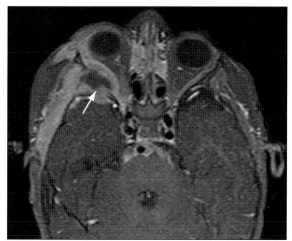

Figure 3. Axial T1-weighted fat-suppressed MR image through the brain after administration of intravenous contrast agent reveals heterogeneous enhancement of lesion (*arrow*).

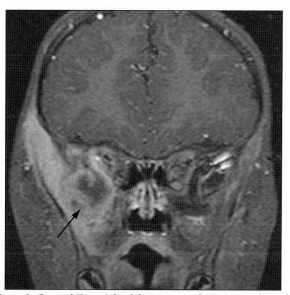

Figure 4. Coronal T1-weighted fat-suppressed MR image through the brain after administration of intravenous contrast agent reveals heterogeneous enhancement of retro-orbital mass within sphenoid bone (*arrow*).

Case 188

DEMOGRAPHICS/CLINICAL HISTORY

The patient is an 11-year-old boy with left hip pain.

FINDINGS

An anteroposterior radiograph of the pelvis (Fig. 1) shows a lucent lesion within the left sacrum. Magnetic resonance imaging (MRI) of the pelvis performed several days later reveals a multiloculated, cystic, expansile lesion within the left sacrum, which is dark on T1-weighted images (Fig. 2), is bright on T2-weighted images with multiple fluid-fluid levels (Fig. 3), and shows areas of internal enhancement after contrast agent administration (Fig. 4).

DISCUSSION

Definition/Background

Aneurysmal bone cyst (ABC) is a rare bone lesion that consists of blood-filled spaces; it may be a primary lesion, or secondarily arise within a preexisting bone lesion (approximately one third of ABCs arise within a preexisting lesion). The sexes are affected with nearly equal frequencies, with a peak incidence in the second decade of life.

Characteristic Clinical Features

ABC may involve any bone, although there is a propensity to involve the metaphyses of the long bones and the posterior elements of the spine. Presenting symptoms include pain and swelling.

Characteristic Radiologic Findings

Radiographic features of ABC include an eccentrically based, lytic lesion causing bony expansion.

Less Common Radiologic Manifestations

MRI shows multiple cystic cavities within the lesion with fluid-fluid levels and perilesional edema.

Differential Diagnosis

- Giant cell tumor
- Fibrous dysplasia
- Simple bone cyst
- Hemophilic pseudotumor
- Metastasis
- Telangiectatic osteosarcoma

Discussion

Giant cell tumor of bone most often occurs after skeletal maturity and appears as a lucent lesion within an epiphysis. Simple bone cysts most commonly occur in the metaphyses of the long bones, may contain septations, and are asymptomatic unless complicated by fracture. Metastasis may be secondary to many different primary neoplasms.

Diagnosis

Aneurysmal bone cyst (ABC)

Suggested Readings

Mahnken AH, Nolte-Ernsting CC, Wildberger JE, et al: Aneurysmal bone cyst: Value of MR imaging and conventional radiography. Eur Radiol 13:1118-1124, 2003.

Maiya S, Davies M, Evans N, et al: Surface aneurysmal bone cysts: A pictorial review. Eur Radiol 12:99-108, 2002.

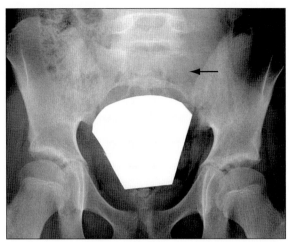

Figure 1. Anteroposterior radiograph of pelvis reveals lucent lesion in left sacrum (*arrow*).

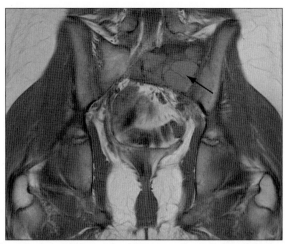

Figure 2. Coronal T1-weighted MR image through the pelvis shows well-circumscribed lesion with relatively low T1 signal (*arrow*).

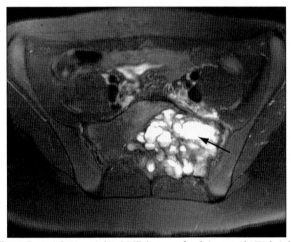

Figure 3. Axial T2-weighted MR image of pelvis reveals T2 bright lesion adjacent to left sacroiliac joint with multiple air-fluid levels (*arrow*).

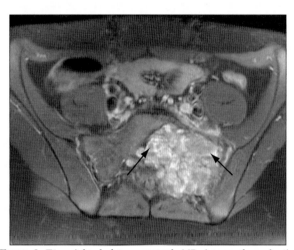

Figure 4. T1-weighted fat-suppressed MR image through the pelvis after intravenous contrast agent administration shows enhancement of multiple septations (*arrows*).

Case 189

DEMOGRAPHICS/CLINICAL HISTORY

The patient is a 13-year-old boy with a palpable lump on the right arm.

FINDINGS

Plain radiographs of the right humerus (Figs. 1 and 2) reveal a pedunculated, bony lesion arising from the anterolateral aspect of the proximal humerus. An axial T1-weighted image from a magnetic resonance imaging (MRI) examination shows the lesion to be contiguous with the marrow cavity of the humerus, and the mass has a thin, cartilaginous cap (Fig. 3).

DISCUSSION

Definition/Background
Osteochondromas are the most common of all bone tumors, and account for 10% to 15% of all bone tumors.

Characteristic Clinical Features
Most osteochondromas are asymptomatic and are discovered incidentally during childhood. New onset of pain related to an osteochondroma raises concern for malignant transformation.

Characteristic Radiologic Findings
Plain radiographs reveal a bony outgrowth, typically within the metaphyses of the long bones, which is projecting away from the joint. MRI reveals the continuity of the lesion with the underlying marrow cavity; on T2-weighted images, the cartilaginous cap shows high signal intensity.

Differential Diagnosis
- Chondrosarcoma
- Parosteal chondroma
- Trevor disease
- Parosteal osteosarcoma

Discussion
A chondrosarcoma is a malignant, cartilage-producing tumor. A parosteal chondroma is a surface variant of an enchondroma that is located beneath the periosteum and external to the cortex of the bone. In contrast to osteochondroma, the underlying cortex of the native bone appears scalloped and sclerotic. Trevor disease is also known as dysplasia epiphysealis hemimelica and is characterized by osteochondromas arising from the epiphyses, in contrast to the metaphyses. A parosteal osteosarcoma is a specific type of surface osteosarcoma with low malignant potential compared with other osteosarcomas.

Diagnosis
Osteochondroma

Suggested Readings
Brien EW, Mirra JM, Luck JV Jr: Benign and malignant cartilage tumors of bone and joint: Their anatomic and theoretical basis with an emphasis on radiology, pathology, and clinical biology, II: Juxtacortical cartilage tumors. Skeletal Radiol 28:1, 1999.

Woertler K: Benign bone tumors and tumor-like lesions: Value of cross-sectional imaging. Eur Radiol 13:1820, 2003.

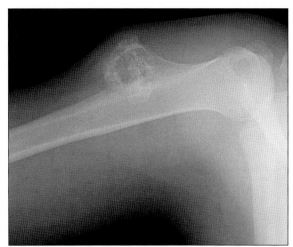

Figure 1. Lateral plain radiograph of right humerus reveals pedunculated, bony lesion arising from anterolateral aspect of proximal humerus.

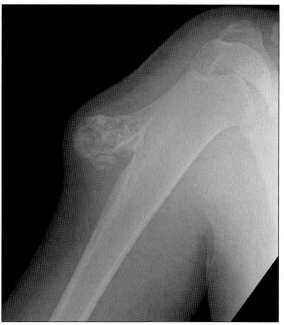

Figure 2. Anteroposterior plain radiograph of right humerus reveals pedunculated, bony lesion arising from anterolateral aspect of proximal humerus.

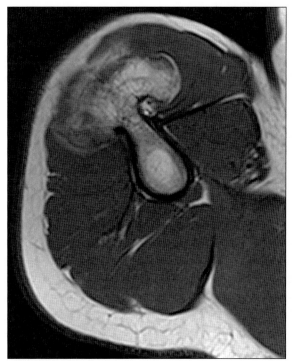

Figure 3. Axial T1-weighted MR image shows lesion to be contiguous with marrow cavity of humerus. The mass has a thin, cartilaginous cap.

Case 190

DEMOGRAPHICS/CLINICAL HISTORY

The patient is a 5-year-old girl with precocious puberty.

FINDINGS

A plain radiograph of the left hip (Fig. 1) reveals coxa vara deformity of the left hip and abnormal ground-glass opacity and a pathologic fracture through the left femoral neck. Computed tomography (CT) scans of the head (Figs. 2 and 3) show ground-glass expansion of the base of the skull, involving the sphenoid bone and maxillas. A radiograph of the left hand (Fig. 4) submitted for bone age analysis reveals the patient's bone age (approximately 12 years) to be far advanced relative to her chronologic age (5 years).

DISCUSSION

Definition/Background

Fibrous dysplasia is more common in girls than in boys. This patient presented early (5 years) compared with the typical age of presentation (second decade of life) likely because she had McCune-Albright syndrome, and the precocious puberty was the initial reason for seeking medical attention.

Characteristic Clinical Features

Although not all patients with fibrous dysplasia have other associated abnormalities, this patient had McCune-Albright syndrome (fibrous dysplasia, precocious puberty, café au lait spots). Most cases of fibrous dysplasia are monostotic, and these patients usually present with bone pain. Patients with polyostotic disease more often have an underlying syndrome, such as McCune-Albright syndrome.

Characteristic Radiologic Findings

Imaging studies show intramedullary bony expansion with ground-glass opacity within the bones. The femur is a common location for fibrous dysplasia to occur, and the coxa vara deformity that results is commonly referred to as a "shepherd's crook."

Differential Diagnosis

- Enchondromatosis
- Fibrous cortical defect
- Osteofibrous dysplasia
- Osteosarcoma (low-grade)

Discussion

A fibrous cortical defect is the most common benign tumor of bone, which is most often identified in the metaphyses of the long bones.

Diagnosis

Fibrous dysplasia

Suggested Readings

DiCaprio MR, Enneking WF: Fibrous dysplasia: Pathophysiology, evaluation, and treatment. J Bone Joint Surg Am 87:1848-1864, 2005.

Kransdorf MJ, Moser RP Jr, Gilkey FW: Fibrous dysplasia. RadioGraphics 10:519-537, 1990.

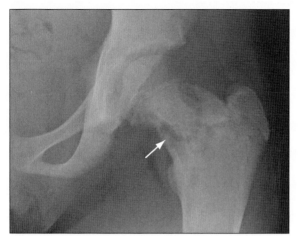

Figure 1. Anteroposterior radiograph of left hip shows coxa vara and abnormal ground-glass opacity within left femoral neck. There also is pathologic fracture through the femoral neck (*arrow*).

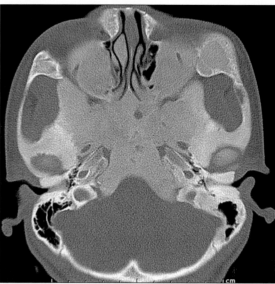

Figure 2. Axial CT scan through the brain shows ground-glass expansion of bones of the skull base, involving sphenoid bone, maxilla, and zygomatic arches bilaterally.

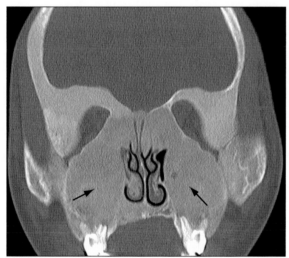

Figure 3. Coronal reformatted image from CT scan through the brain shows near-complete obliteration of maxillary sinuses by bony expansion (*arrows*), and involvement of the orbits bilaterally.

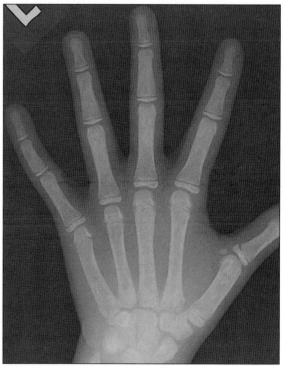

Figure 4. Anteroposterior radiograph of the left hand submitted for bone age analysis shows that the patient's bone age (approximately 12 years) is far advanced relative to her chronologic age (5 years).

Case 191

DEMOGRAPHICS/CLINICAL HISTORY

The patient is a 3-year-old girl with a limp and anterior leg swelling.

FINDINGS

A plain radiograph of the leg (Fig. 1) shows a lucent lesion within the anterior tibia that causes anterior tibial bowing. An axial image from a computed tomography (CT) scan through the lower leg (Fig. 2) confirms the intracortical location of the lesion and the cortical expansion. Contrast-enhanced T1-weighted magnetic resonance imaging (MRI) (Fig. 3) shows enhancement of the lesion with evidence of a single, thin septation.

DISCUSSION

Definition/Background

Osteofibrous dysplasia is a sporadic disease that most often occurs in the first decade of life.

Characteristic Clinical Features

Patients often present with a painless deformity affecting an extremity.

Characteristic Radiologic Findings

Plain radiographs show an eccentric, lucent, relatively well-defined lesion within the anterior cortex of the tibia, which leads to expansion of the cortex. There is associated cortical thickening and anterior bowing.

Differential Diagnosis
- Adamantinoma
- Fibrous dysplasia (pediatric)

Discussion

Adamantinoma is a rare, malignant-behaving lesion of bone that may be indistinguishable from osteofibrous dysplasia radiographically.

Diagnosis

Osteofibrous dysplasia

Suggested Readings

Campbell CJ, Hawk T: A variant of fibrous dysplasia (osteofibrous dysplasia). J Bone Joint Surg Am 64:231-236, 1982.

Levine SM, Lambiase RE, Petchprapa CN: Cortical lesions of the tibia: Characteristic appearances at conventional radiography. Radio-Graphics 23:157-177, 2003.

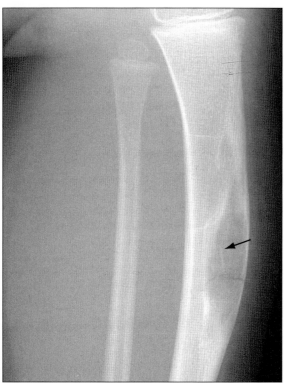

Figure 1. Lateral radiograph of lower leg shows eccentrically based, lucent lesion within the anterior, proximal tibia (*arrow*); there is also anterior tibial bowing.

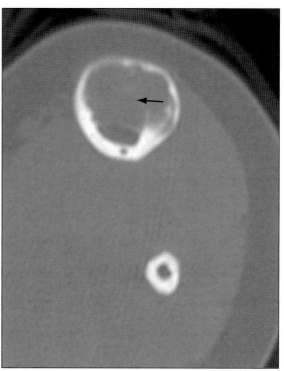

Figure 2. Axial CT image through the lower leg shows anterior cortical location of lesion (*arrow*) that is causing posterior cortical expansion replacing the intramedullary cavity.

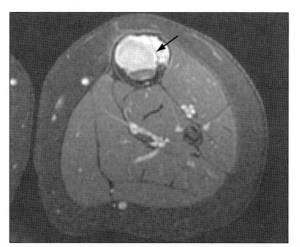

Figure 3. Axial T1-weighted fat-suppressed image from MRI examination through the lower leg after administration of intravenous contrast agent shows enhancement of lesion, with evidence of thin internal septation (*arrow*).

Case 192

DEMOGRAPHICS/CLINICAL HISTORY

The patient is a 3-year-old girl with prominent cheeks.

FINDINGS

Axial and coronal reformatted images from a computed tomography (CT) (Figs. 1 and 2) scan through the mandible show multiple expansile, lucent lesions replacing nearly the entire mandible.

DISCUSSION

Definition/Background
Cherubism is a benign childhood disease characterized by progressive, nontender enlargement of the jaw beginning around age 2 to 3 years.

Characteristic Clinical Features
Patients present early in childhood (2 to 3 years old) with painless progressive enlargement of the mandible bilaterally that gives the face a "cherubic" appearance.

Characteristic Radiologic Findings
CT shows expansile remodeling of the bones, often with a mildly sclerotic matrix and cortical thinning. The lesions are limited to the mandible and maxilla.

Differential Diagnosis
- Craniofacial fibrous dysplasia
- Brown tumors of hyperparathyroidism
- Jaffe-Campanacci syndrome

Discussion
Fibrous dysplasia is a benign lesion of bone with a ground-glass matrix that appears similar to the lesions in cherubism, although genetic analysis has revealed that cherubism and fibrous dysplasia are not the same. Brown tumors are expansile, lucent lesions of the bone that occur in the setting of hyperparathyroidism, and that are often located in the hands. Jaffe-Campanacci syndrome is a syndrome characterized by multiple lucent bone lesions that are nonossifying fibromas in association with mental retardation, hypogonadism or cryptorchidism, café au lait spots, and ocular and cardiovascular abnormalities.

Diagnosis
Cherubism

Suggested Reading
Beaman FD, Bancroft LW, Peterson JJ, et al: Imaging characteristics of cherubism. AJR Am J Roentgenol 182:1051-1054, 2004.

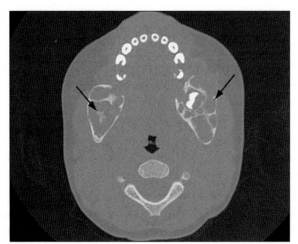

Figure 1. Axial CT image through the mandible shows multiple expansile, lucent lesions replacing nearly the entire mandible (*arrows*).

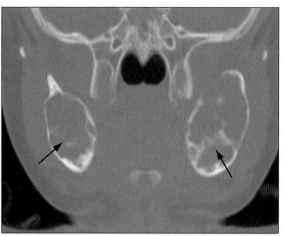

Figure 2. Coronal reformatted CT image through the mandible shows multiple expansile, lucent lesions replacing nearly the entire mandible (*arrows*).

Case 193

DEMOGRAPHICS/CLINICAL HISTORY

The patient is a 5-year-old boy with neck pain.

FINDINGS

A lateral radiograph of the cervical spine (Fig. 1) shows a lucent, expansile lesion in the C2 spinous process. Axial computed tomography (CT) image through the C2 spinous process (Fig. 2) better shows the expansile lytic lesion with internal matrix. Axial T1-weighted magnetic resonance imaging (MRI) (Fig. 3) before contrast agent administration shows the soft tissue mass replacing the spinous process of C2, and infiltration of the fat of the posterior paravertebral soft tissues. Homogeneous enhancement of the mass can be seen on postcontrast axial T1-weighted fat-saturated MRI (Fig. 4). The posterior paravertebral soft tissues show enhancement without a focal mass, reflecting inflammation.

DISCUSSION

Definition/Background
Osteoblastoma is a benign, osteoid-producing tumor that is commonly found in the posterior elements of the spine.

Characteristic Clinical Features
Patients typically present with pain with or without scoliosis. They may have nerve root symptoms if the mass encroaches the neural foramen.

Characteristic Radiologic Findings
On radiographs, an osteoblastoma can be seen as an expansile, lucent lesion, typically in the posterior elements. CT better delineates the well-defined lesion, with a rim of bony sclerosis surrounding the lytic expansile mass and internal calcified matrix. MRI shows enhancement of the mass and often shows adjacent bony and soft tissue inflammation. Osteoblastomas have been associated with aneurysmal bone cysts, and cystic compartments with fluid-fluid levels may be seen in those cases.

Less Common Radiologic Manifestations
Osteoblastomas are rarely within the vertebral bodies, but it does occur.

Differential Diagnosis
- Aneurysmal bone cyst
- Osteosarcoma

Discussion
Aneurysmal bone cysts have many septations with fluid-fluid levels, and they can be associated with osteoblastomas, but they do not have the same enhancement as osteoblastomas. Osteosarcomas tend to have a more aggressive appearance with less definition, more osteoid formation, and a soft tissue mass.

Diagnosis
Osteoblastoma of the spine

Suggested Readings
Ozkal E, Erongun U, Cakir B, et al: CT and MR imaging of vertebral osteoblastoma: A report of two cases. Clin Imaging 20:37-41, 1996.

Shaikh MI, Saifuddin A, Pringle J, et al: Spinal osteoblastoma: CT and MR imaging with pathological correlation. Skeletal Radiol 28:33-40, 1999.

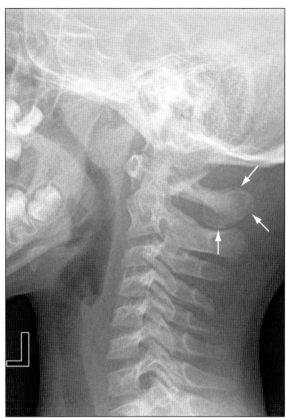

Figure 1. Lateral radiograph of cervical spine shows lucent, expansile lesion in C2 spinous process (*arrows*).

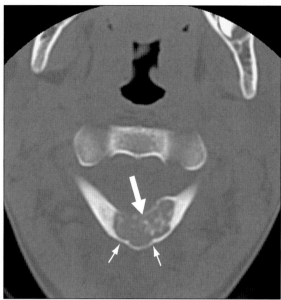

Figure 2. Axial CT image through C2 spinous process better shows expansile lytic lesion (*small arrows*) with internal matrix (*large arrow*).

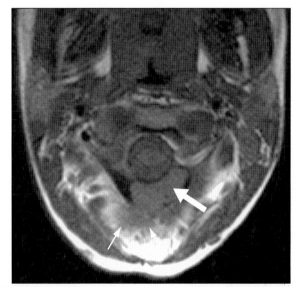

Figure 3. Axial T1-weighted MR image before contrast agent administration shows soft tissue mass (*large arrow*) replacing spinous process of C2. *Small arrows* in posterior paravertebral soft tissues show infiltration of the fat.

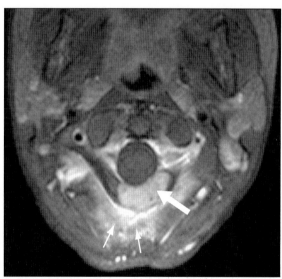

Figure 4. Postcontrast axial T1-weighted fat-saturated MR image shows homogeneous enhancement of mass (*large arrow*). Posterior paravertebral soft tissues show enhancement without a focal mass (*small arrows*), indicating inflammation.

Case 194

DEMOGRAPHICS/CLINICAL HISTORY

The patient is a 5-year-old boy with a lucent lesion incidentally noticed on radiographs of the hip.

FINDINGS

An anteroposterior radiograph of the left hip (Fig. 1) shows abnormal lucent lesions within the femoral neck, proximal femoral shaft, and superior pubic ramus. Anteroposterior radiographs of both hands (Figs. 2 and 3) show multiple lucent lesions within the metacarpals and phalanges, associated soft tissue masses, and cortical irregularity.

DISCUSSION

Definition/Background

Enchondromatosis, also called Ollier disease, is a nonheritable disease with enchondromas of multiple bones. It is more common in boys.

Characteristic Clinical Features

The hands are most commonly involved with the disease, although any bone with a physis can be affected. Early onset may lead to skeletal deformity and limb shortening.

Characteristic Radiologic Findings

Radiographic features of Ollier disease include multiple, expansile, lucent bony lesions.

Differential Diagnosis

- Maffucci syndrome

Discussion

Maffucci syndrome, sometimes called Kast syndrome, consists of multiple enchondromas with associated cutaneous or visceral hemangiomas, which help to differentiate it from Ollier disease.

Diagnosis

Enchondromatosis

Suggested Readings

Al-Ismail K, Torreggiani WC, Munk PL, et al: Ollier's disease in association with adjacent fibromatosis. Skeletal Radiol 31:479-483, 2002.

Brien EW, Mirra JM, Kerr R: Benign and malignant cartilage tumors of bone and joint: Their anatomic and theoretical basis with an emphasis on radiology, pathology, and clinical biology, 1: The intramedullary cartilage tumors. Skeletal Radiol 26:325-352, 1997.

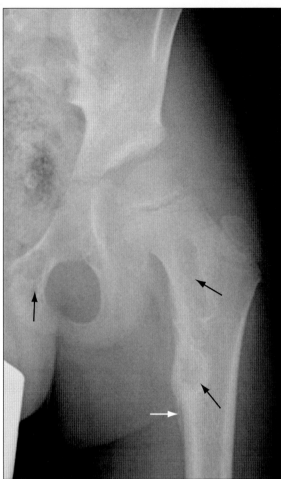

Figure 1. Anteroposterior radiograph of left hip reveals multiple lucent lesions within proximal femur and superior pubic ramus (*black arrows*). Periosteal new bone formation along proximal femur after pathologic fracture is visible (*white arrow*).

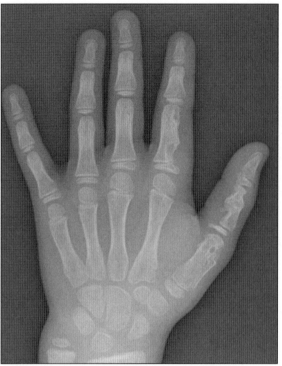

Figure 2. Anteroposterior radiograph of left hand reveals multiple lucent lesions affecting phalanges and metacarpals with associated cortical irregularity and soft tissue masses.

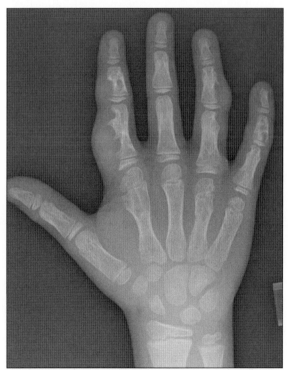

Figure 3. Anteroposterior radiograph of right hand reveals multiple lucent lesions affecting phalanges and metacarpals with associated cortical irregularity and soft tissue masses.

Case 195

DEMOGRAPHICS/CLINICAL HISTORY

The patient is a 4-year-old boy who fell and injured the left knee 4 days ago.

FINDINGS

A plain radiograph of the knee reveals bony exostoses arising from the medial femoral condyle and medial tibial plateau (Fig. 1). Magnetic resonance imaging (MRI) of the knee reveals the lesions to be contiguous with the epiphyses, and shows the presence of overlying cartilage (Fig. 2).

DISCUSSION

Definition/Background

Trevor disease is a rare childhood disorder characterized by overgrowth of the epiphyseal cartilage in long bones, which affects boys more commonly than girls. Patients typically present within the first decade of life with pain or swelling. The patient in this case had no prior history of knee problems.

Characteristic Clinical Features

This patient underwent resection of the intra-articular osteochondroma from the left femur for relief of symptoms. Symptomatic lesions seen in Trevor disease are treated with resection. If there are no symptoms referable to a lesion, the lesion is treated conservatively.

Characteristic Radiologic Findings

Plain radiographs reveal an irregular, lobulated, calcific mass associated with one side (medial or lateral) of the epiphysis of a long bone, commonly in the lower extremity. Medial involvement is more common than lateral involvement. The affected ossification center usually appears prematurely.

Less Common Radiologic Manifestations

MRI is useful for delineating the extent of epiphyseal involvement.

Differential Diagnosis

- Osteochondroma
- Myositis ossificans
- Tumoral calcinosis

Discussion

Tumoral calcinosis refers to deposition of masslike calcifications in the soft tissues adjacent to joints. It is a benign condition of unknown pathogenesis, and patients most often present with a painless mass.

Diagnosis

Trevor disease

Suggested Readings

Glick R, Khaldi L, Ptaszynski K, et al: Dysplasia epiphysealis hemimelica (Trevor disease): A rare developmental disorder of bone mimicking osteochondroma of long bones. Hum Pathol 38:1265-1272, 2007.

Iwasawa T, Aida N, Kobayashi N, et al: MRI findings of dysplasia epiphysealis hemimelica. Pediatr Radiol 26:65-67, 1996.

Lang IM, Azouz EM: MRI appearances of dysplasia epiphysealis hemimelica of the knee. Skeletal Radiol 26:226-229, 1997.

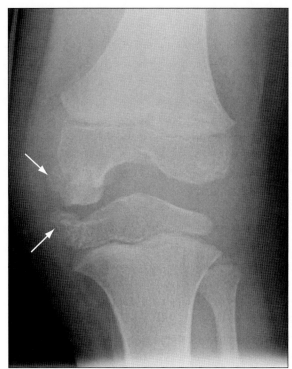

Figure 1. Anteroposterior radiograph of left knee reveals exostosis arising from medial condyle of distal femur and a second lesion arising from proximal tibial epiphysis (*arrows*).

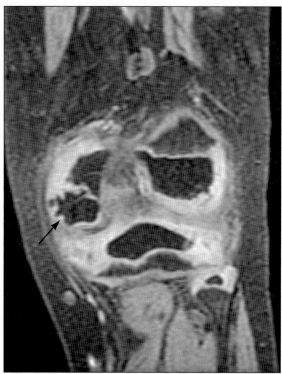

Figure 2. Coronal spoiled gradient-recalled-echo MRI sequence through lesion arising from medial femoral condyle reveals that lesion is contiguous with medial femoral condyle, is isointense in signal as adjacent condyle, and has overlying cartilage (*arrow*).

Case 196

DEMOGRAPHICS/CLINICAL HISTORY

The patient is an 11-year-old boy with left arm pain.

FINDINGS

A plain radiograph of the left humerus (Fig. 1) reveals a sessile, broad-based bony lesion arising from the posterior aspect of the proximal humerus. Magnetic resonance imaging (MRI) (Figs. 2 and 3) shows the lesion to be contiguous with the marrow cavity of the humerus, and the mass has a thin, cartilaginous cap.

DISCUSSION

Definition/Background

Osteochondromas are the most common of all bone tumors; they account for 10% to 15% of bone tumors.

Characteristic Clinical Features

Most osteochondromas are asymptomatic and are discovered incidentally during childhood. New onset of pain related to an osteochondroma raises concern about malignant transformation.

Characteristic Radiologic Findings

Plain radiographs reveal a bony outgrowth, typically within the metaphyses of the long bones, which projects away from the joint. MRI reveals the continuity of the lesion with the underlying marrow cavity. On T2-weighted MR images, the cartilaginous cap shows high signal intensity.

Differential Diagnosis

- Chondrosarcoma
- Parosteal chondroma
- Trevor disease
- Parosteal osteosarcoma

Discussion

A chondrosarcoma is a malignant, cartilage-producing tumor. A parosteal chondroma is a surface variant of an enchondroma that is located beneath the periosteum and external to the cortex of the bone. In contrast to osteochondroma, the underlying cortex of the native bone appears scalloped and sclerotic.

Diagnosis

Osteochondroma

Suggested Readings

Brien EW, Mirra JM, Luck JV Jr: Benign and malignant cartilage tumors of bone and joint: Their anatomic and theoretical basis with an emphasis on radiology, pathology, and clinical biology, II: Juxtacortical cartilage tumors. Skeletal Radiol 28:1-20, 1999.

Woertler K: Benign bone tumors and tumor-like lesions: Value of cross-sectional imaging. Eur Radiol 13.1020 1835, 2003.

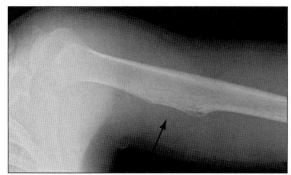

Figure 1. Lateral radiograph of humerus shows broad-based bony lesion arising from posterior aspect of proximal humerus (*arrow*).

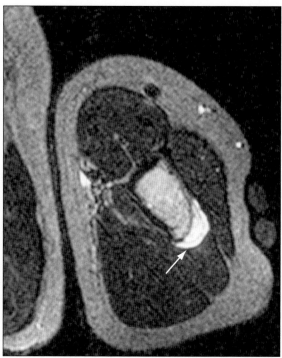

Figure 2. Axial fast spin-echo inversion recovery MR image through lesion shows that mass is contiguous with marrow cavity of humerus. A thin, cartilaginous cap that has bright signal intensity (*arrow*) is apparent.

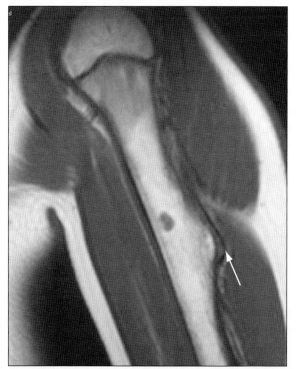

Figure 3. Sagittal T1-weighted MR image through humerus shows that lesion is predominantly isointense in signal to underlying marrow cavity except for low signal intensity cartilage cap (*arrow*).

Case 197

DEMOGRAPHICS/CLINICAL HISTORY

The patient is a 13-year-old boy with right-sided hip pain.

FINDINGS

A plain radiograph of the right hip (Fig. 1) reveals a well-circumscribed lucent lesion within the femoral epiphysis. A computed tomography (CT) scan through the lesion in the right femoral head (Fig. 2) shows a well-circumscribed, round lesion with internal calcifications. On magnetic resonance imaging (MRI), the lesion contains several punctate foci of low T1 (Fig. 3) and T2 signal (Fig. 4).

DISCUSSION

Definition/Background
Chondroblastoma is a rare primary tumor of bone with an incidence of less than 1% of primary bone tumors. It is usually cured with conservative measures.

Characteristic Clinical Features
Patients with chondroblastoma present with pain, likely secondary to the strong inflammatory response invoked by the tumor.

Characteristic Radiologic Findings
The foci of low T2 signal on MRI are likely accounted for by areas of calcification or highly cellular chondroid matrix. Typical MRI findings also include prominent bone marrow edema, which often is misleading and raises concern for a more aggressive lesion.

Less Common Radiologic Manifestations
On plain radiography and CT, punctate calcifications may be detected within the lesion. Periosteal reaction also may be an associated finding.

Differential Diagnosis
- Brodie abscess
- Giant cell tumor

Discussion
Giant cell tumor is an uncommon osseous tumor that most often occurs after skeletal maturity. Giant cell tumors are located within the epiphyses, usually abutting the joint surfaces.

Diagnosis
Chondroblastoma

Suggested Readings
Kaim AH, Hugli R, Bonel HM, et al: Chondroblastoma and clear cell chondrosarcoma: Radiological and MRI characteristics with histopathological correlation. Skeletal Radiol 31:88-95, 2002.

Weatherall PT, Maale GE, Mendelsohn DB, et al: Chondroblastoma: Classic and confusing appearance at MR imaging. Radiology 190:467-474, 1994.

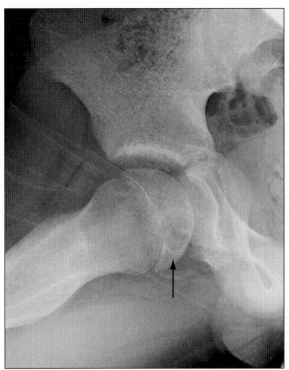

Figure 1. Frog-leg lateral radiograph of right hip shows well-defined lucent lesion within femoral epiphysis, which abuts physis (*arrow*).

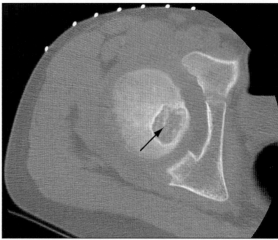

Figure 2. Axial image from CT scan through right hip better shows well-defined margins of lesion and presence of internal chondroid matrix with tiny punctate calcifications (*arrow*). (The grid marks on the patient's skin relate to the fact that this study was performed in preparation for a biopsy of the lesion).

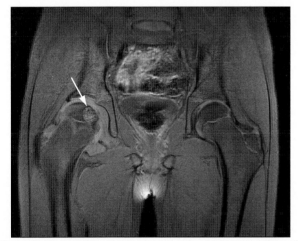

Figure 3. Coronal T1-weighted fat-suppressed MR image through hips and pelvis shows increased signal within lesion with punctate areas of low signal intensity (*arrow*).

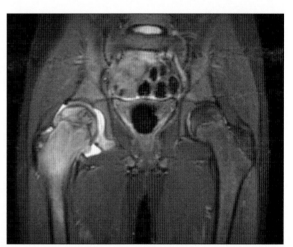

Figure 4. Coronal short tau inversion recovery (STIR) sequence from MRI examination through hips reveals substantial amount of bone marrow edema within femoral head and neck surrounding lesion.

Case 198

DEMOGRAPHICS/CLINICAL HISTORY

The patient is a 3-year-old boy with right thigh pain, mostly at night, which responds to ibuprofen (Motrin), who has started limping secondary to the pain.

FINDINGS

A plain radiograph of the hips and pelvis (Fig. 1) reveals a subtle lucency within the right medial femoral neck with an internal sclerotic focus. A bone scan (Fig. 2) reveals increased uptake of radiotracer in the same region along the right medial femoral neck. Computed tomography (CT) (Figs. 3 and 4) confirms the findings, and shows the lucent lesion in the femoral neck and the central sclerotic focus, which represents osteoid osteoma.

DISCUSSION

Definition/Background

Osteoid osteoma most commonly occurs in male patients, such as the patient in this case. This patient presented at a young age (3 years old); most patients are 10 to 20 years old.

Characteristic Clinical Features

Patients with osteoid osteoma commonly present with a history of nighttime pain that is relieved by nonsteroidal anti-inflammatory drugs.

Characteristic Radiologic Findings

The classic appearance of an osteoid osteoma, as in this case, is a lucent lesion (which represents the nidus of the osteoid osteoma) surrounded by sclerotic bone. There is often a central sclerotic focus within the nidus, as in this case, although this is not required. Osteoid osteomas commonly occur in the femoral neck.

Differential Diagnosis

- Osteoblastoma
- Osteomyelitis
- Stress fracture

Discussion

A stress fracture is an injury of overuse, typically seen in athletes or patients who are highly active. Although a fracture lucency may be detected on radiographs or CT, which should suggest the diagnosis, often only a dense sclerotic reaction with new periosteal bone formation is present, making this entity difficult to distinguish from osteoid osteoma.

Diagnosis

Osteoid osteoma

Suggested Readings

Kayser F, Resnick D, Haghighi P, et al: Evidence of the subperiosteal origin of osteoid osteomas in tubular bones: Analysis by CT and MR imaging. AJR Am J Roentgenol 170:609-614, 1998.

Kransdorf MJ, Stull MA, Gilkey FW, et al: Osteoid osteoma. Radio-Graphics 11:671-696, 1991.

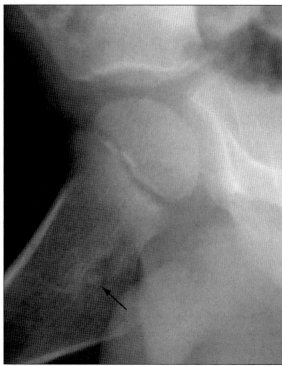

Figure 1. Frog-leg lateral radiograph of right hip reveals subtle sclerotic focus along medial aspect of femoral neck with central sclerotic focus (*arrow*).

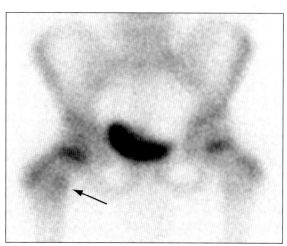

Figure 2. Bone scan performed after administration of an intravenous radiolabeled tracer shows increased uptake within right femoral neck, corresponding to site of abnormality on plain radiograph (*arrow*).

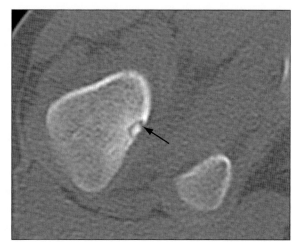

Figure 3. Axial image from CT scan through right femoral neck clearly shows well-defined lucency with central sclerotic focus (*arrow*).

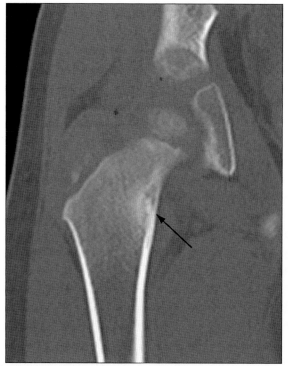

Figure 4. Coronal reformatted image from CT scan through right femur shows abnormal lucent lesion (*arrow*).

Case 199

DEMOGRAPHICS/CLINICAL HISTORY

The patient is a 2-year-old boy with left calf pain that began 2 months ago, but acutely worsened in the past week.

FINDINGS

Plain radiographs of the lower extremities show diffuse osteopenia with metaphyseal lucent bands (Fig. 1) and periosteal new bone formation (Fig. 2). Magnetic resonance imaging (MRI) of the lower extremities reveals a highly cellular bone marrow that is uniformly dark on T1-weighted sequences (Fig. 3) and bright on T2-weighted sequences (Fig. 4).

DISCUSSION

Definition/Background
This patient presented with left calf pain that began 2 months ago, but acutely worsened in the past week. The pain was accompanied by limping and dragging of the left leg and caused the child to awaken at night. Peripheral smear was consistent with acute lymphoblastic leukemia.

Characteristic Clinical Features
Patients may complain of nonspecific bone pain, and radiographs are often normal.

Characteristic Radiologic Findings
Radiographs are often normal, although in some cases imaging reveals the characteristic metaphyseal lucencies associated with the disease.

Differential Diagnosis
- Extramedullary hematopoiesis

Diagnosis
Bone changes in leukemia

Suggested Readings
Gallagher DJ, Phillips DJ, Heinrich SD: Orthopedic manifestations of acute pediatric leukemia. Orthop Clin North Am 27:635-644, 1996.
Rogalsky RJ, Black GB, Reed MH: Orthopaedic manifestations of leukemia in children. J Bone Joint Surg Am 68:494-501, 1986.

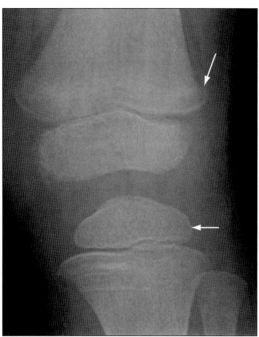

Figure 1. Anteroposterior radiograph of left knee reveals subtle metaphyseal lucencies (*arrows*) within distal femur, proximal tibia, and fibula, which can be seen in the setting of leukemia.

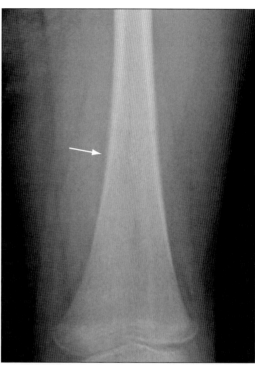

Figure 2. Magnified anteroposterior radiograph of distal femur reveals subtle periosteal new bone formation (*arrow*).

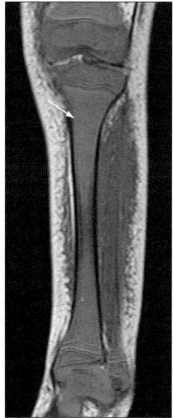

Figure 3. Coronal T1-weighted MR image of lower extremity shows diffuse signal abnormality within intramedullary portions of visualized bones consistent with leukemic infiltration (*arrow*).

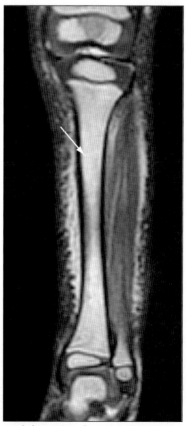

Figure 4. Coronal fast spin-echo inversion recovery MR image through lower leg shows diffuse high signal filling marrow spaces (*arrow*), consistent with leukemic infiltration.

Case 200

DEMOGRAPHICS/CLINICAL HISTORY

The patient is a 5-year-old girl, otherwise healthy, noted to have a mass in the posterior right thigh.

FINDINGS

Magnetic resonance imaging (MRI) of the right thigh shows a well-circumscribed, round mass within the adductor muscles (Figs. 1-4). The mass is bright on T2-weighted MRI (see Fig. 1) and isointense to muscle on T1-weighted MRI with internal T1-bright foci (see Fig. 2).

DISCUSSION

Definition/Background
The mass in this healthy patient is asymptomatic.

Characteristic Clinical Features
The mass was resected, and the patient is disease-free 1 year after excision. MRI showed no recurrence.

Characteristic Radiologic Findings
Imaging shows a well-circumscribed mass with fat signal intensity in some areas.

Less Common Radiologic Manifestations
In some cases, such as this one, there is little fat signal within the lesion.

Differential Diagnosis
- Lipoma
- Liposarcoma

Discussion
A lipoma is a benign mass composed nearly entirely of fat, typically located within the soft tissues. A liposarcoma is a malignant mass that contains various amounts of fat.

Diagnosis
Lipoblastoma

Suggested Readings

Moholkar S, Sebire NJ, Roebuck DJ: Radiological-pathological correlation in lipoblastoma and lipoblastomatosis. Pediatr Radiol 36:851-856, 2006.

Murphey MD, Carroll JF, Flemming DJ, et al: From the archives of the AFIP: Benign musculoskeletal lipomatous lesions. RadioGraphics 24:1433-1466, 2004.

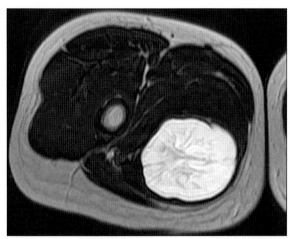

Figure 1. Axial T2-weighted MR image through the right thigh shows well-circumscribed mass within adductor muscles that has homogeneous bright signal.

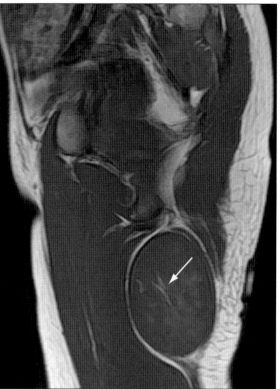

Figure 2. Sagittal T1-weighted MR image reveals well-circumscribed mass within right thigh that is isointense to muscle with areas of increased signal intensity within (arrow).

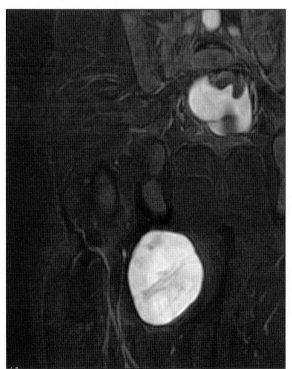

Figure 3. Coronal short tau inversion recovery (STIR) MR image shows well-circumscribed mass within adductor muscles with increased signal intensity relative to surrounding muscles.

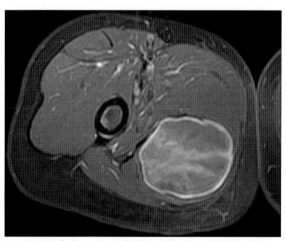

Figure 4. Axial fat-saturated T1-weighted MR image through lesion after intravenous gadolinium administration reveals heterogeneous enhancement of mass.

Case 201

DEMOGRAPHICS/CLINICAL HISTORY

The patient is an 8-year-old boy with ankle pain and swelling.

FINDINGS

Plain radiographs of the ankle show a permeative pattern of lytic destruction involving the distal shaft of the fibula (Fig. 1). Magnetic resonance imaging (MRI) of the ankle reveals a soft tissue mass involving the distal tibia, but excluding the distal epiphysis (Figs. 2 and 3). This mass enhances after gadolinium administration (Fig. 4).

DISCUSSION

Definition/Background

Each of the Ewing family of tumors, including Ewing sarcoma, extraosseous Ewing sarcoma, primitive neuroectodermal tumors, and Askin tumor of the thorax, has a reciprocal translocation of chromosomes 11 and 22.

Characteristic Clinical Features

Patients commonly present with pain.

Characteristic Radiologic Findings

Ewing sarcoma most often occurs in the lower extremity and favors the metadiaphysis of long bones. An "onion skin" periosteal reaction commonly is associated with Ewing sarcoma.

Less Common Radiologic Manifestations

The imaging appearance of the tumor may be lytic, mixed lytic and blastic, or sclerotic. A soft tissue mass usually is identified, although not in all cases.

Differential Diagnosis

- Osteosarcoma (pediatric)
- Osteomyelitis (pediatric)

Diagnosis

Ewing sarcoma

Suggested Readings

Bloem JL, Blemm RG, Taminiau AH, et al: Magnetic resonance imaging of primary malignant bone tumors. RadioGraphics 7:425-445, 1987.

Meyer JS, Mackenzie W: Malignant bone tumors and limb-salvage surgery in children. Pediatr Radiol 34:606-613, 2004.

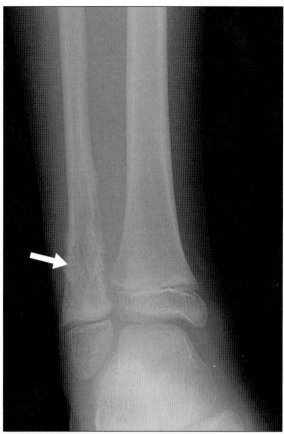

Figure 1. Anteroposterior view of ankle reveals permeative pattern of lytic bone destruction involving distal fibula (*arrow*).

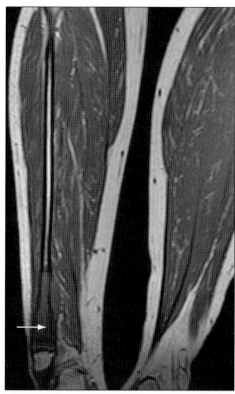

Figure 2. Coronal T1-weighted MR image of ankle reveals abnormal process of marrow replacement involving distal fibular meta-diaphysis, causing bony destruction and expansion (*arrow*).

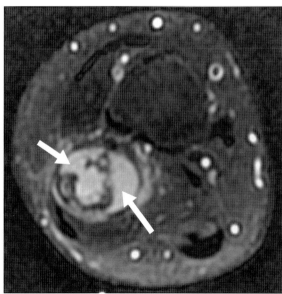

Figure 3. Axial T2-weighted fat-saturated MR image of ankle shows abnormal high signal intensity within distal fibula, which is associated with cortical breakthrough (*long arrow*), and extraosseous soft tissue mass (*short arrow*).

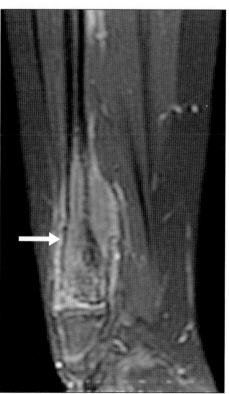

Figure 4. Coronal T1-weighted MR image with fat suppression after administration of intravenous gadolinium reveals enhancement of mass (*arrow*).

Case 202

DEMOGRAPHICS/CLINICAL HISTORY

The patient is a 9-year-old girl with intermittent left leg pain for the past several months and increased left calf and knee pain after a fall, with no past history of trauma.

FINDINGS

A plain radiograph of the knee (Fig. 1) reveals an ill-defined, lytic lesion within the distal femoral metaphysis, with cortical destruction and periosteal reaction. Magnetic resonance imaging (MRI) of the lesion shows multiple, fluid-filled cavities with fluid-fluid levels (Fig. 2) and enhancing septations (Fig. 3).

DISCUSSION

Definition/Background
Telangiectatic osteosarcoma is an unusual subtype of osteosarcoma that makes up approximately 12% of all osteosarcomas. It occurs with a male-to-female ratio of 2:1. Most patients are 10 to 20 years old at presentation.

Characteristic Clinical Features
The symptoms are nonspecific, but include pain in the involved limb.

Characteristic Radiologic Findings
Plain radiographs show a metaphyseal lesion with geographic bone destruction with a wide zone of transition, periosteal reaction, and cortical destruction. MRI reveals areas of hemorrhage as foci of high signal intensity on all pulse sequences and shows fluid levels.

Differential Diagnosis
- Aneurysmal bone cyst (ABC)
- Osteosarcoma

Discussion
Aneurysmal bone cysts are benign, expansile, osteolytic lesions. They are associated with trauma in many cases, but they are a component of or arise in a bone tumor in about one third of cases. Although any bone may be affected, the most common site is the metaphyseal region of the knee. Radiographic findings include an eccentric, central, or subperiosteal lesion that appears cystic or lytic; expansion of the surrounding bone with a blown-out, ballooned, or soap-bubble appearance; an eggshell-like bony rim surrounding the lesion; blood-filled cystic spaces; and, rarely, partially ossified septa. Telangiectatic osteosarcoma has a rim of tumor cells that surrounds the cystic spaces; an aneurysmal bone cyst does not. On computed tomography (CT), the tissue rim shows typically nodular enhancement after intravenous administration of contrast agent.

Osteosarcoma is the most common primary malignant bone tumor in children and adolescents. Approximately 75% of all osteosarcomas are the classic type, and telangiectatic osteosarcoma, considered to be a variant of the classic form, accounts for 0.4% to 12% of cases in various series. Telangiectatic osteosarcoma usually appears radiographically as a lytic mass lesion in the metaphyseal portion of the long bones. It has dilated, blood-filled vascular spaces lined by malignant osteoblasts, which are separated by fibrous septa that contain the malignant cells, multinucleated giant cells, and tumor osteoid. On conventional radiographs, pure lytic lesions define these tumors.

Diagnosis
Telangiectatic osteosarcoma

Suggested Readings

Murphey MD, wan Jaovisidha S, Temple HT, et al: Telangiectatic osteosarcoma: Radiologic-pathologic comparison. Radiology 229:545-553, 2003.
Weiss A, Khoury JD, Hoffer FA, et al: Telangiectatic osteosarcoma: The St. Jude Children's Research Hospital's experience. Cancer 109:1627-1637, 2007.

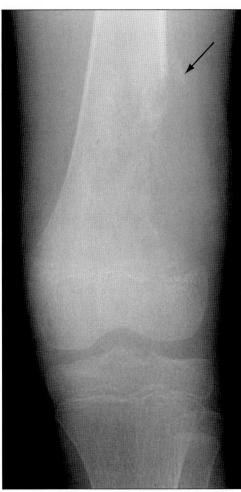

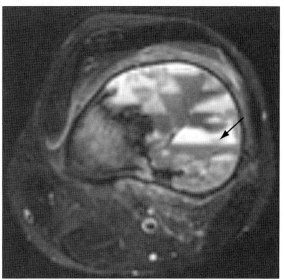

Figure 2. Axial T2-weighted fat-suppressed MR image through distal femur reveals lesion with multiple cystic cavities with fluid-fluid levels (*arrow*).

Figure 1. Anteroposterior radiograph of knee reveals lytic metaphyseal lesion with wide zone of transition, cortical destruction, and periosteal reaction (*arrow*).

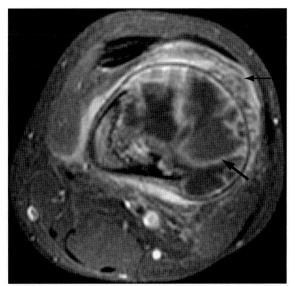

Figure 3. Axial T1-weighted fat-suppressed MR image through distal femur after intravenous gadolinium administration reveals enhancement of multiple septations (*large arrow*) and enhancement in surrounding soft tissues (*small arrow*).

Case 203

DEMOGRAPHICS/CLINICAL HISTORY

The patient is a 16-year-old boy with leg pain after a fall.

FINDINGS

A plain radiograph of the knee (Fig. 1) shows a permeative pattern of bone destruction in the proximal tibia with abnormal osseous mineralization within the soft tissues. Computed tomography (CT) of the tibia (Fig. 2) better illustrates the degree of cortical destruction in the tibia and shows a soft tissue mass posteriorly with osseous mineralization. Magnetic resonance imaging (MRI) of the knee and upper leg reveals the extent of the mass, which is heterogeneous on T2-weighted imaging (Fig. 3), and shows areas of nonenhancement consistent with necrosis (Fig. 4).

DISCUSSION

Definition/Background

Osteosarcoma is the most common malignant bone tumor in children. It most often occurs in children and young adults 15 to 25 years old.

Characteristic Clinical Features

Patients often present with pain or a limp. In some cases, a mass is palpable.

Characteristic Radiologic Findings

In cases of conventional osteosarcoma, plain radiographs show a large, mixed sclerotic and lytic lesion located within the metaphyses of the long bones. There typically is cortical disruption and periosteal new bone forming a Codman triangle.

Differential Diagnosis

- Ewing sarcoma
- Primary lymphoma of bone
- Langerhans cell histiocytosis

Diagnosis

Osteosarcoma

Suggested Readings

Murphey MD, Robbin MR, McRae GA, et al: The many faces of osteosarcoma. RadioGraphics 17:1205-1231, 1997.
Suresh S, Saifuddin A: Radiological appearances of appendicular osteosarcoma: A comprehensive pictorial review. Clin Radiol 62:314-323, 2007.

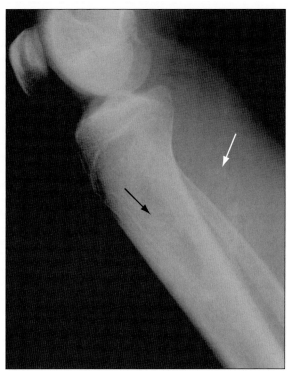

Figure 1. Lateral radiograph of knee shows ossific mineralization within soft tissues of posterior leg (*white arrow*) and permeative pattern of bone destruction in proximal tibia (*black arrow*).

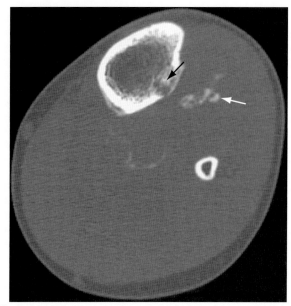

Figure 2. Axial CT image through the knee and lower leg shows osseous matrix within posterior soft tissues of calf (*white arrow*) and bony destruction (*black arrow*).

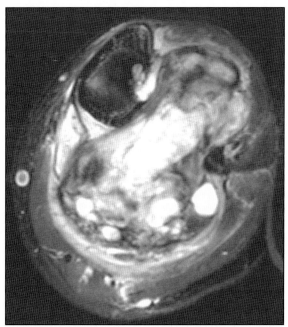

Figure 3. Axial T2-weighted fat-suppressed MR image through the lower leg shows large mass involving tibia and extending into posterior soft tissues with heterogeneous signal and with many areas of bright signal intensity.

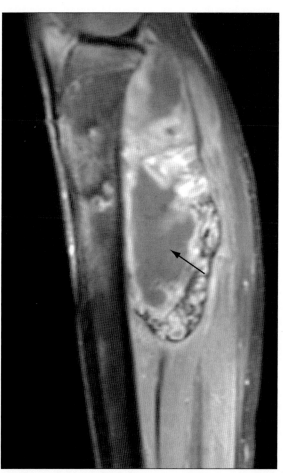

Figure 4. Axial T1-weighted fat-suppressed MR image through lower leg after administration of intravenous contrast agent shows heterogeneous enhancement of mass, with large area of nonenhancement that indicates necrosis (*arrow*).

Case 204

DEMOGRAPHICS/CLINICAL HISTORY

The patient is a 13-year-old boy with a left chest wall mass.

FINDINGS

An axial fluid-sensitive sequence from a magnetic resonance imaging (MRI) examination of the chest (Fig. 1) shows a large, multilobulated, infiltrative lesion within the left chest wall adjacent to the axilla with heterogeneously bright signal characteristics. An axial T1-weighted MR image of the chest (Fig. 2) shows a large soft tissue mass within the left chest wall deep to the pectoralis muscle. A sagittal T1-weighted MR image of the chest with fat suppression after intravenous gadolinium administration (Fig. 3) shows a large, enhancing, infiltrative soft tissue mass within the left chest wall.

DISCUSSION

Definition/Background

Synovial sarcoma most often is diagnosed in adults older than 40 years, but nearly half of cases occur in children. It is one of the most common soft tissue sarcomas.

Characteristic Clinical Features

Patients most often present with pain, which may be long-standing. In other instances, a palpable mass is the presenting symptom.

Characteristic Radiologic Findings

MRI is the modality of choice to evaluate synovial sarcoma. Although imaging appearances vary, the mass is commonly intermediate to low signal on T1-weighted images and bright on T2-weighted images, and often has well-circumscribed margins.

Less Common Radiologic Manifestations

In approximately 30% of patients, plain radiographs show soft tissue calcifications.

Differential Diagnosis

- Rhabdomyosarcoma
- Desmoid

Discussion

Rhabdomyosarcoma is a malignant soft tissue neoplasm in children that is often found in the extremities and may be locally invasive. Desmoid is a benign neoplasm composed of fibrous tissue, which may be locally invasive and often occurs in the extremities. In some cases, desmoid tumors form as a response to previous trauma.

Diagnosis

Synovial sarcoma

Suggested Readings

McCarville MB, Spunt SL, Skapek SX, et al: Synovial sarcoma in pediatric patients. AJR Am J Roentgenol 179:797, 2002.

Murphey MD, Gibson MS, Jennings BT, et al: From the archives of the AFIP: Imaging of synovial sarcoma with radiologic-pathologic correlation. RadioGraphics 26:1543, 2006.

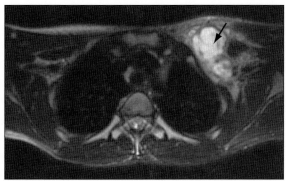

Figure 1. Axial fluid-sensitive sequence from MRI of the chest shows large, multilobulated, infiltrative lesion within left chest wall with heterogeneously bright signal characteristics (*arrow*).

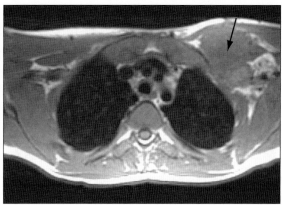

Figure 2. Axial T1-weighted MR image of chest shows large soft tissue mass within left chest wall deep to pectoralis muscle (*arrow*).

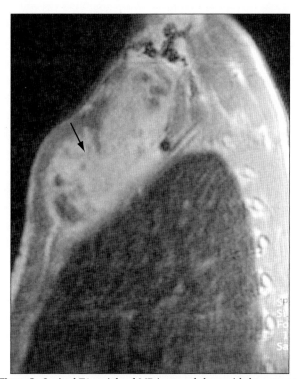

Figure 3. Sagittal T1-weighted MR image of chest with fat suppression after intravenous gadolinium administration shows large, enhancing, infiltrative soft tissue mass within left chest wall (*arrow*).

Case 205

DEMOGRAPHICS/CLINICAL HISTORY

The patient is a 14-year-old girl with chest wall pain.

FINDINGS

Anteroposterior and lateral radiographs of the chest (Figs. 1 and 2) show abnormal soft tissue density within the left lower lobe with a meniscus sign, indicating a pleural effusion. Axial images from a contrast-enhanced computed tomography (CT) scan of the chest (Figs. 3 and 4) show a large pleural effusion and soft tissue masses lining the chest wall.

DISCUSSION

Definition/Background

Askin tumor is a primitive neuroectodermal tumor that arises from the chest wall in children and young adults.

Characteristic Clinical Features

Patients present with chest wall pain or a chest wall mass, or both.

Characteristic Radiologic Findings

CT is the modality of choice for imaging Askin tumors. On CT, the mass appears as a unilateral soft tissue mass involving the chest wall. When the mass has invaded the pleura, pleural effusions often are seen.

Less Common Radiologic Manifestations

Invasion into the lung, ribs, and chest wall musculature can be seen in the setting of Askin tumor, and lung metastases and mediastinal lymphadenopathy may occur.

Differential Diagnosis

- Rhabdomyosarcoma
- Neuroblastoma
- Lymphoma

Diagnosis

Askin tumor

Suggested Readings

Sallustio G, Pirronti T, Lasorella A, et al: Diagnostic imaging of primitive neuroectodermal tumour of the chest wall (Askin tumour). Pediatr Radiol 28:696-702, 1998.

Winer-Muram HT, Kauffman WM, Gronemeyer SA, et al: Primitive neuroectodermal tumors of the chest wall (Askin tumors): CT and MR findings. AJR Am J Roentgenol 161:265-268, 1993.

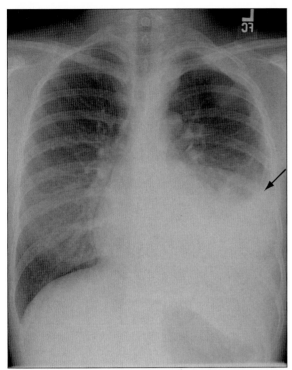

Figure 1. Anteroposterior radiograph of chest shows abnormal soft tissue density occupying left lower lung with meniscus sign (*arrow*).

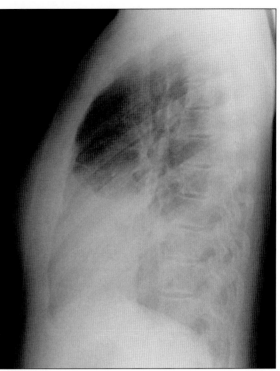

Figure 2. Lateral radiograph of chest shows abnormal soft tissue density within left lower lobe and lingula.

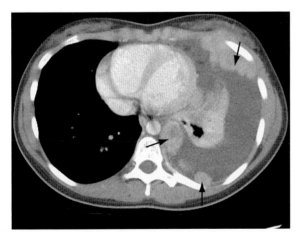

Figure 3. Axial contrast-enhanced CT image of chest through the level of the ventricles shows large pleural effusion and multiple soft tissue masses lining chest wall (*arrows*).

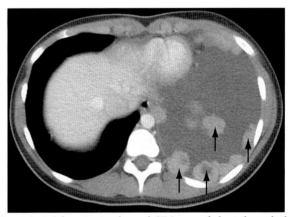

Figure 4. Axial contrast-enhanced CT image of chest through the level of the liver dome shows large pleural effusion and multiple soft tissue masses lining chest wall (*arrows*).

Case 206

DEMOGRAPHICS/CLINICAL HISTORY

The patient is an 11-year-old boy with leg pain.

FINDINGS

A lateral radiograph of the knee (Fig. 1) shows a mixed lytic and sclerotic pattern of bone destruction in the distal femoral metaphysis associated with abnormal periosteal reaction. Anterior and posterior projection images from a bone scan performed with technetium 99m (^{99m}Tc)–labeled MDP (Fig. 2) shows abnormal increased tracer uptake in the distal left femoral metaphysis. Coronal T1-weighted magnetic resonance imaging (MRI) of the femur with fat suppression after intravenous contrast agent administration (Fig. 3) reveals abnormal enhancement within the bone marrow and surrounding soft tissues. Areas of nonenhancement within the mass represent necrotic foci.

DISCUSSION

Definition/Background

Osteosarcoma is the most common malignant bone tumor in children. It occurs most often in adolescents and young adults 15 to 25 years old.

Characteristic Clinical Features

Patients often present with pain or limp.

Characteristic Radiologic Findings

Plain radiographs in cases of conventional osteosarcoma show a large, mixed sclerotic and lytic lesion located within the metaphyses of the long bones. There is typically cortical disruption and periosteal new bone formation forming a Codman triangle.

Differential Diagnosis

- Ewing sarcoma
- Primary lymphoma of bone
- Langerhans cell histiocytosis

Discussion

Ewing sarcoma is a primary bone neoplasm in the same family as the primitive neuroectodermal tumor family of neoplasms. It commonly occurs in the diaphyses of long bones, and associated soft tissue mass is common. Primary lymphoma in bone is rare. The imaging features of primary lymphoma of bone mimic osteosarcoma and are often indistinguishable from it. Langerhans cell histiocytosis is a spectrum of disorders ranging from a solitary bone lesion (eosinophilic granuloma) to a multisystem, disseminated disorder. Bone lesions have aggressive and nonaggressive imaging features.

Diagnosis

Osteosarcoma

Suggested Readings

Murphey MD, Robbin MR, McRae GA, et al: The many faces of osteosarcoma. RadioGraphics 17:1205-1231, 1997.
Suresh S, Saifuddin A: Radiological appearances of appendicular osteosarcoma: A comprehensive pictorial review. Clin Radiol 62:314-323, 2007.

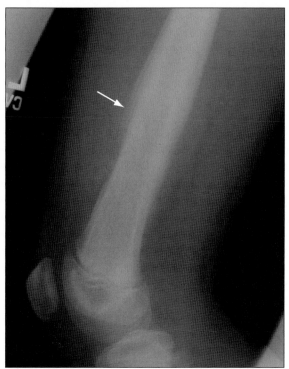

Figure 1. Lateral radiograph of knee shows mixed lytic/sclerotic pattern of bone destruction in distal femoral metaphysis associated with abnormal periosteal reaction (*arrow*).

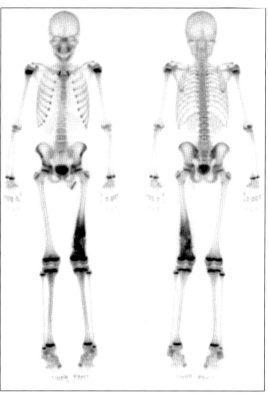

Figure 2. Anterior and posterior projection images from bone scan performed with ^{99m}Tc-labeled MDP show abnormal increased tracer uptake in distal left femoral metaphysis.

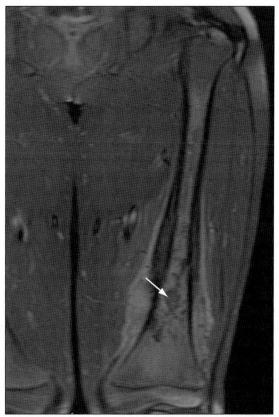

Figure 3. Coronal T1-weighted MR image of femur with fat suppression after intravenous contrast agent administration reveals abnormal enhancement within bone marrow and surrounding soft tissues. Areas of nonenhancement within mass represent necrotic foci (*arrow*).

Case 207

DEMOGRAPHICS/CLINICAL HISTORY

The patient is a 3-year-old girl with a progressively painful right foot mass.

FINDINGS

Magnetic resonance imaging (MRI) of the right foot (Figs. 1-3) shows a lobular mass insinuating between the first and second metatarsals. The mass is low signal on T1-weighted images, is bright on T2-weighted images, and enhances avidly and homogeneously after administration of intravenous contrast agent.

DISCUSSION

Characteristic Clinical Features

This patient is being treated with weekly vinblastine and methotrexate.

Characteristic Radiologic Findings

These tumors have a variable MRI appearance. This particular lesion was well defined and nodular.

Differential Diagnosis

- Neurofibroma
- Synovial cell sarcoma
- Rhabdomyosarcoma

Diagnosis

Desmoid tumor, extra-abdominal

Suggested Readings

Bixby SD, Hettmer S, Taylor GA, Voss SD: Synovial sarcoma in children: imaging features and common benign mimics. AJR Am J Roentgenol, *in press*.

Humar A, Chou S, Carpenter B: Fibromatosis in infancy and childhood: The spectrum. J Pediatr Surg 28:1446-1450, 1993.

Kingston CA, Owens CM, Jeanes A, et al: Imaging of desmoids fibromatosis in pediatric patients. AJR Am J Roentgenol 178:191-199, 2002.

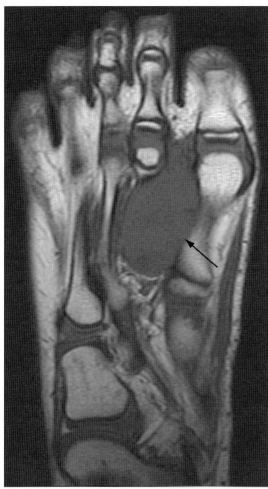

Figure 1. Coronal T1-weighted MR image of right foot shows lobular mass (*arrow*) situated between first and second metatarsals that is low in signal relative to surrounding muscle.

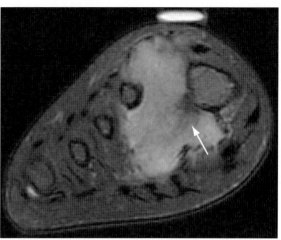

Figure 2. Axial fat-saturated T2-weighted MR image of right foot shows that mass (*arrow*) is well defined and bright, and displaces surrounding tendons.

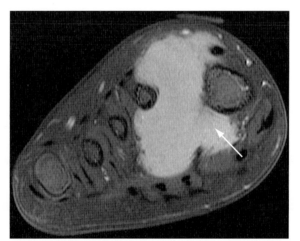

Figure 3. Axial fat-saturated T1-weighted MR image of foot after intravenous administration of gadolinium reveals avid, homogeneous enhancement of mass (*arrow*).

Case 208

DEMOGRAPHICS/CLINICAL HISTORY

The patient is an 18-year-old man who was playing basketball when another player collided into the lateral aspect of his thigh.

FINDINGS

Plain radiographs of the thigh show dense, sheetlike calcifications within the vastus lateralis muscle of the left thigh (Figs. 1 and 2).

DISCUSSION

Definition/Background

Myositis ossificans is most common in adolescents, particularly individuals involved in athletics.

Characteristic Clinical Features

This patient complained of pain in his thigh, a palpable mass, and limited range of motion at the knee joint. Myositis ossificans is most often a post-traumatic condition, as in this case, secondary to a direct insult.

Characteristic Radiologic Findings

In the subacute phase of this lesion (as in this case, 5 weeks after the initial injury), plain radiographs show dense, sheetlike calcifications within the muscle with a distinct cleavage plain between the lesion and the underlying bone.

Less Common Radiologic Manifestations

Computed tomography (CT) often shows a lucent center to the lesion with a rim of calcification.

Differential Diagnosis

- Tumoral calcinosis

Discussion

Tumoral calcinosis is a rare condition characterized by calcific deposits in the soft tissues near major joints.

Diagnosis

Myositis ossificans

Suggested Readings

Gindele A, Schwamborn D, Tsironis K, et al: Myositis ossificans traumatica in young children: Report of three cases and review of the literature. Pediatr Radiol 30:451, 2000.

Shirkhoda A, Armin AR, Bis KG, et al: MR imaging of myositis ossificans: Variable patterns at different stages. J Magn Reson Imaging 5:287, 1995.

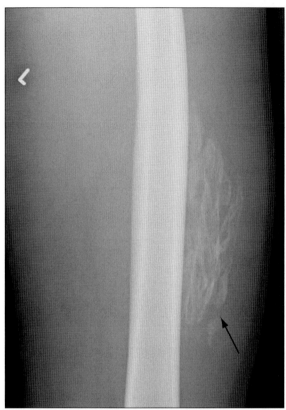

Figure 1. Lateral radiograph of midshaft of left femur reveals dense, sheetlike layers of heterotopic bone within region of vastus lateralis muscle (*arrow*), which are separate from the underlying bone.

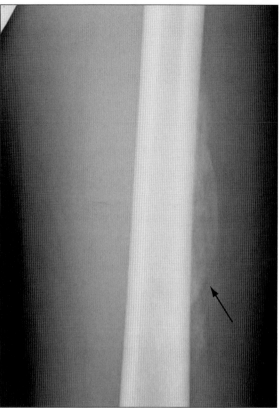

Figure 2. Anteroposterior radiograph of femur shows smooth heterotopic bone formation within vastus lateralis muscle (*arrow*).

Case 209

DEMOGRAPHICS/CLINICAL HISTORY

The patient is an 18-month-old girl with a bump on the dorsum of the foot.

FINDINGS

An anteroposterior radiograph of the foot (Fig. 1) shows normal anatomy. Focused ultrasound of the dorsum of the foot (Fig. 2) shows a hypoechoic lesion within the subcutaneous soft tissues. Magnetic resonance imaging (MRI) of the foot shows a lesion in the dorsum of the foot that has bright signal on fluid-sensitive sequences (Fig. 3) and enhances after administration of intravenous contrast agent (Fig. 4).

DISCUSSION

Definition/Background

Granuloma annulare is a rare group of dermatoses that consists of localized, generalized, and subcutaneous types. Subcutaneous granuloma annulare is a benign condition that often affects young, otherwise healthy children.

Characteristic Clinical Features

Patients present with a painless, nonmobile mass in the lower extremity.

Characteristic Radiologic Findings

MRI is useful in the work-up of subcutaneous granuloma annulare. Most lesions are located in the pretibial subcutaneous tissues and are poorly defined. Although imaging features vary, most lesions are isointense to muscle on T1-weighted images, have variable signal on T2-weighted images, and enhance after contrast agent administration.

Less Common Radiologic Manifestations

Although lesions are commonly located in the pretibial subcutaneous soft tissues, they may also occur in other locations, as in this case.

Differential Diagnosis

- Hemangioma
- Lymphangioma
- Fibroma
- Foreign body reaction
- Fat necrosis
- Vascular malformation

Discussion

Hemangioma is a benign tumor of endothelial cells that usually is self-involuting and may be associated with skin discoloration if it is close to the skin surface. Lymphangioma is a type of lymphatic malformation composed of anomalous lymphatic channels or cavities that do not communicate normally with the main lymphatic system. Fibroma is a benign tumor composed of fibrous or connective tissue. A foreign body reaction describes an inflammatory response or granuloma formation around an irritant, such as a foreign body. Fat necrosis often manifests as a palpable lump, often over bony protuberances, and it is most likely related to post-traumatic necrosis of subcutaneous adipose tissue. Vascular malformation comprises several types of vascular anomalies, including venous malformations, lymphatic malformations, and arteriovenous malformations, which form as a result of anomalous vascular or lymphatic channels.

Diagnosis

Subcutaneous granuloma annulare

Suggested Readings

Chung S, Frush DP, Prose NS, et al: Subcutaneous granuloma annulare: MR imaging features in six children and literature review. Radiology 210:845-849, 1999.

Kransdorf MJ, Murphey MD, Temple HT: Subcutaneous granuloma annulare: Radiologic appearance. Skeletal Radiol 27:266-270, 1998.

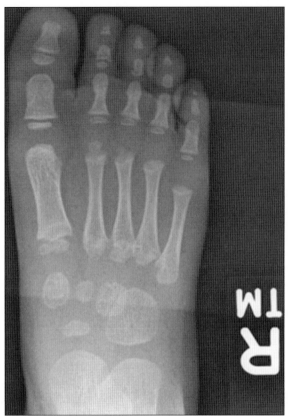

Figure 1. Anteroposterior radiograph of foot shows normal bony contour and mineralization, and no abnormal soft tissue calcifications.

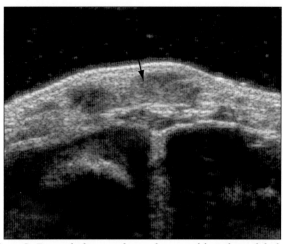

Figure 2. Focused ultrasound over dorsum of foot shows lobular, hypoechoic mass (*arrow*) within subcutaneous soft tissues.

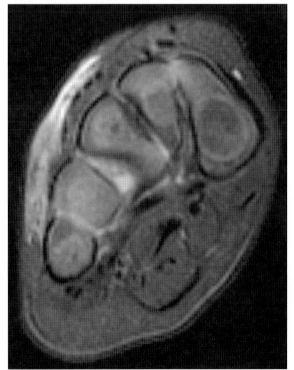

Figure 3. Axial fast spin-echo inversion recovery MR image shows abnormal bright signal within subcutaneous soft tissues of foot that corresponds to lesion.

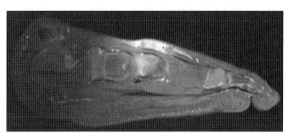

Figure 4. Sagittal T1-weighted MR image of foot with fat suppression and after administration of intravenous contrast agent shows enhancement of subcutaneous soft tissue mass on dorsum of foot.

Case 210

DEMOGRAPHICS/CLINICAL HISTORY

The patient is a 3-month-old girl with irritability and leg swelling.

FINDINGS

An anteroposterior (AP) radiograph of the lower leg (Fig. 1) shows periosteal new bone formation along the entire fibular shaft, medially and laterally. Several months later, an AP radiograph of the lower leg (Fig. 2) shows progressive expansion of the fibula with a lamellated appearance secondary to incorporation of the periosteal new bone. There is also periosteal new bone formation along the tibial shaft.

DISCUSSION

Definition/Background

Caffey disease is also known as infantile cortical hyperostosis. Average age of onset is approximately 9 weeks of age; boys and girls are affected equally.

Characteristic Clinical Features

Patients present with irritability, swelling, and cortical thickening of the underlying bone. Caffey disease is usually a self-limited disorder.

Characteristic Radiologic Findings

Radiographs show hyperostosis within the tubular bones of the skeleton, most prominent within the ribs. Mandibles, clavicles, and ulnas are the bones most frequently involved.

Differential Diagnosis

- Trauma
- Osteomyelitis
- Scurvy
- Congenital syphilis

Discussion

Fractures related to trauma may be associated with periosteal new bone formation as they heal, which may be mistaken for the cortical hyperostosis of Caffey disease. Infection of the bone as seen in infantile osteomyelitis may also manifest with periosteal new bone formation along the affected bone. Scurvy is caused by a deficiency of vitamin C, which may be associated with subperiosteal hemorrhages and periosteal new bone formation. Congenital syphilis is manifested by multiple bone involvement, predominantly affecting the metaphyses, although when the diaphyses are affected, periosteal new bone formation may be a feature of the disease.

Diagnosis

Caffey disease

Suggested Readings

Katz JM, Kirkpatrick JA, Papanicolaou N, et al: Case report 139: Infantile cortical hyperostosis (Caffey disease). Skeletal Radiol 6:77-80, 1981.

Langer R, Kaufmann HJ: Case report 363: Infantile cortical hyperostosis (Caffey disease ICH) iliac bones, femora, tibiae and left fibula. Skeletal Radiol 15:377-382, 1986.

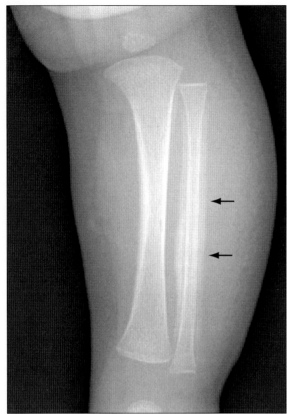

Figure 1. AP radiograph of lower leg shows periosteal new bone formation along entire fibular shaft, medially and laterally (*arrows*).

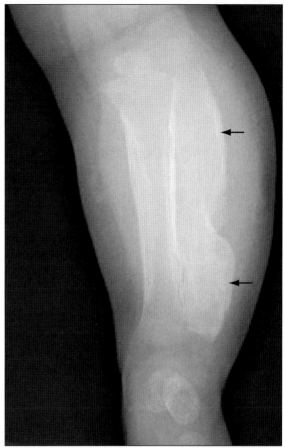

Figure 2. AP radiograph of lower leg several months later shows progressive expansion of fibula with lamellated appearance secondary to incorporation of periosteal new bone (*arrows*). There is also periosteal new bone formation along the tibial shaft.

Case 211

DEMOGRAPHICS/CLINICAL HISTORY

The patient is a newborn girl with positive Barlow and Ortolani maneuvers on physical examination of bilateral hips.

FINDINGS

Ultrasound examination of the hips performed shortly after birth (Figs. 1 and 2) shows shallow acetabula bilaterally. Both femoral heads are laterally partially dislocated. A plain radiograph of the pelvis (Fig. 3) shows superolateral subluxation of the femoral heads. Magnetic resonance imaging (MRI) of the pelvis performed after an attempt at closed reduction in the operating room (Fig. 4) reveals persistent posterior subluxation of bilateral femoral heads.

DISCUSSION

Definition/Background

Developmental dysplasia of the hip is most frequently encountered in female infants, as in this case. This patient was born via cesarean section for breech presentation. Breech positioning also is a risk factor.

Characteristic Clinical Features

The diagnosis is often made on the basis of a "hip clunk" or "click" heard on physical examination when the hips are stressed (Ortolani and Barlow maneuvers). In this infant, the hips were frankly dislocatable.

Characteristic Radiologic Findings

In infants younger than 6 months old, ultrasound is the imaging study of choice. At ultrasound, the alpha angle, which is related to the angle of inclination of the superior acetabulum, is less than 60 degrees, and the femoral head is less than 50% covered by the superior acetabulum.

Differential Diagnosis

- Proximal femoral deficiency
- Arthrogryposis
- Myelomeningocele

Discussion

Patients with neuromuscular disorders such as myelomeningocele and arthrogryposis have abnormal hips at birth, which may appear similar to developmental dysplasia of the hip, but are usually much more severe because the disease process occurred early on in gestation.

Diagnosis

Developmental dysplasia of the hip

Suggested Readings

Gerscovich EO: A radiologist's guide to the imaging in the diagnosis and treatment of developmental dysplasia of the hip, II: Ultrasonography: Anatomy, technique, acetabular angle measurements, acetabular coverage of femoral head, acetabular cartilage thickness, three-dimensional technique, screening of newborns, study of older children. Skeletal Radiol 26:447-456, 1997.

Murray KA, Crim JR: Radiographic imaging for treatment and follow-up of developmental dysplasia of the hip. Semin Ultrasound CT MR 22:306-340, 2001.

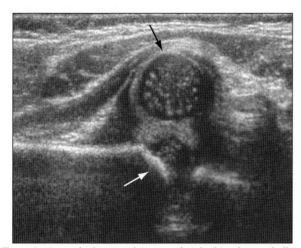

Figure 1. Coronal ultrasound image of right hip shows shallow acetabulum (*white arrow*) with alpha angle measurement less than 60 degrees. The femoral head (*black arrow*) is partially dislocated laterally.

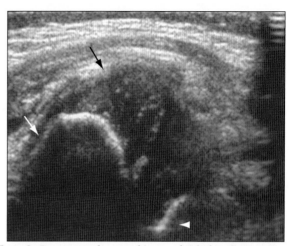

Figure 2. Transverse ultrasound image of right hip shows posterolateral subluxation of femoral head (*black arrow*) with respect to acetabulum. Femoral neck is denoted by *white arrow,* and ischium is denoted by *arrowhead.*

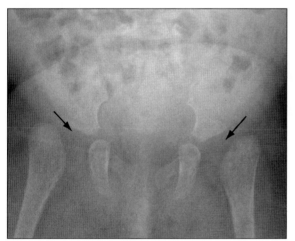

Figure 3. Plain radiograph of pelvis performed at 3 months of age shows that femoral heads are not yet ossified, but their expected position (*arrows*) lies outside normal location.

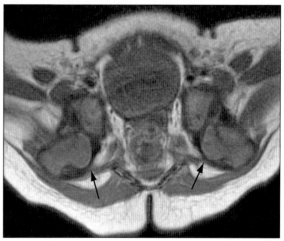

Figure 4. Axial proton density MR image through the hips after attempt at closed hip reduction at age 6 months. Both femoral heads are posteriorly dislocated (*arrows*).

Case 212

DEMOGRAPHICS/CLINICAL HISTORY

The patient is an 8-month-old girl with known left brachial plexus birth palsy.

FINDINGS

Magnetic resonance imaging (MRI) of the brachial plexus was performed, including imaging of both shoulder joints (Figs. 1-3). On MRI, the affected left humeral head is hypoplastic (see Fig. 1) and posteriorly partially dislocated (see Fig. 3). The glenoid is retroverted (see Fig. 3), and the shoulder girdle muscles are hypoplastic (see Fig. 1). The contralateral (right) side is normal.

DISCUSSION

Definition/Background

This patient had a vaginal delivery with suction assistance. She had a flail extremity at birth, but was able to generate a grip. On examination, there is C5-C7 weakness.

Characteristic Clinical Features

The abnormality was noted at birth. MRI was performed for preoperative evaluation to assess the degree of muscle atrophy and glenoid dysplasia.

Characteristic Radiologic Findings

The humeral head is hypoplastic, often posteriorly partially dislocated, and the glenoid is abnormal in contour with loss of its normal concave surface.

Differential Diagnosis

- Clavicle fracture

Discussion

During birth, infants may sustain a fracture to the clavicle, which may manifest with a deformity on the ipsilateral side.

Diagnosis

Erb palsy

Suggested Readings

Poyhia TH, Nietosvaara YA, Remes VM, et al: MRI of rotator cuff muscle atrophy in relation to glenohumeral joint incongruence in brachial plexus birth injury. Pediatr Radiol 35:4402-4409, 2005.

Waters PM, Smith GR, Jaramillo D: Glenohumeral deformity secondary to brachial plexus birth palsy. J Bone Joint Surg Am 80:668-677, 1998.

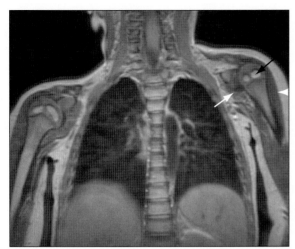

Figure 1. Coronal proton density MR image through both shoulders reveals left humeral head to be superiorly positioned with respect to the right. Left humeral head is hypoplastic (*black arrow*), and muscles of shoulder girdle, including deltoid and pectoralis major, are atrophied (*white arrows*).

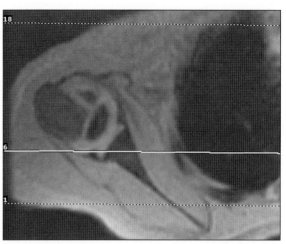

Figure 2. Axial multiple planar gradient-recalled-echo MR image through normal right shoulder reveals humeral head to be appropriately positioned with respect to glenoid. Glenoid has normal concave contour.

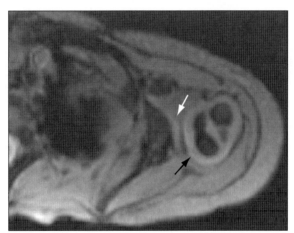

Figure 3. Axial multiple planar gradient-recalled-echo MR image through affected left shoulder reveals hypoplastic humeral head is posteriorly partially dislocated with respect to glenoid (*black arrow*). Glenoid is dysplastic with loss of its normal, concave contour (*white arrow*).

Case 213

DEMOGRAPHICS/CLINICAL HISTORY

The patient is a child born with a left lower extremity deformity.

FINDINGS

Plain radiographs of the left femur (Figs. 1 and 2) show near-complete absence of the femur except for a small, rudimentary femoral head, and a small portion of the distal epiphysis.

DISCUSSION

Characteristic Clinical Features

Deformity is present from birth. This patient was managed with a leg prosthesis.

Characteristic Radiologic Findings

Radiographs show various degrees of absence or hypoplasia of the femur.

Diagnosis

Proximal focal femoral deficiency

Suggested Readings

Hillmann JS, Mesgarzadeh M, Revesz G, et al: Proximal femoral focal deficiency: Radiologic analysis of 49 cases. Radiology 165:769-773, 1987.

Levinson ED, Ozonoff MB, Royen PM: Proximal femoral focal deficiency (PFFD). Radiology 125:197-203, 1977.

Maldjian C, Patel TY, Klein RM, et al: Efficacy of MRI in classifying proximal focal femoral deficiency. Skeletal Radiol 36:215-220, 2007.

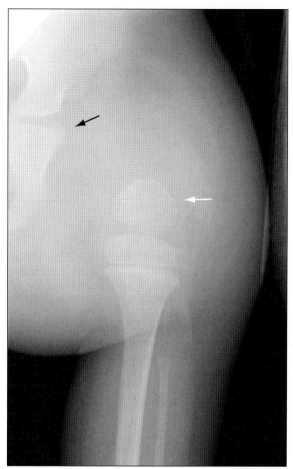

Figure 1. Anteroposterior radiograph of left hip and proximal leg reveals hypoplasia of left acetabulum with hypoplasia of left femur. Small, ossified femoral head is present within acetabulum (*black arrow*), and distal femoral epiphysis, which articulates with tibia (*white arrow*).

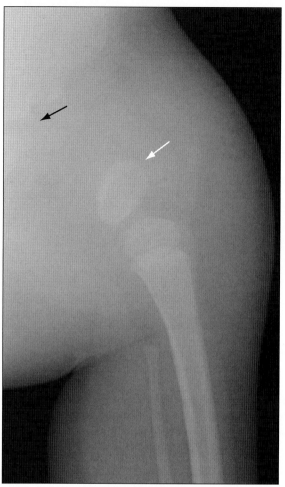

Figure 2. Lateral radiograph of left leg shows similar findings (*arrows*). Fibula also is abnormally shortened in this patient.

Case 214

DEMOGRAPHICS/CLINICAL HISTORY

The patient is a 6-year-old girl with leg-length discrepancy and a known diagnosis of fibular hemimelia.

FINDINGS

Radiographs of the lower leg (Figs. 1 and 2) show absence of the fibula except for a small portion of the distal fibula near the ankle.

DISCUSSION

Characteristic Clinical Features

This patient also has absence of the anterior and posterior cruciate ligaments of the knee and an equinus deformity at the ankle, which are known associations. She has a significant leg-length discrepancy because the tibia of the affected side is shorter than the tibia of the unaffected leg.

Characteristic Radiologic Findings

Radiographs show partial or complete absence of the fibula with associated shortening of the tibia.

Differential Diagnosis

- Fibula-femur-ulna complex
- Camptomelic dysplasia
- Tibial hemimelia

Discussion

Fibula-femur-ulna complex is a rare type of short-limbed dwarfism. Camptomelic dysplasia is an autosomal dominant disorder associated with shortening of all the extremities. Tibial hemimelia refers to complete or incomplete absence of the tibia, and is less common than fibular hemimelia.

Diagnosis

Fibular hemimelia

Suggested Readings

Abel DE, Hertzberg BS, James AH: Antenatal sonographic diagnosis of isolated bilateral fibular hemimelia. J Ultrasound Med 21:811-815, 2002.

Uffelman H, Woo R, Richards DS: Prenatal diagnosis of bilateral fibular hemimelia. J Ultrasound Med 19:341-344, 2000.

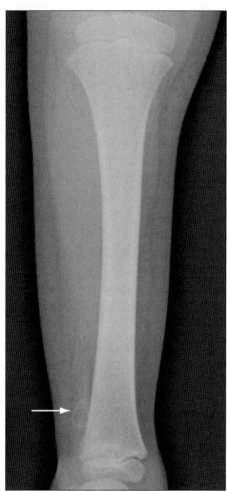

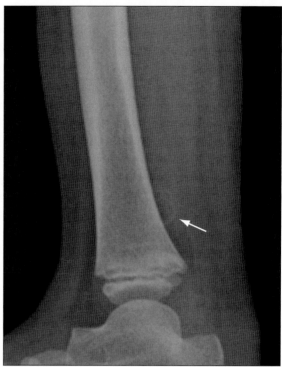

Figure 2. Lateral radiograph of right leg also shows near-total absence of fibula. Small, rudimentary fibular fragment projects posterior to distal tibia (*arrow*).

Figure 1. Anteroposterior radiograph of lower right leg shows near-complete absence of fibula. Only a small portion of the distal fibula is present (*arrow*).

Case 215

DEMOGRAPHICS/CLINICAL HISTORY

The patient is a 1-month-old infant with right upper extremity deformity and no history of perinatal or postnatal complications.

FINDINGS

An anteroposterior radiograph of the right hand (Fig. 1) shows mild broadening of the metacarpals, but otherwise the bones are normal. Magnetic resonance imaging (MRI) of the distal forearm (Fig. 2) and hand (Fig. 3) shows significant muscular atrophy involving the volar aspect of the arm, wrist, and hand.

DISCUSSION

Definition/Background
Constriction band syndrome is a sporadic condition with an incidence between 1:1200 and 1:15,000 live births. The etiology is unknown.

Characteristic Clinical Features
On physical examination, this patient had a hypoplastic right arm associated with an amniotic band along the anterior aspect of the right mid-humerus. The fingers were short, and there was no active wrist flexion or finger flexion.

Characteristic Radiologic Findings
The severity of the imaging findings varies depending on the nature of the amniotic band. The most severe abnormality is a complete limb amputation.

Less Common Radiologic Manifestations
In mild cases, only a small groove or ring in the soft tissues is appreciated on physical examination, a finding that may be missed entirely at imaging or detected only with three-dimensional ultrasound prenatal imaging.

Differential Diagnosis
- Adams-Oliver syndrome

Discussion
Adams-Oliver syndrome is an autosomal dominant condition in which limb defects are associated with scalp and skull defects.

Diagnosis
Constriction band syndrome

Suggested Readings
Paladini D, Foglia S, Sglavo G, et al: Congenital constriction band of the upper arm: The role of three-dimensional ultrasound in diagnosis, counseling and multidisciplinary consultation. Ultrasound Obstet Gynecol 23:520-522, 2004.

Rypens F, Dubois J, Garel L, et al: Obstetric US: Watch the fetal hands. RadioGraphics 26:811-829, 2006.

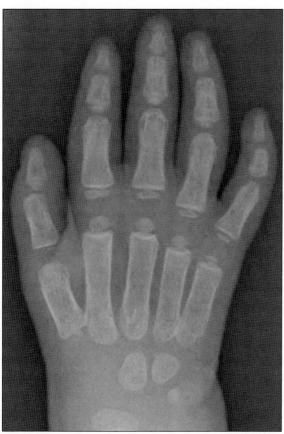

Figure 1. Anteroposterior radiograph of hand shows mild broadening of metacarpals without additional osseous abnormality.

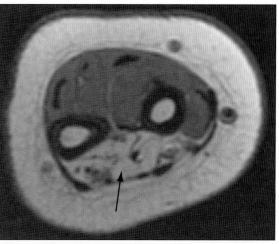

Figure 2. Axial proton density MR image through distal forearm and wrist reveals substantial fatty atrophy of muscle groups along volar aspect of distal forearm (*arrow*).

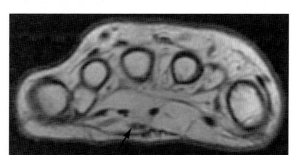

Figure 3. Axial proton density MR image through the level of the hand reveals atrophy of muscles along volar surface of hand (*arrow*).

Case 216

DEMOGRAPHICS/CLINICAL HISTORY

The patient is a 4-month-old girl with congenital clubfeet, in whom no imaging was performed at birth, and who was initially treated with serial casting.

FINDINGS

Anteroposterior (Fig. 1) and lateral (Fig. 2) radiographs of the foot reveal forefoot abduction, hindfoot varus, and hindfoot equinus.

DISCUSSION

Definition/Background

Clubfoot is the most common congenital musculoskeletal defect in North America. The etiology is not well understood.

Characteristic Clinical Features

The foot is in equinus and cavus position. The patient in this case was treated with serial casting, the Denis Browne splint at night, and exercises.

Characteristic Radiologic Findings

Hindfoot varus, hindfoot equinus, and forefoot adduction are seen on imaging.

Differential Diagnosis

- Metatarsus varus
- Skewfoot

Discussion

Metatarsus varus is a common cause of intoeing in young children. The forefoot adduction is isolated, and the midfoot and hindfoot relationships are otherwise normal. In skewfoot, there is forefoot adduction and hindfoot valgus. In contrast to clubfoot, this is not a congenital abnormality.

Diagnosis

Clubfoot, congenital

Suggested Readings

Ippolitio E, Fraracci L, Farsetti P, et al: Validity of the anteroposterior talocalcaneal angle to assess congenital clubfoot correction. AJR Am J Roentgenol 182:1279, 2004.

Radler C, Manner HM, Suda R, et al: Radiographic evaluation of idiopathic clubfeet undergoing Ponseti treatment. J Bone Joint Surg Am 89:1177, 2007.

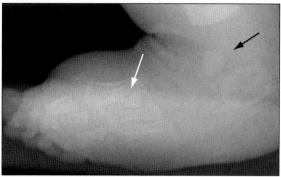

Figure 2. Lateral radiograph of right foot reveals hindfoot varus, with nearly parallel relationship of talus and calcaneus (*black arrow*). Metatarsals have a "stepladder" configuration on lateral projection in light of associated forefoot varus (*white arrow*).

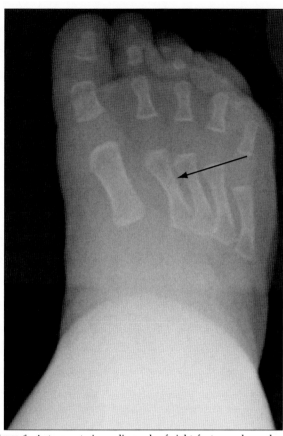

Figure 1. Anteroposterior radiograph of right foot reveals moderate forefoot adduction (*arrow*).

Case 217

DEMOGRAPHICS/CLINICAL HISTORY

The patient is a 13-year-old boy with short fingers.

FINDINGS

A posteroanterior radiograph of the chest (Fig. 1) reveals hyperlucency of the right hemithorax relative to the left side. An anteroposterior radiograph of the hand (Fig. 2) reveals multiple hypoplastic phalanges.

DISCUSSION

Definition/Background

Most cases of Poland syndrome are sporadic and thought to occur because of in utero subclavian artery disruption.

Characteristic Clinical Features

Patients have upper limb anomalies; syndactyly and brachydactyly are the most common. They may have absence or hypoplasia of pectoralis major muscle.

Characteristic Radiologic Findings

Unilateral hyperlucency of the chest is related to the absence of the pectoralis major muscle on that side. Patients have abnormal, short (hypoplastic) phalanges or fused phalanges (syndactyly).

Differential Diagnosis
- Atrophy of the chest wall
- Postmastectomy changes of the chest wall

Discussion

Atrophied chest wall muscle and postmastectomy changes (usually in women) are acquired conditions that may mimic the chest radiographic features of Poland syndrome.

Diagnosis

Poland syndrome

Suggested Readings

Mentzel HJ, Seidel J, Sauner D, et al: Radiological aspects of the Poland syndrome and implications for treatment: A case study and review. Eur J Pediatr 161:455-459, 2002.

Wright AR, Milner RH, Bainbridge LC, et al: MR and CT in the assessment of Poland syndrome. J Comput Assist Tomogr 16:442-447, 1992.

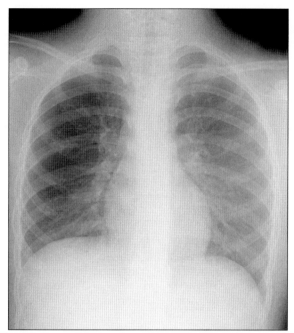

Figure 1. Posteroanterior chest radiograph reveals hyperlucency of right hemithorax.

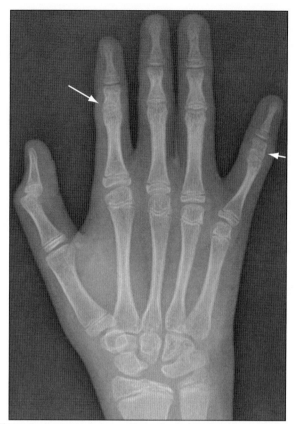

Figure 2. Anteroposterior radiograph of right hand reveals short middle phalanges of second and fifth digits (*arrows*). Abnormalities of carpal bones can be seen.

Case 218

DEMOGRAPHICS/CLINICAL HISTORY

The patient is an 11-year-old girl with bilateral ankle pain (left more than right).

FINDINGS

An oblique, anteroposterior radiograph of the left foot (Fig. 1) reveals elongation of the lateral portion of the navicular bone and the anterior process of the calcaneus. There is cortical irregularity and evidence of a nonosseous calcaneonavicular coalition. Sagittal reformatted computed tomography (CT) scan of the foot (Fig. 2) reveals the nonosseous coalition between the navicular and calcaneus. A coronal reformatted CT image through the ankle in a different patient with ankle pain (Fig. 3) reveals a nonosseous coalition of the medial facet of the talocalcaneal joint.

DISCUSSION

Definition/Background

Most patients present in early adolescence. A precipitating injury often causes patients to undergo imaging evaluation, and the coalition is identified incidentally.

Characteristic Clinical Features

Coalitions most often occur between the calcaneus and the navicular bone (as in this case) and in the medial facet of the talonavicular joint (as in the supplementary case).

Characteristic Radiologic Findings

Calcaneonavicular coalition can be diagnosed on the basis of plain radiographs. The anterior process of the calcaneus is elongated, and there is narrowing of the space between the calcaneus and navicular.

Diagnosis

Tarsal coalition

Suggested Readings

Crim JR, Kjeldsberg KM: Radiographic diagnosis of tarsal coalition. AJR Am J Roentgenol 182:323-328, 2004.
Newman JS, Newberg AH: Congenital tarsal coalition: Multimodality evaluation with emphasis on CT and MR imaging. RadioGraphics 20:321-322, 2000.

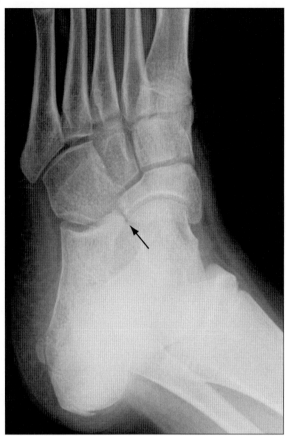

Figure 1. Oblique anteroposterior radiograph of foot shows narrowing of space between navicular and calcaneus, elongation of anterior process of calcaneus (*arrow*), and cortical irregularity involving both bones.

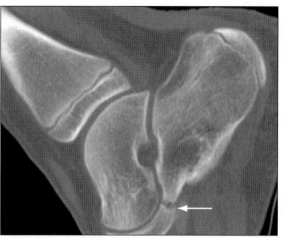

Figure 2. Sagittal reformatted CT scan of foot shows nonosseous calcaneonavicular coalition (*arrow*).

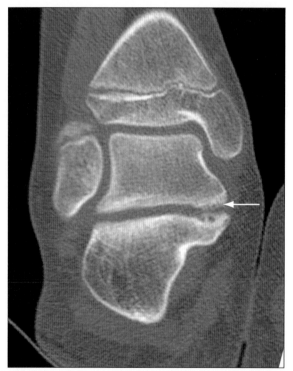

Figure 3. In a different patient, coronal reformatted CT image through ankle reveals nonosseous coalition involving medial facet of talocalcaneal joint (*arrow*).

Case 219

DEMOGRAPHICS/CLINICAL HISTORY

The patient is a 10-year-old child with chronic decreased neck motion.

FINDINGS

A lateral cervical spine radiograph (Fig. 1) shows hypoplasia of the vertebral bodies of C3-C7, with narrowing of the disk spaces and fusion of the spinous processes. Flexion (Fig. 2) and extension (Fig. 3) views demonstrate minimal to no significant motion at the involved levels.

DISCUSSION

Definition/Background
Congenital fusion of the cervical spine is called Klippel-Feil anomaly.

Characteristic Clinical Features
Patients typically have a shortened neck, a low posterior neckline, and decreased range of motion in the affected area.

Characteristic Radiologic Findings
Fusion of two or more cervical vertebrae often causes the affected vertebral bodies to have a diminutive or hypoplastic appearance. Spinal stenosis can affect the involved area. Associations with Sprengel deformity and other congenital anomalies of the ears and kidneys can be seen.

Differential Diagnosis
- Ankylosing spondylitis
- Juvenile idiopathic arthritis

Discussion
Ankylosing spondylitis can cause fusion of the spine. The vertebral bodies are typically normally shaped, however, because ankylosing spondylitis typically affects skeletally mature patients. Juvenile idiopathic arthritis usually does not cause multilevel fusion early in childhood.

Diagnosis
Klippel-Feil syndrome

Suggested Reading
Kaplan KM, Spivak JM, Bendo JA: Embryology of the spine and associated congenital abnormalities. Spine J 5:564-576, 2005.

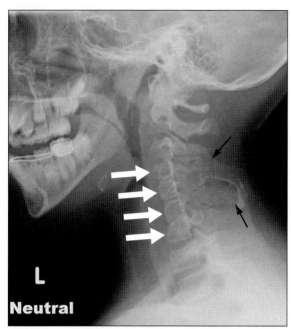

Figure 1. Lateral cervical spine radiograph shows hypoplasia of vertebral bodies of C3-C7 (*white arrows*), with narrowing of the disk spaces and fusion of the spinous processes (*black arrows*).

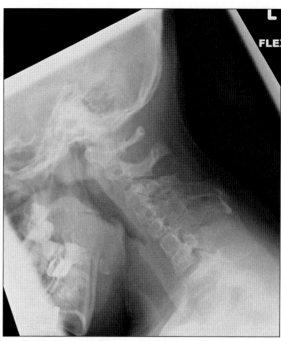

Figure 2. Flexion view shows minimal to no significant motion at involved levels.

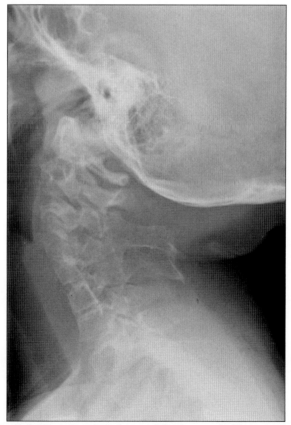

Figure 3. Extension view shows minimal to no significant motion at involved levels.

Case 220

DEMOGRAPHICS/CLINICAL HISTORY

The patient is a 1-year-old child with an incidental finding on radiographs after a fall.

FINDINGS

A frontal view of the neck and upper chest (Fig. 1) shows an omovertebral bone articulating with the left C5 vertebra and a high-riding scapula. A lateral view of the neck and upper chest (Fig. 2) shows the appearance of the omovertebral bone and the high-riding scapula.

DISCUSSION

Definition/Background
Sprengel deformity is the most common congenital malformation of the scapula.

Characteristic Clinical Features
Some patients come to medical attention because of asymmetry of the scapulae as the result of the abnormally high-riding and angulated scapula.

Characteristic Radiologic Findings
The scapula is high-riding in patients with Sprengel deformity. An accessory omovertebral bone may be seen in 50% of patients with Sprengel deformity. Other anomalies associated with Sprengel deformity include segmentation abnormalities of vertebrae and ribs (particularly Klippel-Feil anomaly), renal abnormalities, and hypoplasia of the muscles of the neck and shoulder.

Diagnosis
Sprengel deformity

Suggested Readings
Cho TJ, Choi IH, Chung CY, et al: The Sprengel deformity: Morphometric analysis using 3D-CT and its clinical relevance. J Bone Joint Surg Br 82:711-718, 2000.

Williams MS: Developmental anomalies of the scapula—the "omo"st forgotten bone. Am J Med Genet A 120A:583-587, 2003.

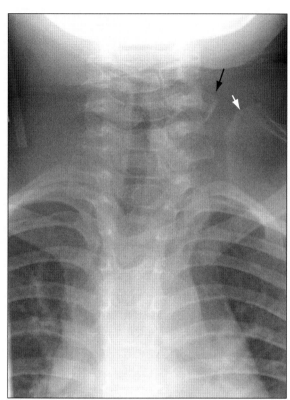

Figure 1. Frontal view of neck and upper chest shows omovertebral bone (*black arrow*) articulating with the left C5 vertebra, and a high-riding scapula (*white arrow*).

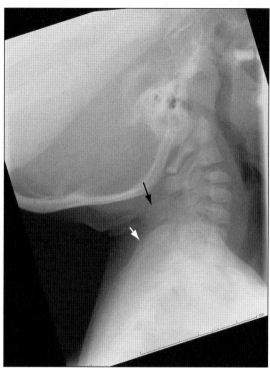

Figure 2. Lateral view of neck and upper chest shows appearance of omovertebral bone (*black arrow*) and high-riding scapula (*white arrow*).

Case 221

DEMOGRAPHICS/CLINICAL HISTORY

The patient is a 9-year-old boy presenting after falling onto an arm.

FINDINGS

Lateral (Fig. 1) and anteroposterior (Fig. 2) radiographs of the elbow show scattered foci of sclerotic bone within the distal humerus and proximal radius and ulna.

DISCUSSION

Definition/Background

Osteopoikilosis is an autosomal dominant condition.

Characteristic Clinical Features

Patients with osteopoikilosis are most often asymptomatic.

Characteristic Radiologic Findings

Radiographs show small foci of bone sclerosis, usually in a round or oval configuration, within areas of cancellous bone.

Less Common Radiologic Manifestations

The lesions may show increased radiotracer uptake on bone scan.

Differential Diagnosis

- Melorheostosis, pediatric
- Enostosis

Discussion

Melorheostosis is a rare and progressive disease characterized by hyperostosis of cortical bone. An enostosis is an isolated sclerotic focus within the bone (i.e., bone island).

Diagnosis

Osteopoikilosis

Suggested Readings

Greenspan A: Sclerosing bone dysplasias—a target-site approach. Skeletal Radiol 20:561-583, 1991.

Jacobson HG: Dense bone—too much bone: Radiological considerations and differential diagnosis. Part 1. Skeletal Radiol 13:1-20, 1985.

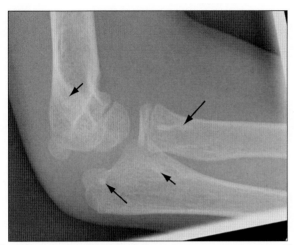

Figure 1. Lateral radiograph of elbow shows many enostoses within distal humerus and proximal radius and ulna (*arrows*).

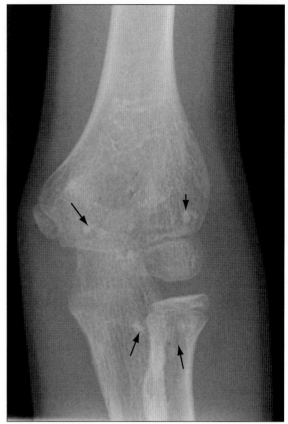

Figure 2. Anteroposterior radiograph of elbow shows many sclerotic foci within bones (*arrows*).

Case 222

DEMOGRAPHICS/CLINICAL HISTORY

The patient is a 5-year-old child with a musculoskeletal abnormality.

FINDINGS

A chest radiograph (Fig. 1) shows absence of the clavicles. A pelvic radiograph (Fig. 2) shows lack of ossification of the pubic bones.

DISCUSSION

Definition/Background

Cleidocranial dysplasia (or cleidocranial dysostosis) is characterized by autosomal dominant genetic inheritance and skeletal abnormalities, including hypoplasia or aplasia of the clavicles and abnormalities of the cranium, including wormian bones and open fontanelles.

Characteristic Clinical Features

Clinical features reflect the underlying skeletal abnormalities, including hyperflexibility resulting from absence or hypoplasia of the clavicles. Cranial abnormalities include brachycephaly, hypertelorism, midface hypoplasia, and open fontanelles. Short stature and abnormal dentition are typically seen. Hearing loss is common.

Characteristic Radiologic Findings

Wormian bones, open fontanelles, aplasia or hypoplasia of the clavicles, and delayed ossification of the pubic bones are common radiologic findings. Brachycephaly, hypertelorism, midface hypoplasia, and supernumerary teeth can also be seen.

Differential Diagnosis

- Acrocephalosyndactyly

Discussion

Acrocephalosyndactylies can have similar craniofacial abnormalities, but the aplasia or hypoplasia of the clavicles is characteristic for cleidocranial dysplasia.

Diagnosis

Cleidocranial dysplasia

Suggested Readings

Gonzalez GE, Caruso PA, Small JE, et al: Craniofacial and temporal bone CT findings in cleidocranial dysplasia. Pediatr Radiol 38:892-897, 2008.

Mundlos S: Cleidocranial dysplasia: Clinical and molecular genetics. J Med Genet 36:177-182, 1999.

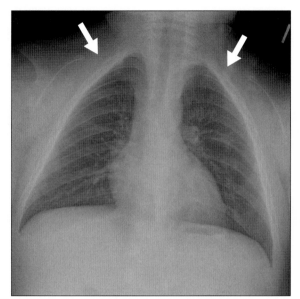

Figure 1. Chest radiograph shows absence of clavicles (*arrows*).

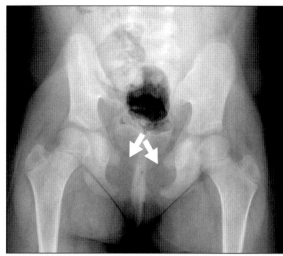

Figure 2. Pelvic radiograph shows lack of ossification of pubic bones (*arrows*).

Case 223

DEMOGRAPHICS/CLINICAL HISTORY

The patient is a 5-year-old boy with an incidental finding on an earlier abdominal radiograph and with no symptoms of hip pain.

FINDINGS

Anteroposterior and frog-leg radiographs of the hips (Figs. 1 and 2) show mild fragmentation and irregularity of the femoral epiphyses bilaterally. The right side is more affected than the left.

DISCUSSION

Definition/Background

Meyer dysplasia is a benign developmental disorder of the hip that is asymptomatic, and that typically occurs in boys younger than 4 years.

Characteristic Clinical Features

Patients are typically asymptomatic.

Characteristic Radiologic Findings

Plain radiographs show a small, irregular femoral epiphysis. The abnormality may be bilateral in half of the cases. The radiographic appearance returns to normal within 2 to 4 years after the diagnosis.

Less Common Radiologic Manifestations

Magnetic resonance imaging (MRI) of the hip reveals normal signal within the epiphyseal fragments.

Differential Diagnosis

- Legg-Calvé-Perthes disease
- Epiphyseal dysplasia
- Sickle cell disease

Discussion

Legg-Calvé-Perthes disease is an idiopathic, avascular necrosis of the femoral head, and it usually occurs in boys 5 to 10 years old. Epiphyseal dysplasia is a skeletal dysplasia characterized by symmetric and bilateral irregularity of the femoral epiphyses. Sickle cell disease can lead to avascular necrosis of the femoral head or heads, which may appear indistinguishable from Meyer dysplasia.

Diagnosis

Meyer dysplasia

Suggested Readings

Khermosh O, Wientroub S: Dysplasia epiphysealis capitis femoris: Meyer's dysplasia. J Bone Joint Surg Br 73:621-625, 1991.

Rowe SM, Chung JY, Moon ES, et al: Dysplasia epiphysealis capitis femoris: Meyer dysplasia. J Pediatr Orthop 25:18-21, 2005.

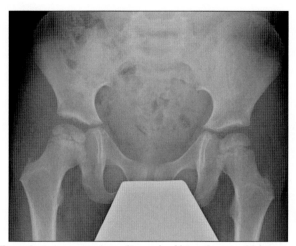

Figure 1. Anteroposterior radiograph of hips shows mild fragmentation and irregularity of femoral epiphyses bilaterally. The right side is affected more than the left.

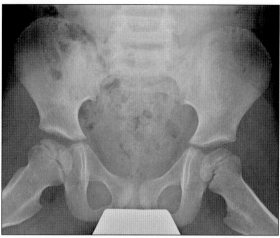

Figure 2. Frog-leg radiograph of hips shows mild fragmentation and irregularity of femoral epiphyses bilaterally. The right side is affected more than the left.

Case 224

DEMOGRAPHICS/CLINICAL HISTORY

The patient is a 4-year-old girl with cleidocranial dysostosis and coxa vara.

FINDINGS

Anteroposterior (Fig. 1) and frog-leg (Fig. 2) radiographs of both hips show abnormal varus angulation of the femoral necks with respect to the femoral shafts, with a head-neck angle approaching 90 degrees. There is irregularity of the proximal femoral physes bilaterally, which appear nearly vertical (see Fig. 1), and the femoral heads are abnormally tall and show a loss of sphericity.

DISCUSSION

Definition/Background

Coxa vara refers to a diminished femoral neck-shaft angle, which may result from various congenital or acquired conditions.

Characteristic Clinical Features

Infants and young children with coxa vara present with an early gait abnormality or an abnormal stance.

Characteristic Radiologic Findings

Radiographs of the pelvis show a decreased femoral neck-shaft angle (≤90 degrees); widening and irregularity of the proximal physis, which is vertically oriented; and an abnormal triangular fragment at the inferior aspect of the femoral physis. The acetabulum is normal.

Differential Diagnosis

- Cleidocranial dysplasia
- Spondyloepiphyseal dysplasia
- Achondroplasia
- Renal osteodystrophy

Discussion

Coxa vara associated with cleidocranial dysplasia is identical to that of idiopathic infantile coxa vara, but there are other skeletal changes, including absence of the clavicles and delayed ossification of the pubic symphysis. Spondyloepiphyseal dysplasia is characterized by multiple epiphyseal abnormalities that are present at birth. Patients with achondroplasia also have coxa vara secondary to a bowed femoral shaft. Renal osteodystrophy, or osteomalacia, manifests with osseous changes, including osteopenia, resorption of bilateral femoral necks, slipped capital femoral epiphyses, and Looser zones in the femoral necks.

Diagnosis

Coxa vara, congenital

Suggested Readings

Pavlov H, Goldman AB, Freiberger RH: Infantile coxa vara. Radiology 135:631-640, 1980.

Weinstein JN, Kuo KN, Millar EA: Congenital coxa vara: A retrospective review. J Pediatr Orthop 4:70-77, 1984.

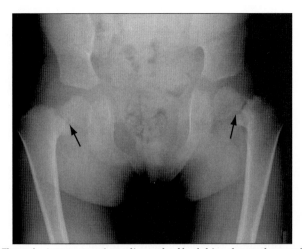

Figure 1. Anteroposterior radiograph of both hips shows abnormal varus angulation of femoral necks with respect to femoral shafts. There is irregularity of proximal femoral physes bilaterally, which are vertically oriented (*arrows*), and femoral heads are abnormally tall and have a loss of sphericity.

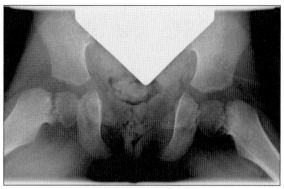

Figure 2. Frog-leg radiograph of both hips shows abnormal varus angulation of femoral necks with respect to femoral shafts. There is irregularity of proximal femoral physes bilaterally, and femoral heads are abnormally tall and have a loss of sphericity.

Case 225

DEMOGRAPHICS/CLINICAL HISTORY

The patient is an 8-year-old girl with worsening spinal curvature.

FINDINGS

Fig. 1 is an anteroposterior radiograph of the entire spine that shows a moderate to severe dextroscoliosis of the thoracic spine with an associated rotary component. There is a compensatory levoscoliosis of the upper thoracic spine. No osseous vertebral anomalies are visualized on the radiograph. Fig. 2 is a lateral radiograph of the entire spine that shows an exaggerated lumbar lordosis and thoracic kyphosis.

DISCUSSION

Definition/Background

Congenital scoliosis is due to a developmental defect in vertebral formation and may be associated with other anomalies, including genitourinary or cardiac defects.

Characteristic Clinical Features

The patient presents with a spinal curvature at a very young age (in infancy), which usually worsens as the child grows.

Characteristic Radiologic Findings

Radiographs not only show the abnormal spinal curvature, but also may reveal abnormalities of the vertebra at the apex of the curve. Absent or fused ribs are an associated finding.

Less Common Radiologic Manifestations

Computed tomography (CT) with three-dimensional reconstructions is often employed in addition to plain radiographs to show best the bony anatomy of the vertebral column.

Differential Diagnosis

- Spondylocostal dysostosis

Discussion

Spondylocostal dysostosis is an inherited vertebral malformation and is exceedingly rare.

Diagnosis

Congenital scoliosis

Suggested Readings

Hedequist D, Emans J: Congenital scoliosis. J Am Acad Orthop Surg 12:266, 2004.
Hedequist D, Emans J: Congenital scoliosis: A review and update. J Pediatr Orthop 27:106, 2007.

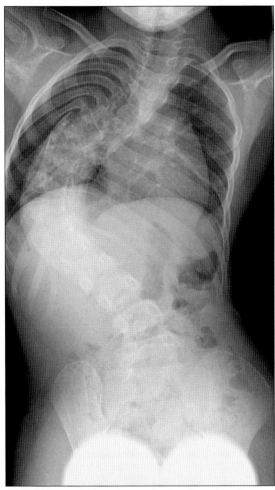

Figure 1. Anteroposterior radiograph of entire spine shows moderate to severe dextroscoliosis of thoracic spine with associated rotary component. There is compensatory levoscoliosis of upper thoracic spine. No vertebral anomalies are present.

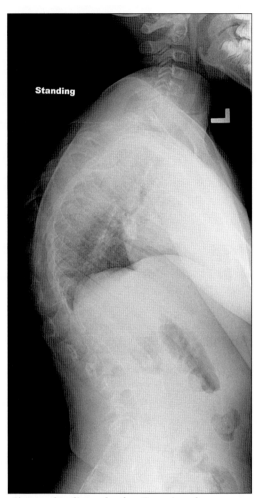

Figure 2. Lateral radiograph of entire spine shows exaggerated lumbar lordosis and thoracic kyphosis.

Case 226

DEMOGRAPHICS/CLINICAL HISTORY

The patient is a 16-year-old boy with hemoglobin SS sickle cell disease.

FINDINGS

Posteroanterior (Fig. 1) and lateral (Fig. 2) radiographs of the chest show central superior and inferior end plate depressions, giving the vertebral bodies a characteristic H-shaped form.

DISCUSSION

Definition/Background
Most children in the United States with sickle cell disease are African American.

Characteristic Clinical Features
Patients often present with bone pain caused by a vaso-occlusive crisis. The vertebral changes seen on the chest radiograph may be asymptomatic and discovered incidentally.

Characteristic Radiologic Findings
Depressed vertebral end plates produce H-shaped vertebral bodies.

Less Common Radiologic Manifestations
Other manifestations include widening of the diploic spaces in the skull, mixed sclerotic and lucent areas within the bones related to infarction, and dactylitis caused by bone infarcts in the hands and feet.

Differential Diagnosis
- Thalassemia
- Hereditary spherocytosis
- Langerhans cell histiocytosis (vertebral plana)
- Leukemia

Discussion
Hereditary spherocytosis is a type of hemolytic anemia that may cause widening of the diploic space in the skull.

Diagnosis
Sickle cell disease: bone changes

Suggested Readings
Ejindu VC, Hine AL, Mashayekhi M, et al: Musculoskeletal manifestations of sickle cell disease. RadioGraphics 27:1005-1021, 2007.
Madani G, Papadopoulou AM, Holloway B, et al: The radiological manifestations of sickle cell disease. Clin Radiol 62:528-538, 2007.

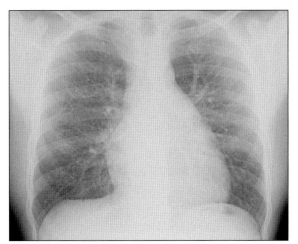

Figure 1. Posteroanterior radiograph of chest shows slightly enlarged cardiac silhouette.

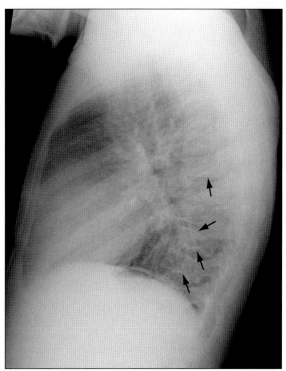

Figure 2. Lateral chest radiograph shows central end plate depressions in many vertebral bodies (*arrows*), giving the vertebrae a characteristic H-shaped form.

Case 227

DEMOGRAPHICS/CLINICAL HISTORY

The patient is an 8-month-old boy with sickle cell disease with swelling and pain in the right foot and left hand.

FINDINGS

Radiographs of the right foot (Fig. 1) and the left hand (Fig. 2) reveal soft tissue swelling, bony expansion, mottled lucencies, and periosteal new bone formation involving the first and second metatarsals (see Fig. 1) and the fourth metacarpal and proximal phalanx (see Fig. 2).

DISCUSSION

Definition/Background

This patient was treated 2 weeks previously for streptococcal meningitis with a 2-week course of ceftriaxone. Hand-foot disease occurs in young children with sickle cell disease.

Characteristic Clinical Features

The patient was admitted with the diagnosis of "dactylitis." An aspiration of the first metatarsal revealed only bloody aspirate.

Characteristic Radiologic Findings

Radiographs show permeative or "moth-eaten" bony destruction involving the small bones of the hands or feet, soft tissue swelling, and periosteal reaction.

Differential Diagnosis
- Osteomyelitis

Diagnosis

Hand-foot syndrome

Suggested Readings

Babhulkar SS, Pande K, Babhulkar S: The hand-foot syndrome in sickle-cell haemoglobinopathy. J Bone Joint Surg Br 77:310-312, 1995.

Silver L, Sarreck R: Bone scan in the hand-foot syndrome. Clin Nucl Med 9:710-711, 1984.

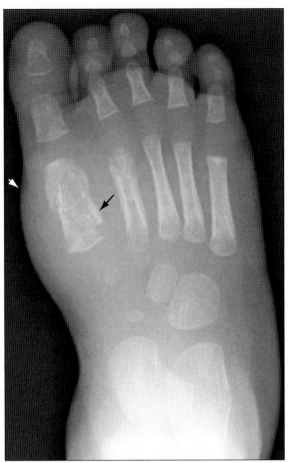

Figure 1. Anteroposterior radiograph of right foot reveals soft tissue swelling (*white arrow*), and "moth-eaten" bony destruction within expanded first metatarsal with periosteal new bone formation (*black arrow*). Similar, although less extensive, changes are noted in the second metatarsal.

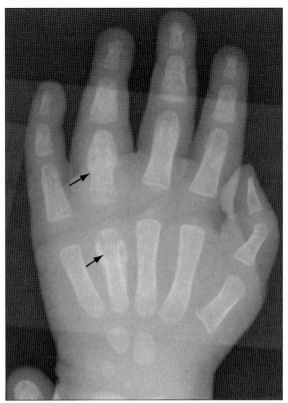

Figure 2. Anteroposterior radiograph of left hand reveals expanded fourth metacarpal and proximal phalanx (*arrows*) with areas of mottled lucency and periosteal new bone formation with surrounding soft tissue swelling.

Case 228

DEMOGRAPHICS/CLINICAL HISTORY

The patient is a 15-year-old boy with β-thalassemia.

FINDINGS

Skull radiographs show widening of the diploic spaces of the skull with a "hair-on-end" appearance (Figs. 1 and 2).

DISCUSSION

Definition/Background

Thalassemia is a heritable hemoglobinopathy that occurs with high frequency in Mediterranean regions. Patients are most severely affected when they are homozygous for the β-thalassemia hemoglobin gene, in which case an excess of insoluble α chains in red blood cells causes intracellular precipitation.

Characteristic Clinical Features

Patients present with anemia and jaundice. Without treatment, life expectancy is only several years.

Characteristic Radiologic Findings

Patients usually present with splenomegaly, which can be detected on abdominal ultrasound or computed tomography (CT). Skeletal radiographs show osteopenia and undertubulation of the shafts of the long bones, and thinning of the bony cortex. The hyperplastic marrow expands the medullary cavities throughout the skeleton, causing a classic "hair-on-end" appearance in the skull.

Less Common Radiologic Manifestations

The ribs appear widened and osteopenic. The classic "rodent facies" appearance is secondary to marrow overgrowth in the maxillary bone, which causes lateral displacement of the orbits and vertical displacement of the central incisors.

Differential Diagnosis

- Sickle cell anemia—acute chest syndrome (pediatric)
- Leukemia, acute lymphoblastic (pediatric)
- Mastocytosis

Discussion

Sickle cell anemia occurs in patients homozygous for the S hemoglobin gene, which causes the red blood cells to assume an abnormal morphology, resulting in obstruction at the capillary level. Osseous abnormalities are largely secondary to infarction and may affect any bone in the body. The skeleton is a common site of involvement in acute leukemic conditions, and osseous lesions are most common in children younger than 5 years. Skeletal radiographs show lucent metaphyseal bands in the long bones, periosteal new bone formation, and diffuse osteoporosis. Mastocytosis is an abnormal proliferation of mast cells that may be systemic or cutaneous. In systemic mastocytosis, skeletal changes include widespread osteosclerosis with focal osteolytic lesions.

Diagnosis

Thalassemia

Suggested Readings

Chan YL, Pang LM, Chik KW, et al: Patterns of bone disease in transfusion-dependent homozygous thalassaemia major: Predominance of osteoporosis and desferrioxamine-induced bone dysplasia. Pediatr Radiol 32:492-497, 2002.

Moseley JR: Skeletal changes in the anemias. Semin Roentgenol 9:169-184, 1974.

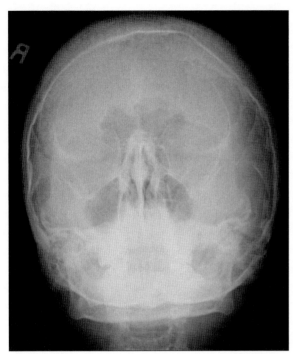

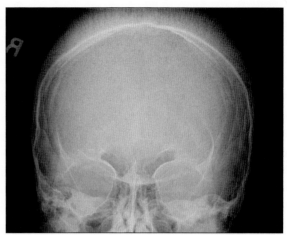

Figure 2. Magnification view from posteroanterior skull radiograph better shows widening of diploic spaces of skull with a "hair-on-end" appearance.

Figure 1. Waters view of the skull shows widening of diploic spaces of the skull with "hair-on-end" appearance related to widened medullary spaces.

Case 229

DEMOGRAPHICS/CLINICAL HISTORY

The patient is a 15-year-old boy with left knee pain.

FINDINGS

Magnetic resonance imaging (MRI) of the left knee shows a large joint effusion with multiple intra-articular rice bodies (Fig. 1) and nodular synovial enhancement (Figs. 2 and 3).

DISCUSSION

Definition/Background

In addition to knee pain, this patient had an elevated erythrocyte sedimentation rate and hypertrophied, inflamed synovium noted at arthroscopy.

Characteristic Clinical Features

This patient was suspected to have an inflammatory arthritis after arthroscopy was performed, and a thickened "shaggy" synovium was encountered. In this case, contrast agent administration was crucial to the MRI diagnosis to illustrate the thickened, enhancing synovium.

Characteristic Radiologic Findings

Imaging findings include synovial enhancement, joint effusion, and multiple intra-articular rice bodies.

Differential Diagnosis

- Septic arthritis
- Lyme arthritis

Discussion

Lyme arthritis is due to infection with a spirochete, *Borrelia burgdorferi*. Imaging features at MRI are similar to idiopathic arthritis, although enlarged popliteal lymph nodes and myositis are seen more often in the presence of Lyme arthritis.

Diagnosis

Juvenile rheumatoid arthritis

Suggested Readings

Gylys-Morin VM, Graham TB, Blebea JS, et al: Knee in early juvenile rheumatoid arthritis: MR imaging findings. Radiology 220:696-706, 2001.

Johnson K: Imaging of juvenile idiopathic arthritis. Pediatr Radiol 36:743-758, 2006.

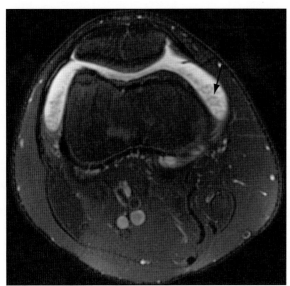

Figure 1. Axial fat-saturated T2-weighted MR image through the knee shows large joint effusion with multiple intra-articular rice bodies (*arrow*).

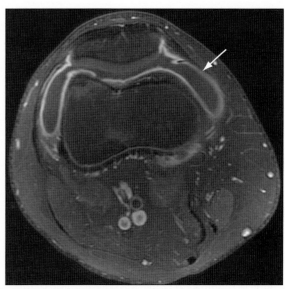

Figure 2. Axial fat-saturated T1-weighted MR image through the knee after administration of intravenous gadolinium reveals diffuse synovial enhancement (*arrow*).

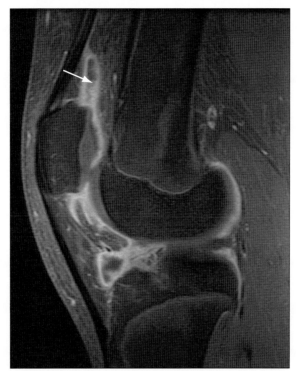

Figure 3. Sagittal fat-saturated T1-weighted MR image through the knee after administration of intravenous gadolinium reveals diffuse, nodular synovial enhancement (*arrow*).

Case 230

DEMOGRAPHICS/CLINICAL HISTORY

The patient is a 17-year-old adolescent with knee pain and swelling after three knee joint aspirations that revealed bloody fluid.

FINDINGS

Magnetic resonance imaging (MRI) evaluation of the knee shows a large joint effusion. On T2-weighted images, there are multiple fronds of low signal intensity synovial tissue within the suprapatellar joint space (Fig. 1). On gradient-recalled-echo MRI sequences, there is signal dropout or "blooming" of the corresponding areas (Fig. 2). After gadolinium administration, there is abnormal nodular synovial enhancement (Fig. 3).

DISCUSSION

Definition/Background
Pigmented villonodular synovitis (PVNS) is more common in adults, although children and adolescents 10 to 20 years old account for 15% of cases.

Characteristic Clinical Features
Patients often present with pain and swelling. Most cases are monarticular, although polyarticular disease can occur in children.

Characteristic Radiologic Findings
Radiographs are often normal, although a joint effusion is usually present. MRI reveals multiple nodular synovial masses with hemosiderin, which causes signal dropout of gradient-recalled-echo images.

Less Common Radiologic Manifestations
In rare cases, PVNS may invade the bone and soft tissues.

Differential Diagnosis
- Juvenile idiopathic arthritis
- Hemophilic arthropathy
- Intra-articular vascular malformation
- Synovial osteochondromatosis

Discussion
Juvenile idiopathic arthritis is the most common form of chronic arthritis in children. Radiographic changes include soft tissue swelling, osteopenia or osteoporosis, joint space narrowing, bony erosions, intra-articular bony ankylosis, periostitis, growth disturbances, epiphyseal compression fracture, joint subluxation, and synovial cysts. PVNS produces hemosiderin deposition in the synovium similar to that of hemophilia. The early changes of effusion and synovitis in hemophilic arthropathy are poorly seen on radiographs, and computed tomography (CT), ultrasound, and MRI can better evaluate masses that develop in a patient with hemophilia. Intra-articular vascular malformations include synovial hemangiomas and arteriovenous malformations. Synovial hemangiomas are rare, benign lesions with increased numbers of blood vessels. They arise from any surface that is lined by synovium and typically occur in young patients. On MRI, hemangiomas have increased signal intensity on T1-weighted and T2-weighted images. MRI and magnetic resonance angiography (MRA) can accurately differentiate hemangiomas from vascular malformations, including arteriovenous malformations. Synovial osteochondromatosis, also called synovial chondromatosis, is a benign condition characterized by synovial membrane proliferation and metaplasia. If the intra-articular fragments are adequately calcified, the diagnosis can be made with plain radiography. For noncalcified fragments, MRI is required to show the nature and extent of disease. Pressure erosions and cyst formation can be seen in adjacent bone, although this is more typical for joints with lax capsules, such as the hip. A similar observation may be found in patients with PVNS.

Diagnosis
Pigmented villonodular synovitis

Suggested Readings
Bravo SM, Winalski CS, Weissman BN: Pigmented villonodular synovitis. Radiol Clin North Am 34:311-326, 1996.

Eckhardt BP, Hernandez RJ: Pigmented villonodular synovitis: MR imaging in pediatric patients. Pediatr Radiol 34:943-947, 2004.

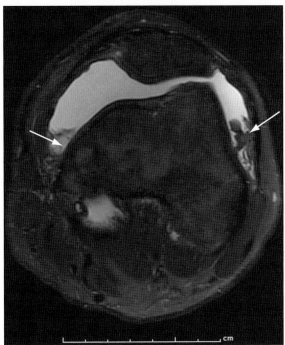

Figure 1. Axial T2-weighted MR image through the knee shows large suprapatellar joint effusion with multiple, nodular, low signal intensity lesions along the synovium projecting within joint (*arrows*).

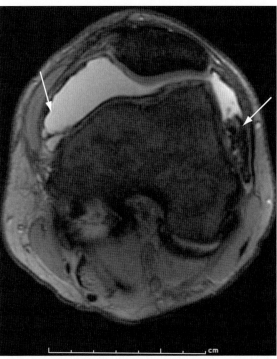

Figure 2. Axial gradient-recalled-echo MR image through the knee shows low signal intensity "blooming" artifact related to hemosiderin deposition along the synovium (*arrows*).

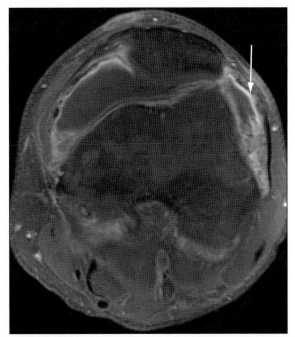

Figure 3. Axial T1-weighted fat-suppressed MR image through the knee after gadolinium administration reveals abnormal nodular synovial enhancement (*arrow*).

Case 231

DEMOGRAPHICS/CLINICAL HISTORY

The patient is a 12-year-old boy with ankle pain and crepitus.

FINDINGS

Coronal and sagittal reformatted images from a computed tomography (CT) scan through the ankle show a round, ossific density within the region of the sinus tarsi (Figs. 1 and 2). A sagittal T1-weighted image from magnetic resonance imaging (MRI) of the ankle shows a round lesion in the sinus tarsi that follows marrow signal consistent with an osseous fragment (Fig. 3).

DISCUSSION

Definition/Background
Synovial osteochondromatosis is a rare disorder in children. It consists of metaplastic transformation of the synovium and formation of osteocartilaginous foci in the joint space.

Characteristic Clinical Features
Synovial osteochondromatosis is typically monarticular and has a predilection for large joints, such as the hip.

Characteristic Radiologic Findings
Plain radiographs show multiple calcified or ossified loose bodies in the joint space, usually of relatively uniform size and shape.

Less Common Radiologic Manifestations
MRI better shows noncalcified or nonossified cartilaginous loose bodies, which appear bright on T2-weighted images. Joint effusion and synovial thickening are typically present.

Differential Diagnosis
- Pigmented villonodular synovitis
- Synovial vascular malformation

Discussion
Pigmented villonodular synovitis consists of multinodular masses within the joint or synovium. The presence of hemosiderin deposition causes signal dropout on T2-weighted MRI. Synovial vascular malformations are benign lesions that most commonly occur in the knee. A lobulated soft tissue mass within the joint is detected on MRI, and the presence of phleboliths is classic.

Diagnosis
Synovial osteochondromatosis

Suggested Readings
McKenzie G, Raby N, Ritchie D: A pictorial review of primary synovial osteochondromatosis: Non-neoplastic soft tissue masses. Br J Radiol 82:775-785, 2009.
Murphey MD, Vidal JA, Fanburg-Smith JC, et al: Imaging of synovial chondromatosis with radiologic-pathologic correlation. RadioGraphics 27:1465-1488, 2007.

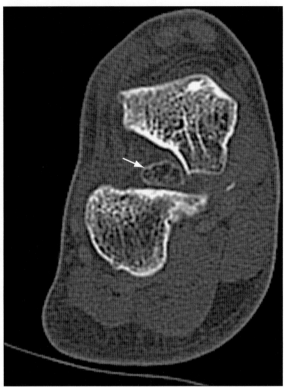

Figure 1. Coronal reformatted image from CT scan through the ankle shows round, ossific density within region of the sinus tarsi (*arrow*).

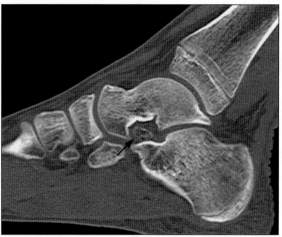

Figure 2. Sagittal reformatted image from CT scan through the ankle shows round, ossific density within region of the sinus tarsi (*arrow*).

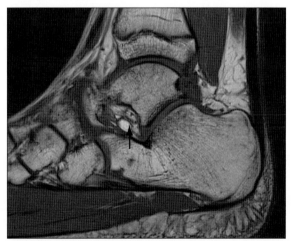

Figure 3. Sagittal T1-weighted MR image of the ankle shows round lesion in sinus tarsi that follows marrow signal consistent with osseous fragment (*arrow*).

Case 232

DEMOGRAPHICS/CLINICAL HISTORY

The patient is a 16-year-old girl with ankle pain and a history of psoriatic arthritis.

FINDINGS

Magnetic resonance imaging (MRI) of the ankle reveals abnormal signal surrounding the medial and lateral tendons on fluid-sensitive sequences (Fig. 1). There is a subtalar joint effusion (Fig. 2), and abnormal enhancement of the tendon sheaths is seen (Fig. 3).

DISCUSSION

Definition/Background

Psoriatic arthritis is seen more often in female patients.

Characteristic Clinical Features

Features of psoriatic disease include arthritis with dactylitis, nail pitting, and a positive family history. The arthritis is often pauciarticular and has a tendency to involve the tendon sheaths.

Characteristic Radiologic Findings

MRI features of the disease include the presence of joint effusion, synovial enhancement, and abnormal enhancement of the tendon sheaths. Osseous erosions may be appreciated on radiographs and on MRI.

Differential Diagnosis

- Juvenile idiopathic arthritis
- Lyme arthritis
- Seronegative spondyloarthropathies

Discussion

Lyme arthritis is caused by infection with the spirochete *Borrelia burgdorferi*. Seronegative spondyloarthropathies are a group of inflammatory arthritides that often affect the axial skeleton and joints.

Diagnosis

Psoriatic arthritis

Suggested Readings

Buchmann RF, Jaramillo D: Imaging of articular disorders in children. Radiol Clin North Am 42:151-168, 2004.

Weishaupt D, Schweitzer ME, Alam F, et al: MR imaging of inflammatory joint diseases of the foot and ankle. Skeletal Radiol 28:663-669, 1999.

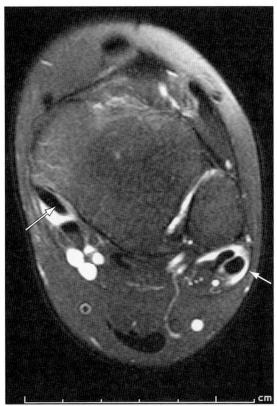

Figure 1. Axial T2-weighted fat-suppressed MR image through the ankle reveals abnormally bright signal intensity surrounding medial and lateral tendons (*arrows*).

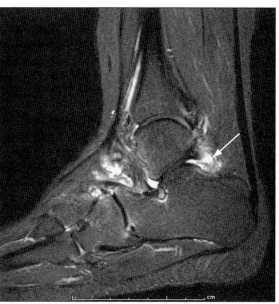

Figure 2. Sagittal T2-weighted fat-suppressed MR image through the ankle shows subtalar joint effusion (*arrow*). There is also abnormal signal anterior to the talus.

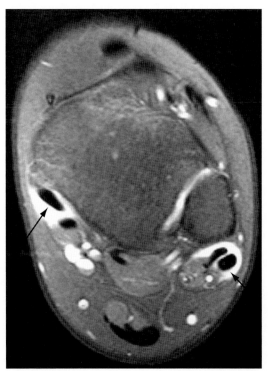

Figure 3. Axial T1-weighted fat-suppressed MR image through the ankle after intravenous administration of contrast agent shows abnormal enhancement of tendon sheaths (*arrows*).

Case 233

DEMOGRAPHICS/CLINICAL HISTORY

The patient is a 17-year-old boy with hemophilia and ankle pain.

FINDINGS

A plain radiograph of the ankle (Fig. 1) shows marked narrowing of the ankle joint space, subchondral bone destruction and cyst formation, and flattening of the talar dome. Axial proton density magnetic resonance imaging (MRI) of the ankle (Fig. 2) shows marked joint space narrowing, flattening of the talar dome, and full-thickness cartilage loss involving the talar and tibial articular surfaces. Sagittal short tau inversion recovery (STIR) image from MRI of the ankle (Fig. 3) shows joint space narrowing associated with bone marrow edema within the periarticular aspects of the distal tibia and talar dome.

DISCUSSION

Definition/Background
Hemophilic arthropathy is an X-linked recessive disorder that leads to abnormal coagulation mechanisms. Hemorrhage into joints causes accelerated arthritis and joint destruction.

Characteristic Clinical Features
Patients are nearly always male. Commonly affected joints include the knee, elbow, and ankle.

Characteristic Radiologic Findings
Plain radiographs show radiodense joint effusions and subchondral sclerosis and cyst formation. The intercondylar notch in the knee is typically widened, and the radial head in the elbow may appear enlarged.

Less Common Radiologic Manifestations
MRI shows the presence of hemarthrosis, synovial thickening with diffuse hemosiderin deposition, and cartilage abnormalities.

Differential Diagnosis
- Neuropathic joint
- Pigmented villonodular synovitis
- Foreign body synovitis

Discussion
A neuropathic joint is the result of a destructive arthropathy related to repetitive trauma or altered sensation (such as occurs in diabetes and children with myelomeningocele). Pigmented villonodular synovitis consists of multilobular synovial masses with hemosiderin deposition causing signal dropout on T2-weighted MRI. Foreign body synovitis is a monarticular arthritis that is associated with a puncture wound. The foreign body may be a thorn or splinter that may be appreciated only on MRI or ultrasound.

Diagnosis
Hemophilic arthropathy

Suggested Readings
Baunin C, Railhac JJ, Younes I, et al: MR imaging in hemophilic arthropathy. Eur J Pediatr Surg 1:358-363, 1991.

Ng WH, Chu WC, Shing MK, et al: Role of imaging in management of hemophilic patients. AJR Am J Roentgenol 184:1619-1623, 2005.

Yulish BS, Lieberman JM, Strandjord SE, et al: Hemophilic arthropathy: Assessment with MR imaging. Radiology 164:759-762, 1987.

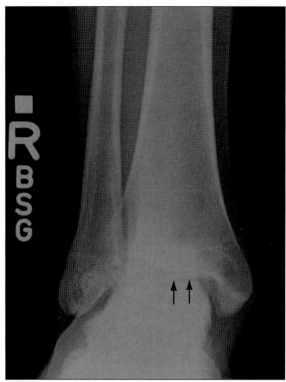

Figure 1. Anteroposterior radiograph of the ankle shows marked narrowing of ankle joint space, subchondral bone destruction and cyst formation, and flattening of the talar dome (*arrows*).

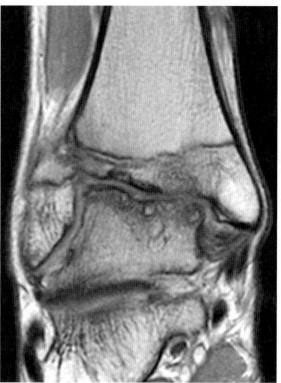

Figure 2. Axial proton density MR image of the ankle shows marked joint space narrowing, flattening of the talar dome, and full-thickness cartilage loss involving the talar and tibial articular surfaces.

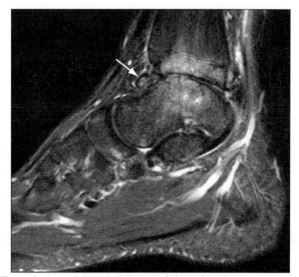

Figure 3. Sagittal STIR MR image of the ankle shows joint space narrowing associated with bone marrow edema within periarticular aspects of distal tibia and talar dome. Synovium is thickened and is diffusely low in signal secondary to hemosiderin deposition (*arrow*).

Case 234

DEMOGRAPHICS/CLINICAL HISTORY

The patient is a 15-year-old boy with a history of hemophilia and a fall.

FINDINGS

Magnetic resonance imaging (MRI) of the pelvis shows a lenticular subperiosteal collection along the inner aspect of the right iliac bone, which is heterogeneous on T1-weighted images (Fig. 1) and heterogeneously bright on T2-weighted images (Fig. 2). After administration of contrast agent, there is peripheral enhancement surrounding the collection and linear areas of central enhancement (Fig. 3). Computed tomography (CT) scan performed 3 weeks later (Fig. 4) shows a sharply defined ossific border surrounding the lesion.

DISCUSSION

Definition/Background

Hemophilic pseudotumor is a rare process that occurs in 1% to 2% of patients with hemophilia. It is caused by repetitive bleeding into bones or soft tissues and usually is related to trauma.

Characteristic Clinical Features

Hemophilic pseudotumor is an encapsulated, slowly growing hematoma that occurs in patients with a coagulation disorder such as hemophilia. The lesions may be osseous, subperiosteal, or soft tissue, depending on the location.

Characteristic Radiologic Findings

Intraosseous pseudotumors produce expansile, lytic lesions of various sizes that simulate bone tumors. Soft tissue pseudotumors manifest with increased attenuation within soft tissue structures, which may or may not contain calcifications.

Less Common Radiologic Manifestations

Subperiosteal pseudotumors (as in this case) manifest with subperiosteal collections that extend into the adjacent soft tissues and produce a periosteal reaction.

Differential Diagnosis

- Ewing sarcoma
- Tuberculosis
- Metastasis
- Aneurysmal bone cyst
- Brown tumor

Discussion

A Brown tumor is a lytic osseous lesion seen in patients with hyperparathyroidism.

Diagnosis

Hemophilic pseudotumor

Suggested Readings

Park JS, Ryu KN: Hemophilic pseudotumor involving the musculoskeletal system: Spectrum of radiologic findings. AJR Am J Roentgenol 183:55-61, 2004.

Stafford JM, James TT, Allen AM, et al: Hemophilic pseudotumor: Radiologic-pathologic correlation. RadioGraphics 23:852-856, 2003.

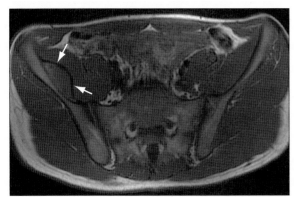

Figure 1. Axial T1-weighted MR image of the pelvis shows subperiosteal collection along inner surface of right iliac bone and projecting into iliacus muscle (*arrows*), producing a heterogeneous signal.

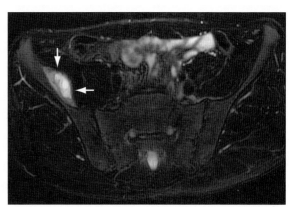

Figure 2. Axial T2-weighted fat-suppressed MR image of the pelvis shows subperiosteal collection along inner surface of right iliac bone (*arrows*), which has a heterogeneous signal, although it contains bright signal intensity centrally.

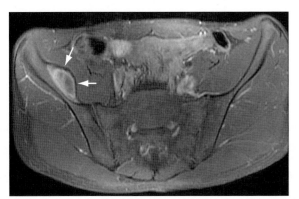

Figure 3. Axial T1-weighted fat-suppressed MR image of the pelvis after administration of intravenous contrast agent shows peripheral enhancement of subperiosteal collection along inner surface of right iliac bone (*arrows*) with areas of fine, linear, central enhancement.

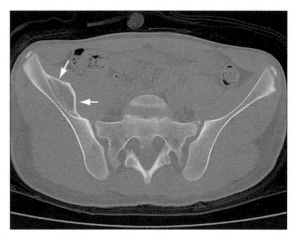

Figure 4. Axial CT scan of the pelvis shows well-circumscribed subperiosteal collection along inner surface of right iliac bone (*arrows*), which contains central areas of calcification.

Case 235

DEMOGRAPHICS/CLINICAL HISTORY

The patient is an 18-year-old woman with frostbite injuries to the left hand after being found unconscious in the snow.

FINDINGS

A plain radiograph of the left hand 1 month after exposure to extreme cold (Fig. 1) shows a contraction deformity of the middle finger without frank osseous injuries. A plain radiograph of the left hand obtained several months after surgical amputation of the left middle finger (Fig. 2) shows a prosthesis in place. There is acro-osteolysis of the distal tufts of the second, fourth, and fifth digits.

DISCUSSION

Definition/Background
Exposure to extremely cold temperatures causes damage to the most distal portions of bones (tips of fingers and toes) secondary to ischemic damage.

Characteristic Clinical Features
Patients present with necrotic damage to the affected digits, usually with loss of the nail of the affected digit and soft tissue damage.

Characteristic Radiologic Findings
Manifestations of damage on plain radiographs occur 6 to 12 months after the injury and include shortening of the phalanges secondary to premature growth plate fusion and amputation of the distal aspects of the phalanges.

Differential Diagnosis
- Hadju-Cheney syndrome
- Scleroderma
- Congenital insensitivity to pain

Discussion
Patients with congenital insensitivity to pain sustain injuries to the extremities identical to patients with frostbite because these patients are often unaware of extreme temperatures in their digits. Patients with scleroderma and other connective tissue disorders may also have acro-osteolysis of the distal phalanges. Patients with Hadju-Cheney syndrome have characteristic bandlike acro-osteolysis of the distal phalanges, in contrast to the terminal acro-osteolysis that occurs in thermal injuries.

Diagnosis
Frostbite

Suggested Readings
McAdams TR, Swenson DR, Miller RA: Frostbite: An orthopedic perspective. Am J Orthop 28:21-26, 1999.
Pulla RJ, Pickard LJ, Carnett TS: Frostbite: An overview with case presentations. J Foot Ankle Surg 33:53-63, 1994.

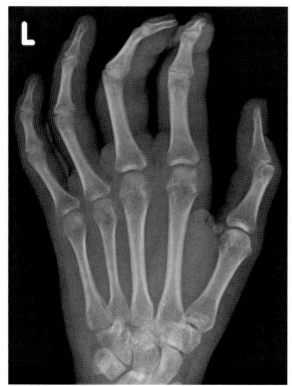

Figure 1. Plain radiograph of the left hand 1 month after injury shows contraction deformity of middle finger without frank osseous injuries.

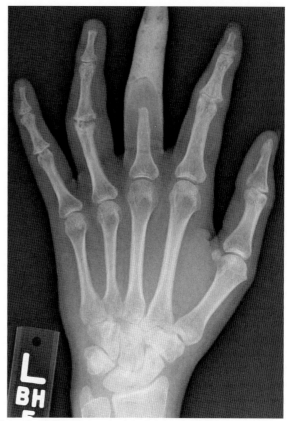

Figure 2. Plain radiograph of the left hand obtained several weeks after surgical amputation of left middle finger shows prosthesis in place. There is acro-osteolysis of the distal tufts of the second, fourth, and fifth digits.

Case 236

DEMOGRAPHICS/CLINICAL HISTORY

The patient is an 8-year-old boy with right hip pain.

FINDINGS

Anteroposterior (Fig. 1) and frog-leg lateral (Fig. 2) radiographs of the hips and pelvis show that the right femoral capital epiphysis is flattened, sclerotic, and fragmented.

DISCUSSION

Definition/Background

Legg-Calvé-Perthes disease occurs in children 4 to 8 years old and is believed to be idiopathic.

Characteristic Clinical Features

Hip pain is a common presenting symptom.

Characteristic Radiologic Findings

Patients may present at different stages of the disease process. By the time the femoral head appears fragmented and sclerotic, this is late-stage disease.

Differential Diagnosis

- Meyer dysplasia
- Avascular necrosis secondary to other causes (e.g., steroid use)

Discussion

When avascular necrosis of the femoral head is not idiopathic, but is secondary to a known cause (e.g., high-dose steroids), the diagnosis is not Legg-Calvé-Perthes disease.

Diagnosis

Legg-Calvé-Perthes disease

Suggested Readings

Connolly LP, Treves ST: Assessing the limping child with skeletal scintigraphy. J Nucl Med 39:1056-1061, 1998.
Wall EJ: Legg-Calvé Perthes' disease. Curr Opin Pediatr 11:76-79, 1999.

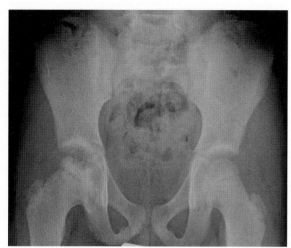

Figure 1. Anteroposterior radiograph of the pelvis reveals sclerosis, fragmentation, and loss of height of right femoral epiphysis. Left hip is normal.

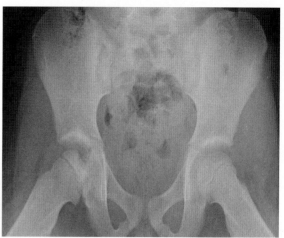

Figure 2. Frog-leg lateral view of the pelvis shows similar findings.

Case 237

DEMOGRAPHICS/CLINICAL HISTORY

The patient is a 9-year-old girl with knee pain.

FINDINGS

Plain radiography of the knee reveals swelling anterior to the tibial tubercle (Fig. 1). Subsequent magnetic resonance imaging (MRI) studies (Figs. 2-4) show increased fluid signal within the soft tissues anterior to the tibial tubercle and abnormal bone marrow signal within the tubercle itself.

DISCUSSION

Definition/Background

Osgood-Schlatter disease commonly is seen in active adolescents, primarily boys.

Characteristic Radiologic Findings

Imaging shows soft tissue swelling at the insertion site of the patellar tendon on the tibial tubercle and marrow edema within the tibial tubercle.

Less Common Radiologic Manifestations

Imaging also shows irregularity and fragmentation of the tibial tubercle.

Differential Diagnosis

- Avulsion of the tibial tubercle

Discussion

An avulsion of the tibial tubercle represents an acute fracture at the insertion site of the patellar tendon.

Diagnosis

Osgood-Schlatter disease

Suggested Readings

Hirano A, Fukubayashi T, Ishii T, et al: Magnetic resonance imaging of Osgood-Schlatter disease: The course of the disease. Skeletal Radiol 31:334-342, 2002.

Rosenberg ZS, Kawelblum M, Cheung YY, et al: Osgood-Schlatter lesion: Fracture or tendonitis? Scintigraphic, CT, and MRI imaging features. Radiology 185:853-858, 1992.

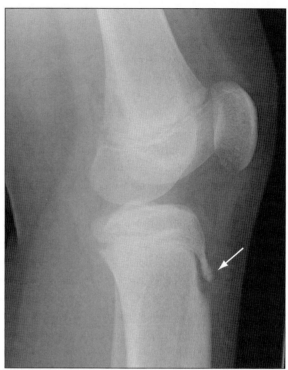

Figure 1. Lateral radiograph of the knee reveals soft tissue swelling anterior to tibial tubercle and thickening of distal patellar tendon (*arrow*).

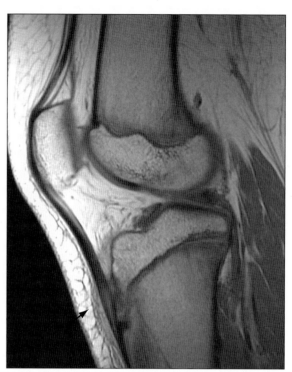

Figure 2. Sagittal T1-weighted MR image reveals abnormal fluid signal anterior to attachment site of patellar tendon at tibial tubercle (*arrow*).

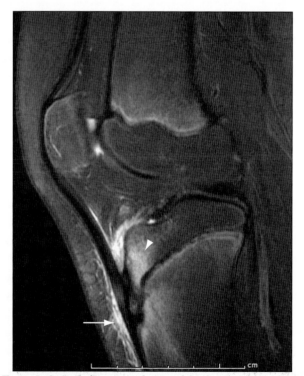

Figure 3. Sagittal fat-saturated T2-weighted MR image shows abnormal fluid signal at attachment of patellar tendon on tibial tubercle (*arrow*) and abnormal bone marrow signal within anterior tibia (*arrowhead*).

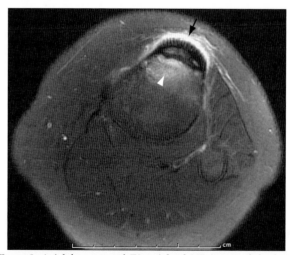

Figure 4. Axial fat-saturated T2-weighted MR image of the knee through the level of patellar tendon insertion on tibial tubercle shows abnormal high signal within soft tissues (*arrow*) and within bone marrow of anterior tibia (*arrowhead*).

Case 238

DEMOGRAPHICS/CLINICAL HISTORY

The patient is a 3-year-old girl with bowed legs.

FINDINGS

A standing anteroposterior radiograph of the lower extremities (Fig. 1) shows asymmetric depression of the proximal, medial portion of the left tibial metaphysis, associated with genu varum. A coronal three-dimensional gradient-recalled-echo sequence from magnetic resonance imaging (MRI) through both knees side-by-side (Fig. 2) shows abnormal bony bridging occurring at the posteromedial aspect of the proximal tibial physis on the left side.

DISCUSSION

Definition/Background

Blount disease, or tibia vara, is a common condition. It is believed to be related to growth suppression at the posteromedial aspect of the proximal tibial physis secondary to stress reaction. Infantile Blount disease is the most common form, but juvenile and late-onset forms also exist.

Characteristic Clinical Features

Patients are often obese and present with bowed legs and gait disturbance.

Characteristic Radiologic Findings

Standing anteroposterior radiographs of both legs show genu varum associated with abnormal depression and irregularity of the posteromedial aspect of the proximal tibial metaphysis. The physis may also appear widened.

Differential Diagnosis
- Physiologic bowing
- Neurofibromatosis
- Rickets

Discussion

Physiologic bowing is thought to be secondary to in utero molding of the lower extremities. This condition usually occurs in children younger than 2 years and corrects when the child begins walking. In contrast to Blount disease, it is usually bilateral. Neurofibromatosis type 1 may cause anterolateral bowing of the tibia in association with hamartomatous fibrous tissue within the bone. Children with rickets may present with bowing of the long bones secondary to the deficient mineralization of osteoid matrix. The physes may also appear widened.

Diagnosis

Blount disease

Suggested Readings

Cheema JI, Grissom LE, Harcke HT: Radiographic characteristics of lower-extremity bowing in children. RadioGraphics 23:871-880, 2003.

Langenskiold A: Tibia vara: A critical review. Clin Orthop Relat Res 246:195-207, 1989.

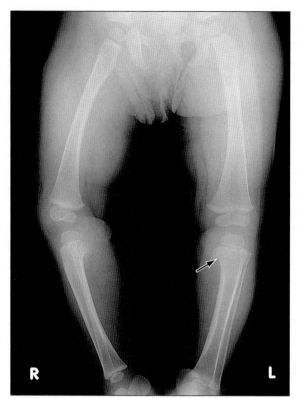

Figure 1. Standing anteroposterior radiograph of lower extremities shows asymmetric depression of proximal, medial portion of left tibial metaphysis (*arrow*), associated with genu varum.

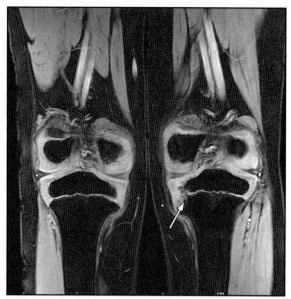

Figure 2. Coronal three-dimensional gradient-recalled-echo sequence from MRI through both knees side-by-side shows abnormal bony bridging occurring at posteromedial aspect of proximal tibial physis on left side (*arrow*).

Case 239

DEMOGRAPHICS/CLINICAL HISTORY

The patient is a 5-year-old girl with foot pain.

FINDINGS

Anteroposterior and lateral radiographs of the foot (Figs. 1 and 2) show flattening, sclerosis, and fragmentation of the tarsal navicular.

DISCUSSION

Definition/Background

Köhler disease is a rare, idiopathic osteochondrosis involving the tarsal navicular bone. It affects children 5 to 6 years old, and boys are affected more frequently than girls.

Characteristic Clinical Features

Patients present with limp, pain, and swelling along the dorsum of the midfoot.

Characteristic Radiologic Findings

Plain radiographs show sclerosis, fragmentation, and flattening of the navicular bone.

Less Common Radiologic Manifestations

Magnetic resonance imaging (MRI) reveals abnormal bone marrow signal, which does not enhance after gadolinium administration, consistent with necrosis.

Differential Diagnosis

- Delayed, irregular ossification of the navicular

Discussion

Delayed, irregular ossification of the navicular is seen in younger children (girls 18 to 24 months old and boys 30 to 36 months old) and may appear bilaterally.

Diagnosis

Köhler disease

Suggested Reading

Khoury J, Jerushalmi J, Loberant N, et al: Köhler disease: Diagnoses and assessment by bone scintigraphy. Clin Nucl Med 32:179-181, 2007.

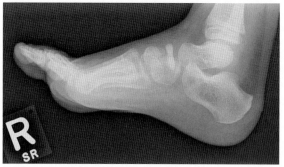

Figure 2. Lateral radiograph of the foot shows flattening, sclerosis, and fragmentation of the tarsal navicular.

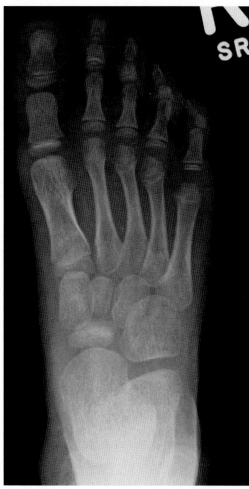

Figure 1. Anteroposterior radiograph of the foot shows flattening, sclerosis, and fragmentation of tarsal navicular.

Case 240

DEMOGRAPHICS/CLINICAL HISTORY

The patient is a 13-year-old boy with a history of acute lymphoblastic leukemia on high-dose steroids with right hip pain.

FINDINGS

A plain radiograph of the pelvis (Fig. 1) is remarkable for osteopenia and an incidental bone island in the right femoral neck. Magnetic resonance imaging (MRI) of the hips and pelvis reveals serpiginous signal abnormality in the proximal femurs on T1-weighted (Fig. 2) and T2-weighted (Fig. 3) images, which enhances after administration of gadolinium (Fig. 4).

DISCUSSION

Definition/Background
The high-dose steroids that are part of many chemotherapy regimens for cancer patients place these patients at risk for osteonecrosis.

Characteristic Clinical Features
In this patient, the bony changes were related to his high-dose steroid regimen, which is a known cause for bone infarction. The presenting symptom is most often hip pain when the changes occur in the proximal femur, such as in this case.

Characteristic Radiologic Findings
The "double-line" sign is the characteristic manifestation of bone infarction on MRI, which consists of serpiginous areas of dark signal intensity adjacent to areas of bright signal.

Differential Diagnosis
- Osteomyelitis
- Chondroblastoma

Discussion
Osteomyelitis also manifests on MRI as abnormal bone marrow signal and enhancement in the epiphyses, although the "double–line" sign of bone infarct should allow differentiation between these two diagnoses. The calcified matrix of a chondroblastoma can appear similar to calcifications within a chronic bone infarct on plain radiographs, although chondroblastomas are commonly epiphyseal lesions, in contrast to bone infarcts, which are often metaphyseal.

Diagnosis
Bone infarct

Suggested Readings
Munk PL, Helms CA, Holt RG: Immature bone infarcts: Findings on plain radiographs and MR scans. AJR Am J Roentgenol 152:547-549, 1989.
Zurlo JV: The double-line sign. Radiology 212:541-542, 1999.

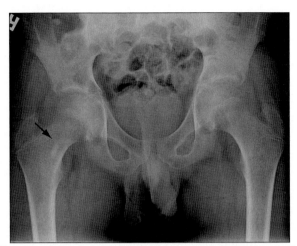

Figure 1. Plain anteroposterior radiograph of the pelvis is remarkable for diffuse osteopenia. Oblong-shaped, sclerotic focus in right femoral neck (*arrow*) is consistent with a bone island.

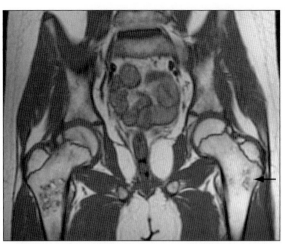

Figure 2. Coronal T1-weighted MR image of both hips reveals serpiginous foci of low signal intensity within bilateral femurs, right more than left (*arrow*).

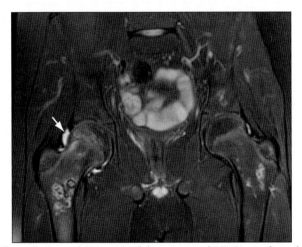

Figure 3. Coronal T2-weighted fat-suppressed MR image through the hips reveals serpiginous areas of low T2 signal surrounded by areas of high T2 signal in proximal femurs. Diffuse bone marrow edema in proximal right femur is manifested as increased signal relative to contralateral hip. There also is a small right hip joint effusion (*arrow*).

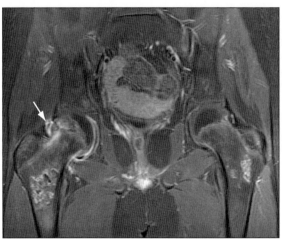

Figure 4. Contrast-enhanced T1-weighted fat-suppressed MR image of both hips shows enhancement surrounding areas of low T1 signal. There also is abnormal bone marrow enhancement in proximal head and neck (*white arrow*) and diffuse synovial enhancement, all likely related to early avascular necrosis of right femoral head.

Case 241

DEMOGRAPHICS/CLINICAL HISTORY

The patient is an 8-year-old girl with bilateral hip pain.

FINDINGS

Anteroposterior (Fig. 1) and frog-leg lateral (Fig. 2) views of the hips reveal asymmetric expansion and irregularity of the left ischiopubic synchondrosis.

DISCUSSION

Definition/Background
The ischiopubic synchondrosis contains cartilage that has a variable ossification pattern and may ossify asymmetrically.

Characteristic Clinical Features
Although patients may complain of pain, this finding on radiographs is usually asymptomatic and incidental.

Characteristic Radiologic Findings
Radiographs show asymmetric enlargement of the ischiopubic synchondrosis on one side relative to the other.

Less Common Radiologic Manifestations
The enlarged ischiopubic synchondrosis may have increased uptake on a radionuclide bone scan.

Differential Diagnosis
- Pelvic osteomyelitis
- Osteosarcoma (Ewing sarcoma)

Discussion
Pelvic osteomyelitis is an infection of the pelvic bones in children that is often centered at the ischiopubic synchondrosis. Often the bone marrow edema and enhancement are not as profound as the adjacent soft tissue abnormality. Ewing sarcoma is a malignant bone tumor that most often affects teenagers. Although the long bones are the most common site of involvement, the pelvis also may be affected.

Diagnosis
Ischiopubic synchondrosis

Suggested Readings
Herneth AM, Philipp MO, Pretterklieber ML, et al: Asymmetric closure of ischiopubic synchondrosis in pediatric patients: Correlation with foot dominance. AJR Am J Roentgenol 182:361, 2004.

Herneth AM, Trattnig S, Bader TR, et al: MR imaging of the ischiopubic synchondrosis. Magn Reson Imaging 18:519, 2000.

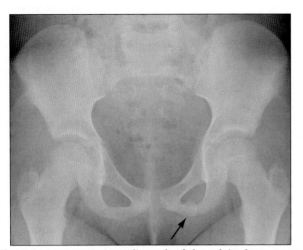

Figure 1. Anteroposterior radiograph of the pelvis shows asymmetric enlargement of left ischiopubic synchondrosis (*arrow*).

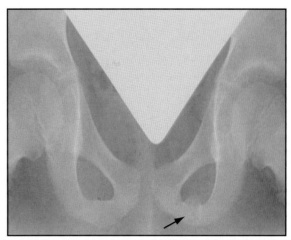

Figure 2. Frog-leg lateral view of both hips shows asymmetric enlargement of left ischiopubic synchondrosis (*arrow*).

Case 242

DEMOGRAPHICS/CLINICAL HISTORY

The patient is a 3-year-old boy with left hip pain and incidental finding on plain radiographs of the knee.

FINDINGS

An anteroposterior radiograph of the left knee (Fig. 1) reveals an oblong lucency projecting in the region of the medial femoral condyle. A lateral radiograph (Fig. 2) shows a cortical defect along the posterior aspect of the condyle. In a different patient, an 8-year-old boy with knee pain, magnetic resonance imaging (MRI) from a three-dimensional spoiled gradient-recalled-echo sequence through the knee (Fig. 3) shows a cortical defect in the posteromedial femoral metaphysis.

DISCUSSION

Definition/Background

This patient presented relatively early (3 years old); this finding is typically identified in patients in the first decade or early second decade of life. Although many patients present with symptoms referable to the knee, the finding is incidental and not related to the symptoms (i.e., this child's hip pain was unrelated to this finding).

Characteristic Clinical Features

This defect is an incidental finding, and not related to the patient's left hip pain.

Characteristic Radiologic Findings

On plain radiographs of the knee, the defect appears as an oblong or round lucent lesion within the medial femoral condyle. A lateral radiograph confirms the posterior location of the lesion.

Differential Diagnosis

- Fibrous cortical defect

Discussion

A fibrous cortical defect is a common pediatric bone tumor (benign), which may be seen in 40% of children. These defects are located within the metaphyses of long bones.

Diagnosis

Distal femoral metaphyseal irregularity

Suggested Readings

Resnick D, Greenway G: Distal femoral cortical defects, irregularities, and excavations. Radiology 143:345-354, 1982.

Yamazaki T, Maruoka S, Takahashi S, et al: MR findings of avulsive cortical irregularity of the distal femur. Skeletal Radiol 24:43-46, 1995.

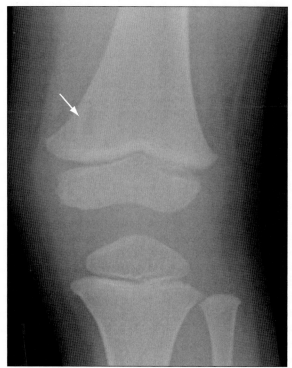

Figure 1. Anteroposterior radiograph of the knee shows oval-shaped lucent lesion projecting over medial femoral condyle (*arrow*).

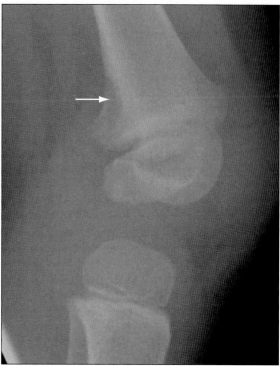

Figure 2. Lateral radiograph of the knee shows posterior cortical defect (*arrow*).

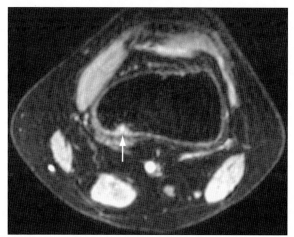

Figure 3. In a different patient, axial reformatted MR image from three-dimensional spoiled gradient-recalled-echo sequence through the knee shows defect within posteromedial cortex of distal femur, which shows high signal (*arrow*).

Case 243

DEMOGRAPHICS/CLINICAL HISTORY

The patient is a 13-year-old boy with knee pain.

FINDINGS

Magnetic resonance imaging (MRI) evaluation of the knee reveals a bilobed fluid collection in the popliteal fossa insinuating between the medial head of the gastrocnemius muscle and the semimembranosus muscle (Figs. 1 and 2), which represents a Baker cyst.

DISCUSSION

Definition/Background
Popliteal, or Baker, cysts may occur at any age. They tend to be more common in boys.

Characteristic Clinical Features
In most cases, a Baker cyst is an isolated finding in children and usually resolves spontaneously.

Characteristic Radiologic Findings
On plain films, a soft tissue mass in the popliteal fossa may be present. On MRI, a Baker cyst appears as a fluid collection between the medial head of the gastrocnemius muscle and the semimembranosus muscle. Baker cysts follow fluid on all sequences, and appear dark on T1-weighted images and bright on T2-weighted images.

Differential Diagnosis
- Hematoma
- Ganglion cyst
- Meniscal cyst

Discussion
A hematoma in the popliteal fossa may appear similar to a Baker cyst; the signal on MRI sequences varies depending on the age of the blood products. A ganglion cyst contains myxomatous debris and may be intra-articular and associated with tendons. A meniscal cyst also follows fluid signal on all sequences and is associated with a tear in the meniscus.

Diagnosis
Baker cyst

Suggested Readings
Janzen DL, Peterfy CG, Forbes JR, et al: Cystic lesions around the knee joint: MR imaging findings. AJR Am J Roentgenol 163:155-161, 1994.
McCarthy CL, McNally EG: The MRI appearance of cystic lesions around the knee. Skeletal Radiol 33:187-209, 2004.

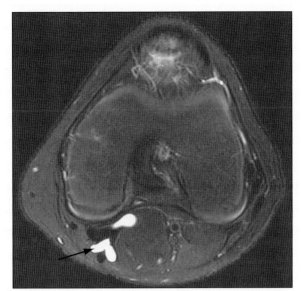

Figure 1. Axial T2-weighted fat-suppressed MR image through the knee shows bilobed fluid collection (*arrow*) insinuating between medial head of gastrocnemius muscle and semimembranosus muscle.

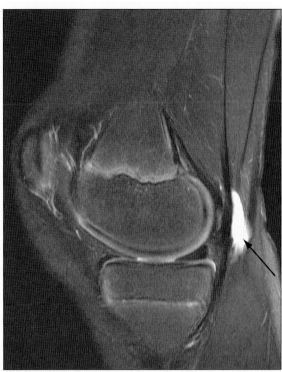

Figure 2. Sagittal T2-weighted fat-suppressed MR image through the knee shows oblong fluid collection (*arrow*) in popliteal fossa adjacent to semimembranosus muscle.

Case 244

DEMOGRAPHICS/CLINICAL HISTORY

The patient is a 17-year-old girl with cervical instability.

FINDINGS

A lateral radiograph (Fig. 1) of the cervical spine performed with the patient in flexion shows an abnormal anterior subluxation of the anterior arch of C1 with respect to the dens, which appears hypoplastic. A C3-C4 fusion can be seen. Axial computed tomography (CT) scan (Fig. 2) through the cervical spine at the level of C1 shows the absence of the odontoid process of C2. Sagittal (Fig. 3) and coronal (Fig. 4) reconstructed CT images of the cervical spine show a small accessory ossicle (i.e., os odontoideum) that has no connection to the body of C2. The body of C2 is directed posteriorly at its superior aspect, causing mild canal narrowing (see Fig. 3).

DISCUSSION

Definition/Background
Os odontoideum is an abnormality of the cervical spine in which the odontoid process is a separate ossicle from the remainder of the body of C2. The abnormality may be congenital or post-traumatic.

Characteristic Clinical Features
The abnormality may be detected incidentally, although patients may also present with spinal instability leading to neurologic impairment.

Characteristic Radiologic Findings
Cervical spine radiographs show an accessory ossicle separate from the body of C2 that projects in the region of the dens. This os odontoideum is often positioned at the base of the clivus. Flexion and extension views reveal abnormal anteroposterior translation of C1 with respect to C2.

Less Common Radiologic Manifestations
Cervical spine magnetic resonance imaging (MRI) may reveal an abnormal signal within the spinal cord at the level of the os odontoideum that is representative of cord edema.

Differential Diagnosis
- C2 fracture

Discussion
A fracture of C2 usually occurs after significant trauma, and it usually appears less well corticated than an os odontoideum, unless it is an old fracture.

Diagnosis
Os odontoideum

Suggested Readings
Choit RL, Jamieson DH, Reilly CW: Os odontoideum: A significant radiographic finding. Pediatr Radiol 35:803-807, 2005.
Klimo P Jr, Kan P, Rao G, et al: Os odontoideum: Presentation, diagnosis, and treatment in a series of 78 patients. J Neurosurg Spine 9:332-342, 2008.

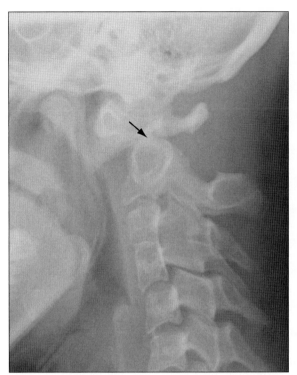

Figure 1. Lateral radiograph of the cervical spine performed with the patient in flexion shows abnormal anterior subluxation of anterior arch of C1 with respect to the dens, which appears hypoplastic (*arrow*). Fusion of C3 and C4 can be seen.

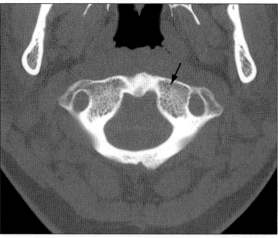

Figure 2. Axial CT image through the cervical spine at the level of C1 (*arrow*) shows absence of odontoid process of C2.

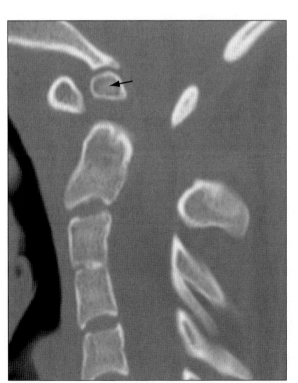

Figure 3. Sagittal reconstructed CT image of the cervical spine shows small accessory ossicle, the os odontoideum (*arrow*), without a connection to the body of C2. The body of C2 is directed posteriorly at its superior aspect, causing mild narrowing of the canal.

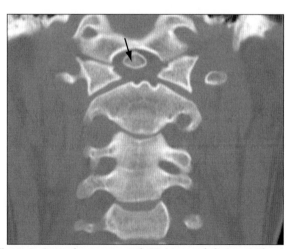

Figure 4. Coronal reconstructed CT image of the cervical spine shows small accessory ossicle, the os odontoideum (*arrow*), without a connection to the body of C2.

Case 245

DEMOGRAPHICS/CLINICAL HISTORY

The patient is a 7-year-old girl with methicillin-resistant *Staphylococcus aureus* septicemia.

FINDINGS

Magnetic resonance imaging (MRI) of the buttock and thigh area (Fig. 1) shows diffusely increased signal intensity within all muscle groups bilaterally. There is a focal area of fluid signal within the left gluteal muscles (Fig. 2). This same area shows peripheral enhancement but without central enhancement after administration of contrast agent, which is consistent with an abscess (Fig. 3).

DISCUSSION

Definition/Background
Pyomyositis refers to an acute infection of skeletal muscle.

Characteristic Clinical Features
Patients may present with fever, pain, and difficulty ambulating.

Characteristic Radiologic Findings
On MRI, the muscles of the buttock and thigh (most commonly affected) have diffusely increased signal intensity on T2-weighted images, and the areas enhance after gadolinium administration.

Less Common Radiologic Manifestations
Rim-enhancing fluid collections may be present when abscesses have developed (as in this case).

Differential Diagnosis
- Dermatomyositis, pediatric
- Trauma
- Myositis ossificans, pediatric

Discussion
Although abnormal fluid signal is seen within the muscle groups of the buttock and thighs in pediatric dermatomyositis, fluid collections are uncommon. Patients who have sustained trauma to the muscle groups of the buttocks and thigh may have diffusely increased muscle signal intensity on T2-weighted MR images.

Diagnosis
Pyomyositis

Suggested Readings
Theodorou SJ, Theodorou DJ, Resnick D: MR imaging findings of pyogenic bacterial myositis (pyomyositis) in patients with local muscle trauma: Illustrative case. Emerg Radiol 14:89-96, 2007.

Yuh WT, Schreiber AE, Montgomery WJ, et al: Magnetic resonance imaging of pyomyositis. Skeletal Radiol 17:190-193, 1988.

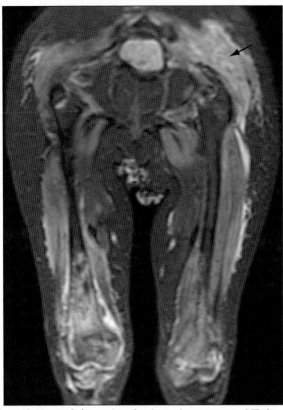

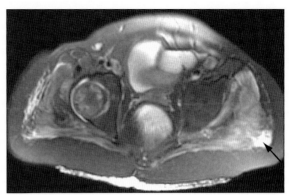

Figure 2. Axial T2-weighted MR image with fat suppression through the level of the femoral heads shows abnormal fluid signal within muscles, including focal area of bright signal intensity within left gluteal muscles (*arrow*).

Figure 1. Coronal fast spin-echo inversion recovery MR image from a study of bilateral hips and thighs shows diffusely increased signal intensity within almost all muscle groups, particularly left gluteal muscles (*arrow*).

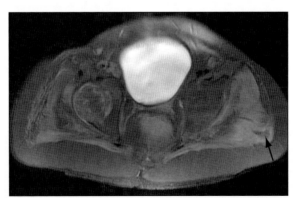

Figure 3. Axial T1-weighted MR image with fat suppression after intravenous administration of contrast agent through the level of the femoral heads shows focal, nonenhancing fluid collection within left gluteal muscles (*arrow*), consistent with abscess.

Case 246

DEMOGRAPHICS/CLINICAL HISTORY

The patient is a 6-year-old girl, previously healthy, who developed a diffuse, erythematous, and painful rash around her face. The rash spread to her arms and legs within a few days. She has also experienced gradual increased weakness. Laboratory studies revealed elevated muscle enzymes.

FINDINGS

Magnetic resonance imaging (MRI) of the hips and thighs was performed. Axial (Fig. 1) and coronal (Fig. 2) short tau inversion recovery (STIR) sequences show diffusely increased signal within the muscles, particularly the vastus lateralis and vastus intermedialis muscles.

DISCUSSION

Characteristic Clinical Features
Proximal lower extremity weakness is a common presenting symptom. This patient was treated with daily steroids and weekly methotrexate injections, and her clinical symptoms improved.

Characteristic Radiologic Findings
MRI is the study of choice to evaluate for changes of dermatomyositis. It reveals diffusely increased signal throughout the muscle on T2-weighted images, thought to be secondary to an underlying vasculitis causing muscle infarction.

Diagnosis
Dermatomyositis

Suggested Readings
Chan WP, Liu GC: MR imaging of primary skeletal muscle diseases in children. AJR Am J Roentgenol 179:989-997, 2002.

Hernandez RJ, Keim DR, Sullivan DB, et al: Magnetic resonance imaging appearance of the muscles in childhood dermatomyositis. J Pediatr 117:546-550, 1990.

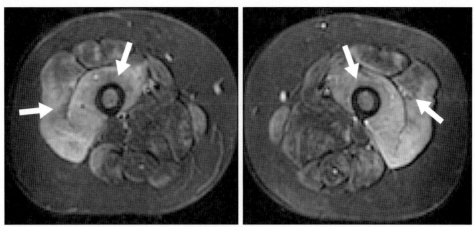

Figure 1. Axial STIR MR image through the thighs reveals bilateral increased signal within all muscle groups, primarily the vastus lateralis and vastus intermedialis (*white arrows*) muscles.

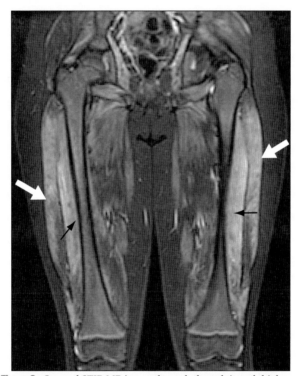

Figure 2. Coronal STIR MR image through the pelvis and thighs reveals abnormal bright signal throughout all muscles, particularly vastus lateralis (*black arrows*) and vastus intermedialis (*white arrows*).

Case 247

DEMOGRAPHICS/CLINICAL HISTORY

The patient is a 17-year-old boy with a 6-month history of pain in the left knee without antecedent trauma or injury, and with a 16-lb weight loss, night sweats, and fevers.

FINDINGS

An anteroposterior radiograph of the distal femur (Fig. 1) reveals diffuse sclerosis, periosteal reaction, and a subtle central lucency within the distal diaphysis. Magnetic resonance imaging (MRI) of the distal femur (Fig. 2) reveals abnormal bone marrow and soft tissue edema. After administration of contrast agent, there is abnormal bone marrow and soft tissue enhancement, with a focal rim-enhancing collection centrally within the distal diaphysis (Figs. 3 and 4).

DISCUSSION

Definition/Background

Osteomyelitis is most often caused by bacterial infection and may occur from hematogenous bacterial spread, adjacent soft tissue infection, a foreign body, or prior trauma or surgery.

Characteristic Clinical Features

Symptoms of bacterial osteomyelitis often include pain in the affected bone and fever, and the patient may have elevated inflammatory markers identified on laboratory studies.

Characteristic Radiologic Findings

On plain radiographs, osteomyelitis manifests as a soft tissue swelling (early) and progresses to a permeative pattern of bone destruction (late). MRI shows areas of abnormal signal intensity, and enhancement within the bone marrow most commonly occurs in the metaphyses of long bones with surrounding abnormal soft tissue edema.

Less Common Radiologic Manifestations

In a long-standing infection, an intraosseous abscess may develop. As bony destruction continues, a thick periosteal sheath (i.e., involucrum) develops, and non-enhancing, devitalized bone (i.e., sequestrum) is seen.

Differential Diagnosis

- Ewing sarcoma
- Osteosarcoma
- Leukemia

Diagnosis

Osteomyelitis

Suggested Readings

Mellada Santos JM: Diagnostic imaging of pediatric hematogenous osteomyelitis: Lessons learned from a multi-modality approach. Eur Radiol 16:2109-2119, 2006.

Morrison WB, Schweitzer ME, Bock GW, et al: Diagnosis of osteomyelitis: Utility of fat-suppressed contrast-enhanced MR imaging. Radiology 189:251-257, 1993.

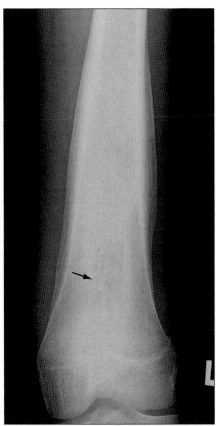

Figure 1. Anteroposterior radiograph of the left distal femur shows diffuse bony sclerosis with mature periosteal new bone formation. Faint, central, irregularly shaped lucency can be appreciated projecting within intramedullary space (*black arrow*).

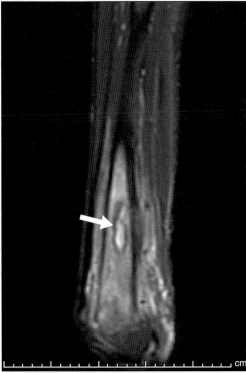

Figure 2. Sagittal short tau inversion recovery (STIR) MR image through the left femur shows diffusely increased bone marrow signal and abnormal signal within surrounding soft tissues. Focal, oblong fluid collection (*arrow*) is identified within distal diaphysis among abnormal bone marrow signals.

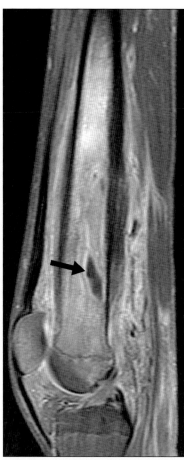

Figure 3. Sagittal T1-weighted fat-suppressed MR image through the distal femur after administration of intravenous gadolinium shows diffuse abnormal bone marrow and soft tissue enhancement. Focal collection within distal diaphysis does not enhance (*arrow*), consistent with abscess.

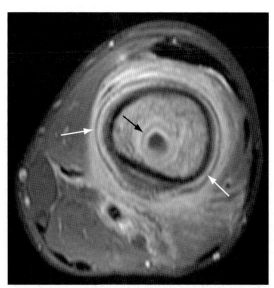

Figure 4. Axial T1-weighted fat-suppressed MR image through the distal femur after administration of intravenous gadolinium shows abnormal enhancement in bone marrow and surrounding soft tissues, diffuse periosteal reaction (*white arrows*), and central nonenhancing collection within medullary cavity (*black arrow*), consistent with abscess.

Case 248

DEMOGRAPHICS/CLINICAL HISTORY

The patient is an 18-month-old girl with knee pain.

FINDINGS

Anteroposterior (Fig. 1) and lateral (Fig. 2) radiographs of the knee show a well-circumscribed, lucent lesion within the distal femoral metaphysis adjacent to the growth plate. Coronal T2-weighted image with fat suppression from magnetic resonance imaging (MRI) examination of the knee (Fig. 3) shows abnormal bright signal in the distal femoral metaphysis corresponding to the lesion noted on prior radiographs.

DISCUSSION

Definition/Background

Brodie abscess is a form of subacute osteomyelitis with a central area of suppurative necrosis well circumscribed by a fibrous rim.

Characteristic Clinical Features

Patients may present with localized pain and limp (when the lower extremity is affected). Fever may also be present.

Characteristic Radiologic Findings

Radiographs show a well-circumscribed lucent lesion, usually within the metaphysis of long bones, with a thin rim of sclerosis.

Less Common Radiologic Manifestations

MRI of Brodie abscess shows a characteristic "penumbra" sign characterized by a peripheral intermediate or bright signal intensity on T1-weighted images relative to the lower signal intensity central abscess cavity and the surrounding lower-signal intensity reactive sclerotic bone.

Differential Diagnosis

- Simple bone cyst
- Osteoid osteoma
- Nonossifying fibroma
- Eosinophilic granuloma

Discussion

A simple bone cyst is a benign, lucent, fluid-containing lesion in the metaphyses of long bones. Osteoid osteoma is a benign osseous neoplasm that is smaller than 1.5 cm in diameter, and that characteristically occurs in the appendicular skeleton. Radiographs of osteoid osteoma show a sclerotic lesion with a characteristic central lucent nidus. Nonossifying fibroma is a common benign, lucent lesion seen in the metaphyses of long bones in children in the second decade. These lesions are usually eccentrically located and appear well defined. Eosinophilic granuloma is characterized by a single or by multiple osseous lucent lesions with a predilection for the calvaria, ribs, and femur. It is the most benign form of the spectrum of Langerhans cell histiocytosis.

Diagnosis

Brodie abscess

Suggested Readings

Davies AM, Grimer R: The penumbra sign in subacute osteomyelitis. Eur Radiol 15:1268-1270, 2005.

Kozlowski K: Brodie's abscess in the first decade of life: Report of eleven cases. Pediatr Radiol 10:33-37, 1980.

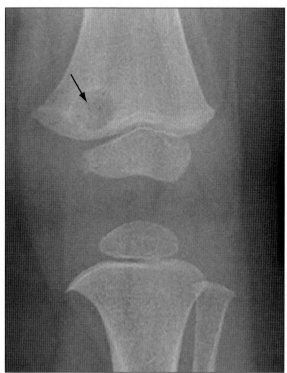

Figure 1. Anteroposterior radiograph of the knee shows well-circumscribed, lucent lesion within distal femoral metaphysis adjacent to growth plate (*arrow*).

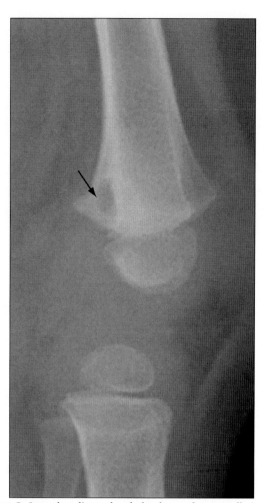

Figure 2. Lateral radiograph of the knee shows well-circumscribed, lucent lesion within distal femoral metaphysis adjacent to growth plate (*arrow*).

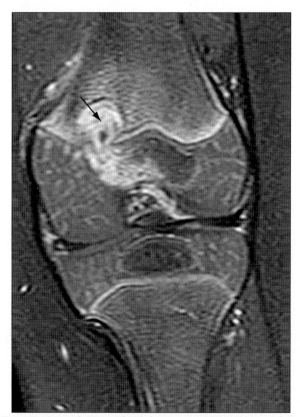

Figure 3. Coronal T2-weighted fat-suppressed MR image of the knee shows abnormal bright signal in distal femoral metaphysis that crosses growth plate into epiphysis, corresponding to lesion noted on prior radiographs (*arrow*).

Case 249

DEMOGRAPHICS/CLINICAL HISTORY

The patient is a 17-year-old boy with epitrochlear and axillary masses.

FINDINGS

Magnetic resonance imaging (MRI) of the left arm (Figs. 1 and 2) shows multiple fluid collections within the axilla and epitrochlear region, with significant surrounding soft tissue edema. There is peripheral enhancement after administration of contrast agent without central enhancement (Fig. 3). Ultrasound confirms the cystic nature of the axillary mass (Fig. 4), consistent with an abscess rather than necrotic lymphadenopathy.

DISCUSSION

Definition/Background

Cat-scratch disease is a benign regional lymphadenitis associated with exposure to cats or cat scratches, and it is caused by bacterial infection.

Characteristic Clinical Features

Most patients describe exposure to a cat, although this history is not elicited in all affected patients. Patients present with painful regional lymphadenopathy, usually occurring on or around the elbow, axilla, head, and neck.

Characteristic Radiologic Findings

Ultrasound, MRI, and computed tomography (CT) findings reveal markedly enlarged lymph nodes with extensive surrounding edema in a lymphatic distribution (i.e., proximal to the site of inoculation).

Less Common Radiologic Manifestations

Necrotic lymph nodes appear as low attenuation collections on CT or bright collections on T2-weighted MRI, which enhance peripherally but not centrally after intravenous administration of contrast agent.

Differential Diagnosis

- Lymphadenitis from other causes
- Rhabdomyosarcoma
- Lymphoma

Diagnosis

Cat-scratch disease

Suggested Readings

Dong PR, Seeger LL, Yao L, et al: Uncomplicated cat-scratch disease: Findings at CT, MR imaging, and radiography. Radiology 195:837-839, 1995.

Holt PD, de Lang EE: Cat scratch disease: Magnetic resonance imaging findings. Skeletal Radiol 24:437-440, 1995.

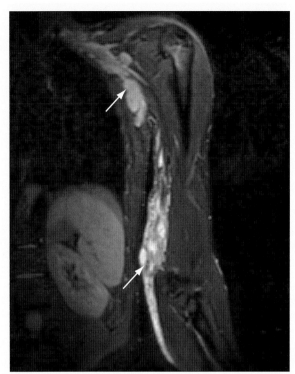

Figure 1. Coronal fluid-sensitive MR image through the left arm shows multiple fluid collections in medial epitrochlear region and axilla (*arrows*) and extensive subcutaneous edema.

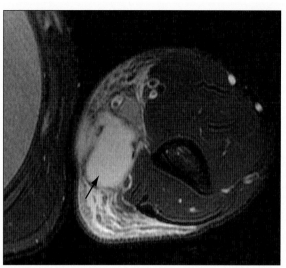

Figure 2. Axial fat-suppressed T2-weighted MR image at the level of the distal humerus shows large, bright lesion within medial epitrochlear region that is consistent with necrotic lymph node (*arrow*). There is extensive surrounding edema.

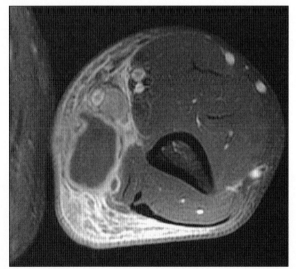

Figure 3. Axial fat-suppressed T1-weighted MR image after administration of intravenous contrast agent shows peripheral enhancement of epitrochlear fluid collection with no central enhancement. There is extensive enhancement of surrounding soft tissue inflammation.

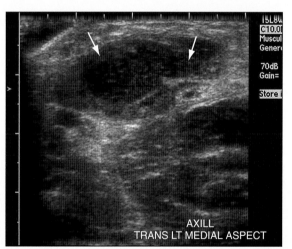

Figure 4. Ultrasound evaluation of axillary mass shows lobular, hypoechoic, fluctuant mass (*arrows*) that is consistent with an abscess rather than suppurative necrotic lymphadenopathy.

Case 250

DEMOGRAPHICS/CLINICAL HISTORY

The patient is an 8-year-old boy with acute onset of hip pain. The boy has no fever, but has a recent history of upper respiratory tract infection.

FINDINGS

Anteroposterior (Fig. 1) and frog-leg lateral (Fig. 2) radiographic views of the pelvis show normal osseous structures, but apparent bulging of the fat planes around the left hip joint. Focused ultrasound examination of bilateral hips (Fig. 3) shows a moderate left-sided hip effusion. A normal physiologic amount of fluid is noted within the right hip.

DISCUSSION

Definition/Background

Transient synovitis is a self-limited inflammatory condition, usually of the hip, that typically affects male patients more often than female patients.

Characteristic Clinical Features

Patients present with acute pain and limp, which lasts less than 2 weeks and resolves on its own. In contrast to septic arthritis of the hip, C-reactive protein level and erythrocyte sedimentation rate are not elevated in many cases, which is often helpful in differentiating between these two entities, although hip aspiration is necessary in some cases.

Characteristic Radiologic Findings

Plain radiographs of the hip are often normal. In some cases, a joint effusion can be appreciated by the displaced fat planes around the hip, although this is insensitive.

Less Common Radiologic Manifestations

Ultrasound of the hip shows a joint effusion. Scintigraphy reveals a slight increase in isotope uptake in the affected hip.

Differential Diagnosis

- Arthritis, septic
- Juvenile spondyloarthropathy

Discussion

Septic arthritis is an infectious arthritis in which there is acute, purulent infection of the joint, commonly caused by *Staphylococcus aureus* bacteria. It may be caused by an adjacent osteomyelitis. Juvenile spondyloarthropathies include juvenile ankylosing spondylitis, reactive arthritis, Reiter syndrome, and juvenile psoriatic arthritis. These disorders consist of synovitis and enthesitis.

Diagnosis

Transient synovitis

Suggested Readings

Caird MS, Flynn JM, Leung YL, et al: Factors distinguishing septic arthritis from transient synovitis of the hip in children. A prospective study. J Bone Joint Surg Am 88:1251-1257, 2006.

Zawin JK, Hoffer FA, Rand FF, et al: Joint effusion in children with an irritable hip: US diagnosis and aspiration. Radiology 187:459-463, 1993.

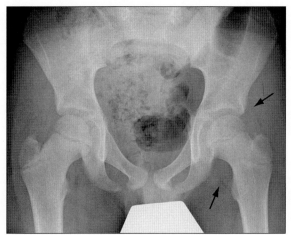

Figure 1. Anteroposterior view of the pelvis shows normal osseous structures, but apparent bulging of fat planes around left hip joint (*arrows*).

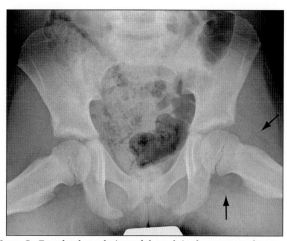

Figure 2. Frog-leg lateral view of the pelvis shows normal osseous structures, but apparent bulging of fat planes around left hip joint (*arrows*).

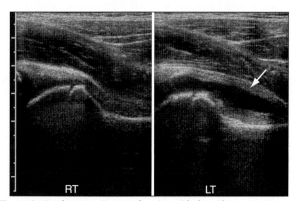

Figure 3. Dual screen image showing side-by-side comparison of longitudinal ultrasound images of bilateral hips. Moderate left-sided hip effusion is present (*arrow*). A normal physiologic amount of fluid is noted within the right hip.

Case 251

DEMOGRAPHICS/CLINICAL HISTORY

The patient is an 11-year-old girl with progressive skeletal deformity and limited range of motion.

FINDINGS

An anteroposterior radiograph of the chest (Fig. 1) shows a severe dextroscoliosis of the thoracic spine, with flexion contractures of the elbows bilaterally. Extensive soft tissue ossification is observed adjacent to the scapula bilaterally. Anteroposterior radiograph of both feet (Fig. 2) shows shortened first metatarsals and proximal first phalanges. A frog-leg view of the pelvis (Fig. 3) shows short, broad femoral necks with small exostoses arising from the necks bilaterally. Lateral radiograph of the elbow (Fig. 4) shows soft tissue mineralization anterior to the distal humerus.

DISCUSSION

Definition/Background

Fibrodysplasia ossificans progressiva, or progressive fibrodysplasia ossificans, an autosomal dominant condition, is a severe, disabling disorder.

Characteristic Clinical Features

Progressive fibrodysplasia ossificans is characterized by a congenital malformation of the great toes, heterotopic ossification in the soft tissues, and temporal progression of osteogenesis.

Characteristic Radiologic Findings

Radiographs of the feet show shortened first metatarsals and proximal phalanges. The great toes may appear to have a single phalanx because of synostosis of the phalanges. The femoral necks are broad and short. Heterotopic bone formation can occur anywhere in the body, although it tends to involve the upper back and neck.

Differential Diagnosis
- Aggressive fibromatosis
- Soft tissue sarcoma
- Myositis ossificans
- Calcified hematoma

Discussion

Aggressive fibromatosis is an infiltrative, benign, mesenchymal tumor that grows rapidly and tends to involve the deep muscles. Soft tissue sarcomas, including rhabdomyosarcoma and fibrosarcoma, are a malignant form of soft tissue tumor in children. Myositis ossificans refers to a form of post-traumatic ossification that occurs in muscle and tends to have characteristic imaging features. Calcifications within a hematoma can be differentiated from the malformations found in progressive fibrodysplasia ossificans.

Diagnosis

Juvenile progressive fibrodysplasia ossificans

Suggested Readings

Kaplan FS, Xu M, Glaser DL, et al: Early diagnosis of fibrodysplasia ossificans progressive. Pediatrics 121:e1295-e1300, 2008.
Mahboubi S, Glaser DL, Shore EM, et al: Fibrodysplasia ossificans progressive. Pediatr Radiol 31:307-314, 2001.

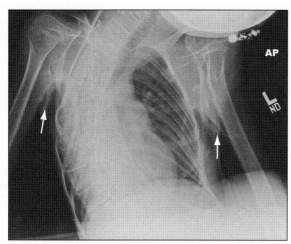

Figure 1. Anteroposterior radiograph of the chest shows severe dextroscoliosis of thoracic spine and flexion contractures of elbows bilaterally. Extensive soft tissue ossification is observed adjacent to scapula bilaterally (*arrows*).

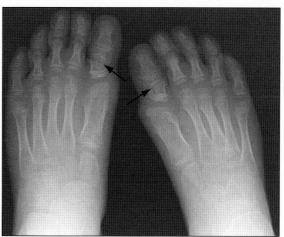

Figure 2. Anteroposterior radiograph of both feet shows shortened first metatarsals and proximal first phalanges (*arrows*).

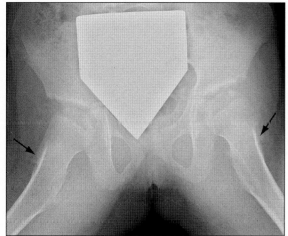

Figure 3. Frog-leg view of the pelvis shows short, broad femoral necks with small exostoses arising from necks bilaterally (*arrows*).

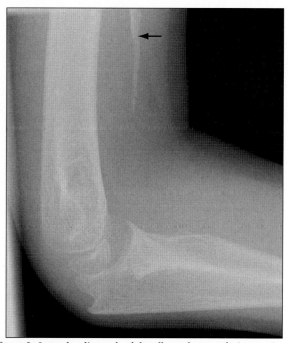

Figure 4. Lateral radiograph of the elbow shows soft tissue mineralization anterior to distal humerus (*arrow*).

Case 252

DEMOGRAPHICS/CLINICAL HISTORY

The patient is a 19-year-old man presenting after renal transplantation for renal failure.

FINDINGS

Radiographs of the ankle (Fig. 1) and foot (Fig. 2) show areas of sclerosis within the metaphyses of the bones. Sagittal reformatted computed tomography (CT) image of the lumbar spine (acquired from CT scan of the abdomen and pelvis) (Fig. 3) shows the classic "rugger jersey" spine.

DISCUSSION

Definition/Background
Patients with renal failure develop bony resorption because of hyperparathyroidism.

Characteristic Clinical Features
Patients universally have chronic renal failure.

Characteristic Radiologic Findings
Radiographs often show evidence of subperiosteal and subchondral bone resorption, particularly in the hands. Radiographs of the skull show a salt-and-pepper pattern, with loss of definition of the inner and outer tables.

Less Common Radiologic Manifestations
Osteosclerosis can manifest as a "rugger jersey" spine. Alternatively, radiographs may show a rickets-like appearance caused by abnormal enchondral ossification. Patients also may have soft tissue calcifications.

Differential Diagnosis
- Rickets
- Hyperparathyroidism

Diagnosis
Renal osteodystrophy

Suggested Readings
Jevtic V: Imaging of renal osteodystrophy. Eur J Radiol 46:85-95, 2003.
Tigges S, Nance EP, Carpenter WA, et al: Renal osteodystrophy: Imaging findings that mimic those of other diseases. AJR Am J Roentgenol 165:143-148, 1995.

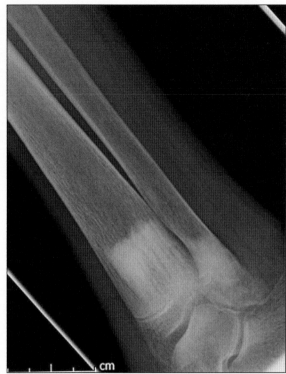

Figure 1. Lateral radiograph of the ankle shows osteosclerosis within metaphyses of tibia and fibula.

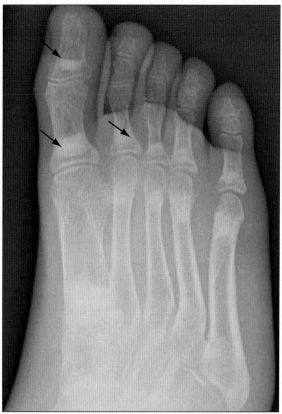

Figure 2. Oblique radiograph of the foot shows sclerosis within proximal metaphyses of phalanges and metatarsals (*arrows*).

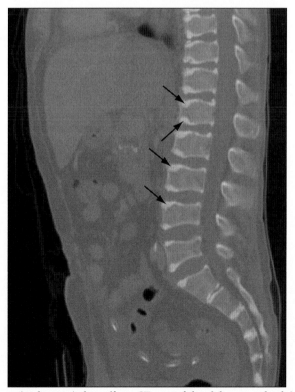

Figure 3. Sagittal reformatted CT image using bone windows (from CT scan of the abdomen and pelvis) shows osseous sclerosis adjacent to vertebral end plates (*arrows*), giving the spine a characteristic "rugger jersey" appearance.

Case 253

DEMOGRAPHICS/CLINICAL HISTORY

The patient is an 11-year-old girl with endocrine abnormalities.

FINDINGS

A frontal view of the left hand (Fig. 1) shows shortening of the third, fourth, and fifth metacarpals. A frontal view of the left foot (Fig. 2) shows shortening of the third, fourth, and fifth metatarsals. Particular shortening of the fourth metatarsal, as seen here, is classically described in pseudohypoparathyroidism.

DISCUSSION

Definition/Background
Pseudohypoparathyroidism is the result of an end organ (kidney and bone) insensitivity to parathyroid hormone.

Characteristic Clinical Features
Clinical features include short stature, round facies, obesity, and mental retardation.

Characteristic Radiologic Findings
Visible radiologic findings include soft tissue calcification and ossification, intracranial basal ganglia calcification, and metacarpal and metatarsal shortening, most commonly of the fourth and fifth digits.

Less Common Radiologic Manifestations
Premature physeal fusion and slipped femoral head epiphyses are additional radiologic findings.

Differential Diagnosis
- Pseudopseudohypoparathyroidism
- Brachydactyly
- Acrodysostosis
- Turner syndrome

Discussion
Pseudopseudohypoparathyroidism is radiographically identical to pseudohypoparathyroidism and is thought to be within the same family of disease. The other entities all may have shortened metacarpals, but do not typically have the additional findings of pseudohypoparathyroidism, such as soft tissue or intracranial calcifications.

Diagnosis
Pseudohypoparathyroidism

Suggested Readings
Adusumilli SK, Brent LH: Bilateral shortening of third and fourth metacarpal bones. J Clin Rheumatol 11:109-111, 2005.
Burnstein MI, Kottamasu SR, Pettifor JM, et al: Metabolic bone disease in pseudohypoparathyroidism: Radiologic features. Radiology 155:351-356, 1985.

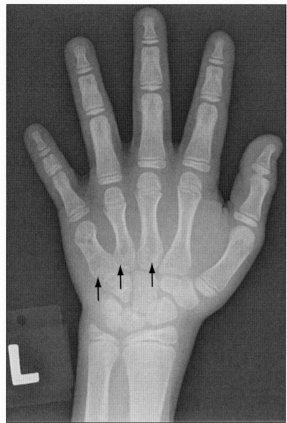

Figure 1. Frontal view of the left hand shows shortening of third, fourth, and fifth metacarpals (*arrows*).

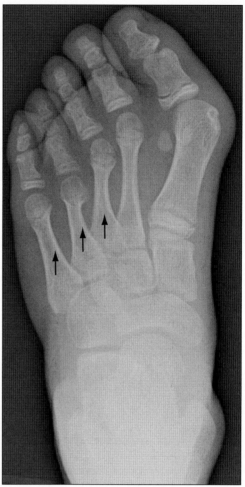

Figure 2. Frontal view of the left foot shows shortening of third, fourth, and fifth metatarsals (*arrows*). Particular shortening of the fourth metatarsal, as seen here, is classically described in pseudo-hypoparathyroidism.

Case 254

DEMOGRAPHICS/CLINICAL HISTORY

The patient is a 16-month-old child with a mass over the right shoulder, which has been present since birth.

FINDINGS

Ultrasound evaluation of the mass on the right shoulder (Fig. 1) reveals a multiseptated, cystic mass within the subcutaneous soft tissues of the right shoulder. Magnetic resonance imaging (MRI) shows a mass along the anterolateral aspect of the right shoulder, superficial to the deltoid muscle, which is low signal on T1-weighted imaging (Fig. 2) and high signal on T2-weighted imaging (Fig. 3), with only minimal septal enhancement after administration of contrast agent (Fig. 4).

DISCUSSION

Definition/Background

Lymphatic malformations form because of a defect in the connection of the lymphatics with the venous system. They may be associated with other syndromes, such as Turner syndrome and Noonan syndrome.

Characteristic Clinical Features

Most lymphatic malformations occur in the head and neck region. They are often present at birth, and sudden enlargement indicates bleeding or infection.

Characteristic Radiologic Findings

On ultrasound, lymphatic malformations are cystic lesions with septations. MRI reveals a cystic mass with low T1 signal and high T2 signal (although this may vary depending on the protein content), and without internal enhancement.

Less Common Radiologic Manifestations

Microcystic lymphatic malformations may appear ill-defined and hyperechoic on ultrasound without discrete cysts identified.

Differential Diagnosis

- Venous malformation
- Hematoma

Discussion

If the mass is new, a resolving hematoma may have imaging features similar to a lymphatic malformation, although usually blood products are identified on MRI.

Diagnosis

Lymphatic malformation

Suggested Readings

Paltiel HJ, Burrows PE, Kozakewich HP, et al: Soft-tissue vascular anomalies: Utility of US for diagnosis. Radiology 214:747, 2000.
Shiels WE 2nd, Kenney BD, Caniano DA, et al: Definitive percutaneous treatment of lymphatic malformation of the trunk and extremities. J Pediatr Surg 43:136, 2008.

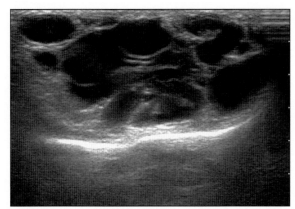

Figure 1. Ultrasound image over the right shoulder reveals anechoic mass with multiple septations within subcutaneous soft tissues.

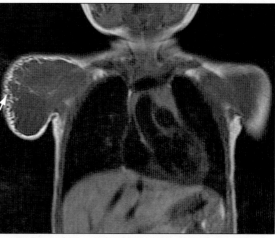

Figure 2. Coronal T1-weighted MR image through the right shoulder reveals that mass is isointense to underlying muscle, and there is reticulation of overlying subcutaneous fat (*arrow*).

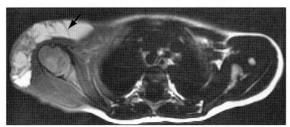

Figure 3. Axial T2-weighted MR image through the right shoulder shows that mass is T2 bright and contains multiple septations (*arrow*).

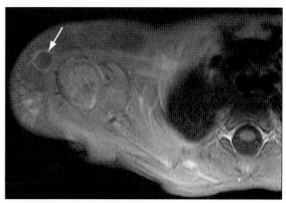

Figure 4. Axial T1-weighted fat-suppressed MR image through the right shoulder reveals mild enhancing thin septations (*arrow*), but no other internal enhancement of mass.

Case 255

DEMOGRAPHICS/CLINICAL HISTORY

The patient is an 11-year-old girl with a known diagnosis of Klippel-Trénaunay syndrome and asymmetric enlargement of her left leg.

FINDINGS

A fluoroscopic spot image of the left lower leg acquired during a venogram (Fig. 1) shows a tangle of enlarged venous channels within the subcutaneous soft tissues of the lower leg. Magnetic resonance imaging (MRI) of both lower extremities reveals that the left leg is slightly larger than the right (Figs. 2 and 3), and it shows multiple dilated venous structures within the soft tissues circumferentially involving the entire leg and deeper muscle groups.

DISCUSSION

Definition/Background
Klippel-Trénaunay syndrome involves enlargement of an extremity with underlying venous, lymphatic, and capillary malformations.

Characteristic Clinical Features
Klippel-Trénaunay syndrome tends to involve only one extremity, although it can occur bilaterally. Prominent superficial varicose veins are often present, and cutaneous lesions suggest a capillary malformation component.

Characteristic Radiologic Findings
Imaging typically shows leg-length discrepancy, soft tissue thickening, calcified phleboliths, and dilated superficial veins.

Less Common Radiologic Manifestations
In some patients, there is segmental absence of the deep venous system.

Differential Diagnosis
- Parkes Weber syndrome

Discussion
Parkes Weber syndrome is similar to Klippel-Trénaunay syndrome except that enlargement of an extremity results from an underlying arteriovenous malformation that is associated with a cutaneous capillary malformation and skeletal or soft tissue hypertrophy.

Diagnosis
Klippel-Trénaunay syndrome

Suggested Readings
James CA, Allison JW, Waner M: Pediatric case of the day. Klippel-Trénaunay syndrome. RadioGraphics 19:1093-1096, 1999.

Kanterman RY, Witt PD, Hsieh PS, et al: Klippel-Trénaunay syndrome: Imaging findings and percutaneous intervention. AJR Am J Roentgenol 167:989-995, 1996.

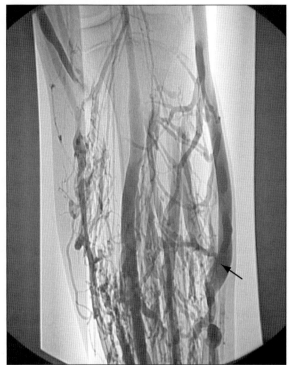

Figure 1. Fluoroscopic spot image of the left leg acquired during a venogram shows large tangle of enlarged venous channels within subcutaneous soft tissues of lower leg. Large, more prominent vein can be seen laterally (*arrow*).

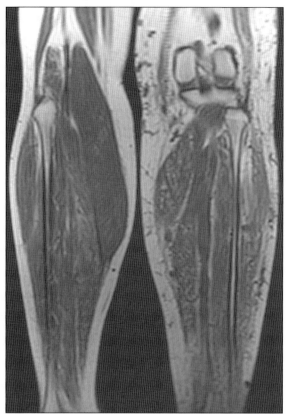

Figure 2. Coronal T1-weighted MRI of both lower extremities reveals that the left leg is slightly larger than the right, and there are multiple dilated venous structures within soft tissues circumferentially.

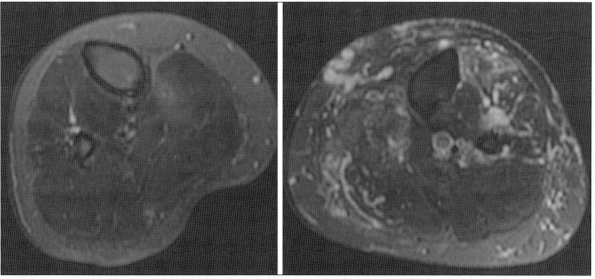

Figure 3. Axial T2-weighted fat-suppressed MRI of both lower extremities reveals that the left leg is slightly larger than the right, and there are multiple dilated venous structures within soft tissues and muscles.

Case 256

DEMOGRAPHICS/CLINICAL HISTORY

The patient is an 8-year-old boy with a palpable lump in the medial left thigh present for 1 year.

FINDINGS

Magnetic resonance imaging (MRI) of the pelvis and proximal thighs (Figs. 1-4) shows an extensive, multiloculated lesion intimately associated with the femoral and iliac vessels that is bright on T2-weighted images (see Figs. 1-3), relatively dark on T1-weighted images, and without enhancement after administration of contrast agent (see Fig. 4).

DISCUSSION

Definition/Background

Lymphatic malformations are often associated with Turner or Noonan syndromes and with other chromosomal abnormalities.

Characteristic Clinical Features

Patients often present with a palpable mass that has suddenly enlarged and become noticeable because of bleeding or infection.

Characteristic Radiologic Findings

Ultrasound reveals multiloculated cystic lesions. There is no flow within the cysts, although blood flow is present within the septations.

Less Common Radiologic Manifestations

MRI shows a multiseptate mass that has low signal intensity on T1-weighted images and high signal intensity on T2-weighted images. Enhancement is seen only within the septa after administration of contrast agent.

Differential Diagnosis

- Venous malformation

Diagnosis

Lymphatic malformation, multiloculated

Suggested Readings

Abernethy LJ: Classification and imaging of vascular malformations in children. Eur Radiol 13:2483-2497, 2003.

Paltiel HJ, Burrows PE, Kozakewich HP, et al: Soft-tissue vascular anomalies: Utility of US for diagnosis. Radiology 214:747-754, 2000.

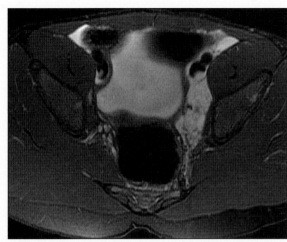

Figure 1. Axial T2-weighted fat-suppressed MR image through the lower pelvis shows a multiloculated lesion that has bright signal characteristics and is tracking along left pelvis adjacent to iliac vessels.

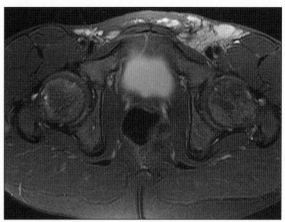

Figure 2. Axial T2-weighted fat-suppressed MR image through the proximal thighs shows extension of bright mass into thigh, where it remains intimately related to the femoral vessels.

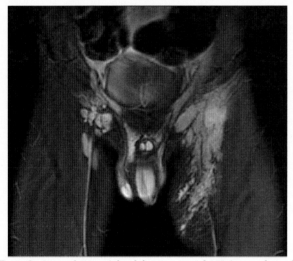

Figure 3. Coronal T2-weighted fat-suppressed MR image through the pelvis and proximal thighs provides a slightly better indication of the extent of mass along femoral vessels, although proximal extent of lesion is not completely imaged.

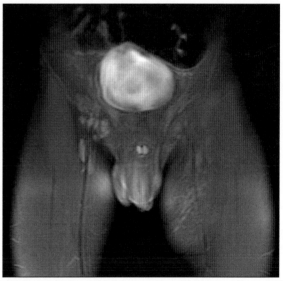

Figure 4. Axial T1-weighted fat-suppressed MR image through the pelvis and proximal thighs after administration of intravenous contrast agent shows no significant enhancement of lesion.

Case 257

DEMOGRAPHICS/CLINICAL HISTORY

The patient is a newborn girl with a raised, strawberry-colored lesion over the back.

FINDINGS

A longitudinal ultrasound image (Fig. 1) shows a well-defined, hypoechoic lesion within the superficial soft tissues of the lower back. Color Doppler ultrasound (Fig. 2) shows a highly vascular lesion with areas of arterial and venous flow.

DISCUSSION

Definition/Background

Hemangiomas are common, benign vascular tumors of infancy that may be cutaneous or located within visceral organs, such as the liver. Most hemangiomas resolve by age 7.

Characteristic Clinical Features

Cutaneous hemangiomas may appear as a reddish discoloration of the skin with an underlying noncompressible papule. When the lesions are located deeper under the skin, there may be no associated skin discoloration.

Characteristic Radiologic Findings

Ultrasound of cutaneous hemangiomas shows a lobular, hypoechoic, solid mass; in some cases, the lesion may appear hyperechoic. Color Doppler ultrasound reveals prominent flow within the lesion.

Differential Diagnosis

- Venous malformation
- Lymphatic malformation
- Arteriovenous malformation

Discussion

A venous malformation is a common childhood vascular malformation that manifests either as a discrete mass or as diffuse varicosity of draining veins. These lesions are compressible, contain slow internal venous flow (unless they are thrombosed), and may contain phleboliths. A lymphatic malformation is a slow-flow lesion that may be microcystic or macrocystic. Lymphatic malformations are formed by the sequestration of primitive lymphatic tissue that does not communicate with the normal lymphatic drainage. An arteriovenous malformation is a high-flow vascular malformation composed of multiple vascular channels with no intervening capillary bed. In contrast to hemangioma, there is no endothelial cell proliferation in arteriovenous malformations.

Diagnosis

Hemangioma

Suggested Readings

Dinehart SM, Kincannon J, Geronemus R: Hemangiomas: Evaluation and treatment. Dermatol Surg 27:475-485, 2001.

Gritzmann N, Hollerweger A, Macheiner P, et al: Sonography of soft tissue masses of the neck. J Clin Ultrasound 30:356-373, 2002.

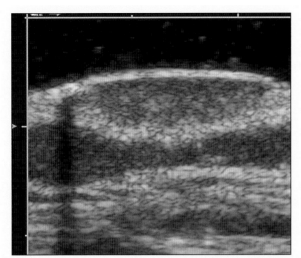

Figure 1. Longitudinal ultrasound image shows well-defined, hypoechoic lesion within superficial soft tissues of lower back.

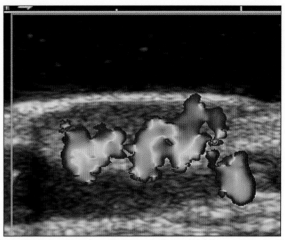

Figure 2. Color Doppler ultrasound shows highly vascular lesion with areas of arterial and venous flow.

Case 258

DEMOGRAPHICS/CLINICAL HISTORY

The patient is a 13-year-old girl with an enlarged, bluish lesion in the web space between the left first and second fingers.

FINDINGS

Axial T2-weighted image with fat suppression from magnetic resonance imaging (MRI) of the left hand (Fig. 1) shows a multilobulated lesion within the web space between the first and second digits that has uniformly bright signal. Coronal fast spin-echo inversion recovery (FSEIR) image from MRI of the hand (Fig. 2) shows similar findings. Coronal maximum intensity projection image from a dynamic enhanced angiographic image during the venous phase of imaging (Fig. 3) shows enhancement of the soft tissue lesion in the left hand and multiple prominent venous channels in the arm. Coronal T1-weighted fat-suppressed MR image after administration of contrast agent shows diffuse, homogeneous enhancement of the lesion (Fig. 4).

DISCUSSION

Definition/Background

Venous malformation is an abnormal collection of venous channels that is characteristically present since birth.

Characteristic Clinical Features

Patients often complain of a soft tissue mass that may have a bluish hue to it. The lesions may become painful if they develop thrombosis or hemorrhage.

Characteristic Radiologic Findings

Lesions are commonly cystic at ultrasound with low-flow vascularity on Doppler evaluation. MRI shows a predominantly T2-bright, well-circumscribed lesion that enhances after administration of contrast agent with prominent venous channels.

Differential Diagnosis

- Hemangioma
- Arteriovenous malformation
- Venolymphatic malformation

Discussion

A hemangioma is a high-flow vascular tumor that has other soft tissue components in addition to vessels. An arteriovenous malformation is an abnormal communication between arteries and veins without an intervening capillary bed. A venolymphatic malformation is a lesion with components of venous malformation and lymphatic malformation.

Diagnosis

Venous malformation

Suggested Readings

Fishman SJ, Mulliken JB: Hemangiomas and vascular malformations of infancy and childhood. Pediatr Clin North Am 40:1177-1200, 1993.
Silverman RA: Hemangiomas and vascular malformations. Pediatr Clin North Am 38:811-834, 1991.

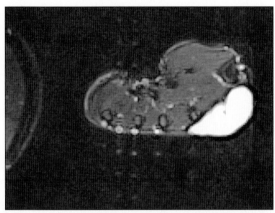

Figure 1. Axial T2-weighted fat-suppressed MR image of the left hand shows multilobulated lesion within web space between first and second digits that has uniformly bright signal.

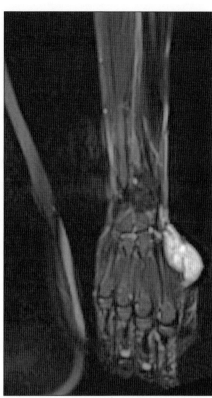

Figure 2. Coronal FSEIR MR image of the hand shows multilobulated lesion within web space between first and second digits that has uniformly bright signal.

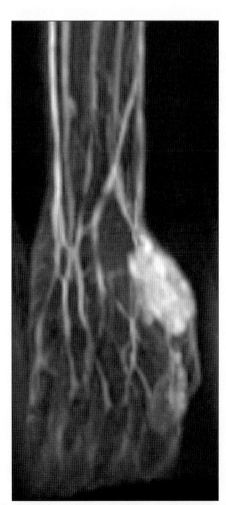

Figure 3. Coronal maximum intensity projection image from dynamic enhanced angiographic image during the venous phase shows enhancement of soft tissue lesion in left hand and multiple prominent venous channels in arm.

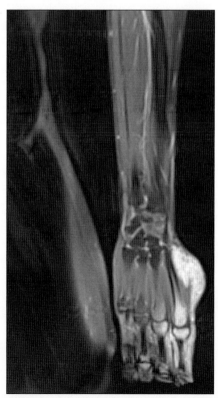

Figure 4. Coronal T1-weighted fat-suppressed MR image after contrast agent administration shows diffuse, homogeneous enhancement of lesion.

Case 259

DEMOGRAPHICS/CLINICAL HISTORY

The patient is a 15-month-old girl with skeletal dysplasia found on prenatal ultrasound.

FINDINGS

An anteroposterior radiograph of the chest, abdomen, and pelvis (Fig. 1) reveals short horizontal ribs, "handlebar" clavicles, horizontal acetabula, and squared-off iliac wings with narrowed sciatic notches. A computed tomography (CT) scan of the chest (Fig. 2) shows bilateral short ribs causing decreased lung volume. A plain radiograph of the chest after placement of bilateral vertebral expandable prosthetic titanium rods (VEPTR) (Fig. 3) shows marked expansion of the thoracic cavity.

DISCUSSION

Definition/Background

Jeune syndrome is a rare skeletal dysplasia (approximately 1:100,000 live births) and has an autosomal recessive inheritance pattern. In addition to skeletal dysplasia, the patient in this case has hepatic fibrosis, has poor weight gain, and requires continuous positive airway pressure at night.

Characteristic Clinical Features

The short, horizontal rib shape leads to limited pulmonary capacity, for which this patient has been treated with oxygen, continuous positive airway pressure, and nebulizers. Patients are often treated with VEPTR for expansion of the thoracic cavity. Hepatic fibrosis and renal failure are known associations.

Characteristic Radiologic Findings

Findings on radiography consist of narrow thoracic cage, rhizomelic brachymelia, short horizontal ribs, "handlebar" clavicles, square-shaped iliac wings, and horizontal acetabular roofs with spur-shaped projections on each side.

Less Common Radiologic Manifestations

This diagnosis also may be suggested at prenatal ultrasound with findings of a narrow thorax, short ribs, and short tubular bones.

Differential Diagnosis

- Ellis-van Creveld syndrome (chondroectodermal dysplasia)

Discussion

Ellis-van Creveld syndrome is a nonlethal skeletal dysplasia characterized by small, short ribs; flared iliac wings; acromelic and mesomelic limb shortening; and polydactyly.

Diagnosis

Jeune syndrome (asphyxiating thoracic dysplasia)

Suggested Readings

Schinzel A, Savoldelli G, Briner J, et al: Prenatal sonographic diagnosis of Jeune syndrome. Radiology 154:777-778, 1985.

Spirt BA, Oliphant M, Gottlieb RH, et al: Prenatal sonographic evaluation of short-limbed dwarfism: An algorithmic approach. RadioGraphics 10:217-236, 1990.

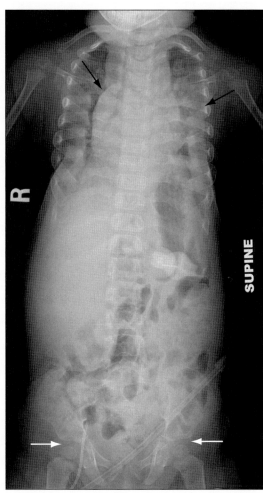

Figure 1. Anteroposterior radiograph of the chest and abdomen reveals short, horizontal, broad ribs (*black arrows*), "handlebar" clavicles, and small intrathoracic cavity. Acetabular roofs are horizontally oriented (*white arrows*), and iliac wings are square.

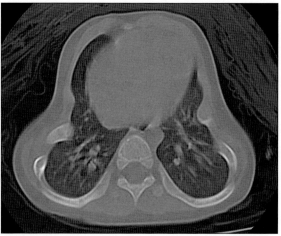

Figure 2. Axial CT scan through the chest shows short, horizontal ribs causing diminished intrathoracic cavity.

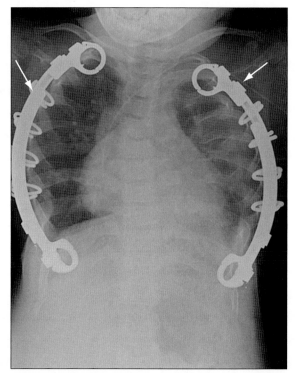

Figure 3. Anteroposterior radiograph of the chest after placement of bilateral VEPTR (*arrows*) reveals improved intrathoracic expansion.

Case 260

DEMOGRAPHICS/CLINICAL HISTORY

The patient is a 12-year-old girl with abdominal pain.

FINDINGS

An anteroposterior radiograph of the abdomen (Fig. 1) reveals progressively narrowed interpediculate distances, slightly flattened vertebral bodies, flared iliac wings that are shaped like elephant ears, narrow sacrosciatic notches, flat acetabular roofs, and short femoral necks.

DISCUSSION

Definition/Background

Achondroplasia is the most common nonlethal skeletal dysplasia. It is an autosomal dominant condition, but there is a high spontaneous mutation rate.

Characteristic Clinical Features

Patients with achondroplasia have short stature and rhizomelic limb shortening.

Characteristic Radiologic Findings

Extremity radiographs reveal rhizomelic limb shortening, although acromelia and mesomelia may also be present; decreased interpediculate distances in the lumbar spine; flattened acetabular roofs in the pelvis; small, shortened ribs in the thorax; and brachydactyly in the hands.

Less Common Radiologic Manifestations

Hydrocephalus is rarely present. Imaging may show a chevron deformity of the knees and prominent deltoid insertion areas in the humeri.

Differential Diagnosis

- Hypochondroplasia

Discussion

Similar to achondroplasia, hypochondroplasia is a developmental disorder caused by an autosomal dominant genetic defect in the fibroblast growth factor receptor 3 gene. Hypochondroplasia is a skeletal dysplasia with many features in common with achondroplasia, although it tends to have milder clinical and radiographic features than seen in cases of achondroplasia.

Diagnosis

Achondroplasia

Suggested Readings

Dominguez R, Talmachoff P: Diagnostic imaging update in skeletal dysplasias. Clin Imaging 17:224-234, 1993.

Lemyre E, Azouz EM, Teebi AS, et al: Bone dysplasia series. Achondroplasia, hypochondroplasia and thanatophoric dysplasia: Review and update. Can Assoc Radiol J 50:185-197, 1999.

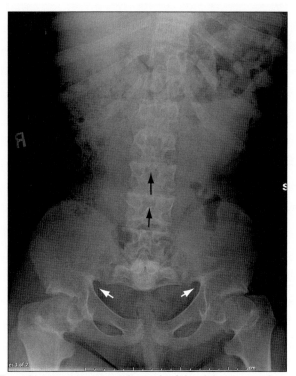

Figure 1. Anteroposterior radiograph of the abdomen reveals progressively narrowed interpediculate distances (*black arrows*), slightly flattened vertebral bodies, flared iliac wings that are shaped like elephant ears, narrow sacrosciatic notches (*white arrows*), flat acetabular roofs, and short femoral necks.

Case 261

DEMOGRAPHICS/CLINICAL HISTORY

The patient is a newborn girl with dysmorphic features who died shortly after birth.

FINDINGS

Postmortem, anteroposterior radiograph (Fig. 1) shows a long, narrow thorax with short ribs; generalized limb shortening (i.e., rhizomelic, mesomelic, and acromelic); and a large skull. Magnification view of the pelvis (Fig. 2) shows platyspondyly; small, flared iliac bones; flat, dysplastic acetabula; telephone receiver–shaped femurs; and round, proximal femoral metaphyses with a medial spike.

DISCUSSION

Definition/Background
Thanatophoric dysplasia is a severe skeletal dysplasia in the achondroplasia group of disorders.

Characteristic Clinical Features
This diagnosis usually is lethal. Very few patients survive beyond the first few days of life, and many are stillborn.

Characteristic Radiologic Findings
Skeletal radiographs show a large skull with a narrow skull base (i.e., kleeblattschädel), a long and narrow thorax with very short ribs; "handlebar" clavicles; telephone receiver–shaped femurs; round, proximal femoral metaphyses with a medial spike; platyspondyly; and small, flared iliac bones with narrow sacrosciatic notches.

Differential Diagnosis
- Achondroplasia
- Hypochondroplasia

Discussion
Achondroplasia is a nonlethal skeletal dysplasia with rhizomelic limb shortening, an enlarged skull, small ribs, elephant ear–shaped iliac wings, and other features. Hypochondroplasia is a common disorder that is almost identical to achondroplasia, but it has milder abnormalities.

Diagnosis
Thanatophoric dysplasia

Suggested Readings
Lemyre E, Azouz EM, Teebi AS, et al: Bone dysplasia series. Achondroplasia, hypochondroplasia and thanatophoric dysplasia: Review and update. Can Assoc Radiol J 50:185-197, 1999.

Wilcox WR, Tavormina PL, Krakow D, et al: Molecular, radiologic, and histopathologic correlations in thanatophoric dysplasia. Am J Med Genet 78:274-281, 1998.

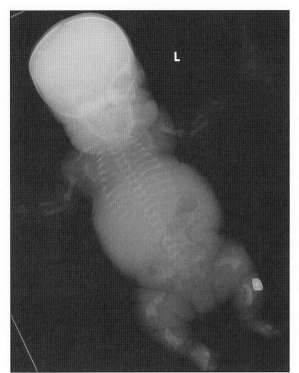

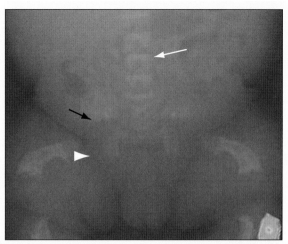

Figure 2. Magnification view of the pelvis shows platyspondyly (*white arrow*); small, flared iliac bones; flat, dysplastic acetabula (*black arrow*); telephone receiver–shaped femurs; and round, proximal femoral metaphyses with a medial spike (*arrowhead*).

Figure 1. Postmortem, anteroposterior radiograph shows long, narrow thorax with short ribs; generalized limb shortening (i.e., rhizomelic, mesomelic, and acromelic); and a large skull.

Case 262

DEMOGRAPHICS/CLINICAL HISTORY

The patient is a 20-month-old boy with broad thumbs and a diagnosis of Rubinstein-Taybi syndrome.

FINDINGS

Anteroposterior radiographs of the left and right hands (Figs. 1 and 2) show broadened thumbs that are radially angulated. The proximal phalanges have a delta configuration. The tufts of the distal phalanges of both thumbs are broadened.

DISCUSSION

Definition/Background

Rubinstein-Taybi syndrome is characterized by mental retardation; characteristic facies; and broad, short terminal phalanges of the thumb and great toe. Most cases are sporadic. Boys and girls are affected equally.

Characteristic Clinical Features

The diagnosis is often made on the basis of the clinical and facial features, rather than on the basis of radiographic findings. Characteristic facial features include a prominent forehead, long eyelashes, thick eyebrows, hypertelorism, low-set ears, and partial ptosis. Other features include cardiac defects, including atrial septal defect, ventricular septal defect, patent ductus arteriosus, and coarctation of the aorta; undescended testicles; and cutaneous features such as spontaneous keloid formation and capillary hemangiomas.

Characteristic Radiologic Findings

Frontal radiographs of the hands and feet reveal shortening and broadening of the first digits. The proximal phalanx often has a delta phalanx configuration.

Less Common Radiologic Manifestations

Scrotal ultrasound examination of boys may reveal undescended testes, and, rarely, a renal anomaly, such as renal agenesis, is identified. The bone age may be delayed.

Diagnosis

Rubinstein-Taybi syndrome

Suggested Readings

Cirillo RL Jr: Pediatric case of the day. Rubinstein-Taybi syndrome. RadioGraphics 17:1604-1605, 1997.
De Silva B: What syndrome is this? Rubinstein-Taybi syndrome. Pediatr Dermatol 19:177-179, 2002.

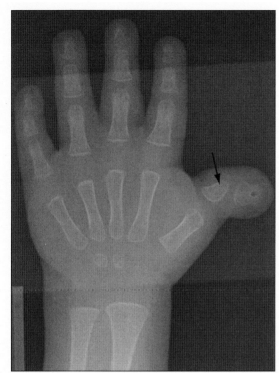

Figure 1. Anteroposterior radiograph of the left hand shows a broadened thumb that is radially angulated. The proximal phalanx has an abnormal delta configuration (*arrow*). The tuft of the distal phalanx is broadened.

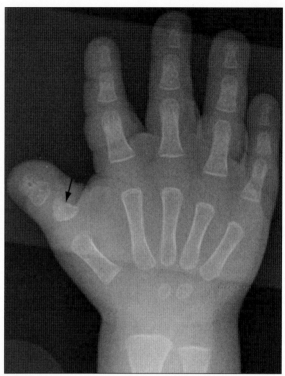

Figure 2. Anteroposterior radiograph of the right hand shows a broadened thumb that is radially angulated. The proximal phalanx has an abnormal delta configuration (*arrow*). The tuft of the distal phalanx is broadened.

Case 263

DEMOGRAPHICS/CLINICAL HISTORY

The patient is a 13-year-old boy with tall stature.

FINDINGS

Sagittal (Fig. 1) and axial (Fig. 2) T2-weighted images from magnetic resonance imaging (MRI) of the lumbar spine in two other patients with Marfan syndrome show dural ectasia in the lower lumbar spine (see Fig. 1) and a lateral meningocele (see Fig. 2).

DISCUSSION

Definition/Background

Marfan syndrome is a multisystemic connective tissue disorder that is autosomal dominant and caused by a mutation on the fibrillin-1 gene on chromosome 15.

Characteristic Clinical Features

Marfan syndrome affects various organ systems, including the cardiovascular, musculoskeletal, central nervous, pulmonary, and ocular systems and the skin. Diagnosis is based on a combination of major and minor clinical features, some of which include dilation with or without dissection of the ascending aorta, mitral valve prolapse, pectus excavatum or carinatum, joint hypermobility, scoliosis, acetabular protrusio, dural ectasia of the spine, and spontaneous pneumothorax.

Characteristic Radiologic Findings

Patients with annuloaortic ectasia have dilation of the aortic root, which is best visualized by computed tomography (CT). CT is also the modality of choice to evaluate for aortic dissection, showing the intimal tear and the true and false lumens of the aorta.

Less Common Radiologic Manifestations

Plain radiographs are satisfactory for showing the degree of spinal scoliosis and the presence of a chest wall deformity, arachnodactyly in the hands, and protrusion acetabula in the pelvis. Dural ectasia (widening of the dural sac with or without nerve root sleeves) often affects the lumbosacral spine and can be noted on radiographs as posterior vertebral body scalloping, but MRI shows this to better advantage and may show an accompanying meningocele or arachnoid cyst.

Differential Diagnosis

- Ehlers-Danlos syndrome

Discussion

Ehlers-Danlos syndrome is a genetic connective system disorder with symptoms that include joint hypermobility and skin elasticity.

Diagnosis

Marfan syndrome

Suggested Reading

Ha HI, Seo JB, Lee SH, et al: Imaging of Marfan syndrome: Multisystemic manifestations. RadioGraphics 27:989-1004, 2007.

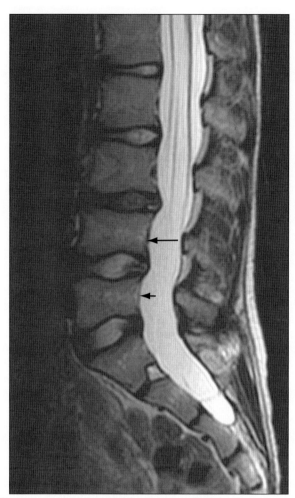

Figure 1. Sagittal T2-weighted MR image of the lumbar spine performed in a patient with Marfan syndrome shows dural ectasia in lower lumbar spine with posterior scalloping of vertebral bodies (*arrows*).

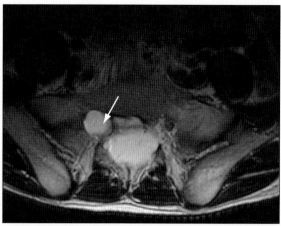

Figure 2. Axial T2-weighted MR image of the lumbar spine performed in a patient with Marfan syndrome shows right lateral meningocele (*arrow*).

Case 264

DEMOGRAPHICS/CLINICAL HISTORY

The patient is a 3-day-old boy with dysmorphic features and heart murmur.

FINDINGS

An anteroposterior (AP) chest radiograph (Fig. 1) shows an enlarged cardiac silhouette and widening of the superior mediastinal contour consistent with dilation of the ascending aorta. An AP radiograph of the hand (Fig. 2) shows elongation of the phalanges of the digits, consistent with arachnodactyly.

DISCUSSION

Definition/Background

Marfan syndrome is a multisystemic connective tissue disorder that is autosomal dominant and that is caused by a mutation on the fibrillin-1 gene on chromosome 15.

Characteristic Clinical Features

Marfan syndrome affects various organ systems, including the cardiovascular, musculoskeletal, central nervous, pulmonary, and ocular systems, and the skin. The diagnosis is based on a combination of major and minor clinical features, some of which include dilation with or without dissection of the ascending aorta, mitral valve prolapse, pectus excavatum or carinatum, joint hypermobility, scoliosis, acetabular protrusion, dural ectasia of the spine, and spontaneous pneumothorax.

Characteristic Radiologic Findings

Patients with annuloaortic ectasia have dilation of the aortic root, which is best visualized on computed tomography (CT). CT is also the modality of choice to evaluate for aortic dissection, showing the intimal tear and the true and false lumens of the aorta.

Less Common Radiologic Manifestations

Plain radiographs show the degree of spinal scoliosis and the presence of a chest wall deformity, arachnodactyly in the hands, and protrusion acetabula in the pelvis. Dural ectasia (widening of the dural sac with or without nerve root sleeves) often affects the lumbosacral spine and can be noted on radiographs as posterior vertebral body scalloping, but magnetic resonance imaging (MRI) shows this to better advantage and may show an accompanying meningocele or arachnoid cyst.

Differential Diagnosis

■ Ehlers-Danlos syndrome

Discussion

Ehlers-Danlos syndrome is a genetic connective system disorder with symptoms that include joint hypermobility and skin elasticity.

Diagnosis

Marfan syndrome

Suggested Reading

Ha HI, Seo JB, Lee SH, et al: Imaging of Marfan syndrome: Multisystemic manifestations. RadioGraphics 27:989-1004, 2007.

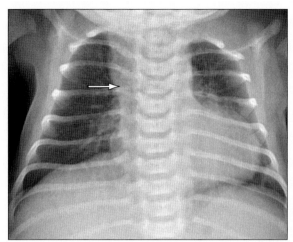

Figure 1. AP chest radiograph shows enlarged cardiac silhouette and widening of superior mediastinal contour consistent with dilation of ascending aorta (*arrow*).

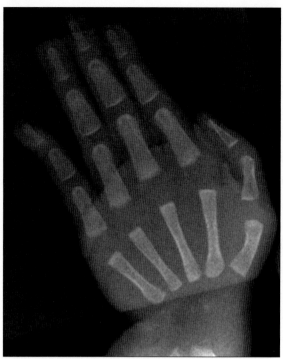

Figure 2. AP radiograph of the hand shows abnormally long and slender digits, consistent with arachnodactyly.

Case 265

DEMOGRAPHICS/CLINICAL HISTORY

The patient is a newborn with a posterior fossa abnormality seen on prenatal ultrasound.

FINDINGS

Sagittal postnatal ultrasound of the head through the anterior fontanelle (Fig. 1) shows hypoplasia of the cerebellar vermis, and coronal ultrasound (Fig. 2) shows cystic space within the posterior fossa. Sagittal T1-weighted magnetic resonance imaging (MRI) (Fig. 3) confirms vermian hypoplasia and a cystic space in the posterior fossa, and shows a normal-sized posterior fossa with appropriate positioning of the torcular. Axial T2-weighted MRI (Fig. 4) shows communication of the fourth ventricle with a retrocerebellar cystic collection.

DISCUSSION

Definition/Background

The Dandy-Walker complex encompasses a spectrum of posterior fossa abnormalities including one or more of the following: vermian hypoplasia, enlarged posterior fossa, and retrocerebellar cystic collection. The presence of all three abnormalities is called the Dandy-Walker malformation; vermian hypoplasia with retrocerebellar cystic collection communicating with the fourth ventricle is often called the Dandy-Walker variant. A megacisterna magna is an enlarged cystic space in the posterior fossa, often detected incidentally, and considered a normal variant.

Characteristic Clinical Features

Dandy-Walker malformations and variants are often detected prenatally. If not, associated central nervous system malformations may be present, and infants present with symptoms such as seizures, developmental delay, or increasing head circumference from hydrocephalus.

Characteristic Radiologic Findings

Variable hypoplasia of the cerebellar vermis, enlargement of the posterior fossa with high positioning of the tentorium and torcular, and retrocerebellar cystic collections are part of the spectrum. The retrocerebellar cystic collection is typically seen in communication with the fourth ventricle.

Less Common Radiologic Manifestations

Associated findings vary widely and include ventriculomegaly, cardiac anomalies, hypogenesis of the corpus callosum, encephaloceles, cortical malformations, migrational anomalies, and schizencephaly.

Differential Diagnosis

- Other causes of cystic posterior fossa masses—arachnoid cysts, epidermoids, neuroepithelial cysts.
- Other causes of vermian hypoplasia/aplasia—Joubert syndrome

Discussion

Epidermoids have slightly different density and intensity characteristics than cerebrospinal fluid, and typically have restricted diffusion on MRI. Arachnoid cysts are extremely difficult to differentiate from a megacisterna magna; however, if the cystic collection enlarges, an arachnoid cyst can be diagnosed. Joubert syndrome has aplasia or severe hypoplasia of the vermis and is associated with other abnormalities of the cerebellar nuclei and often other abnormalities in the kidneys, eyes, liver, or digits. A "bat wing" appearance of the fourth ventricle and "molar tooth" appearance of the midbrain and superior cerebellar peduncles are classic imaging findings of Joubert syndrome on axial MRI.

Diagnosis

Dandy-Walker variant

Suggested Readings

Ecker JL, Shipp TD, Bromley B, Benacerraf B: The sonographic diagnosis of Dandy-Walker and Dandy-Walker variant: Associated findings and outcomes. Prenat Diagn 20:328, 2000.

Harper T, Fordham LA, Wolfe HM: The fetal Dandy Walker complex: Associated anomalies, perinatal outcome and postnatal imaging. Fetal Diagn Ther 22:277, 2007.

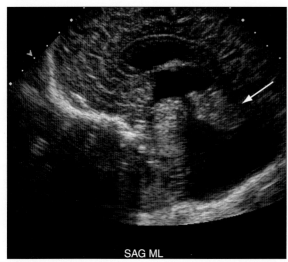

Figure 1. Postnatal sagittal ultrasound of the head through the anterior fontanelle shows hypoplasia of cerebellar vermis (*arrow*).

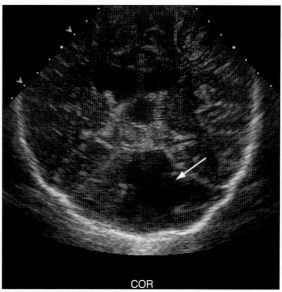

Figure 2. Coronal ultrasound shows cystic collection within retro-cerebellar posterior fossa (*arrow*).

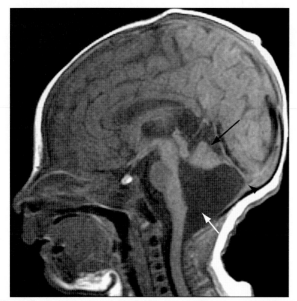

Figure 3. Sagittal T1-weighted MR image shows vermian hypoplasia (*white arrow*), cystic collection in posterior fossa (*black arrow*), and normal-sized posterior fossa with appropriate positioning of torcular (*arrowhead*).

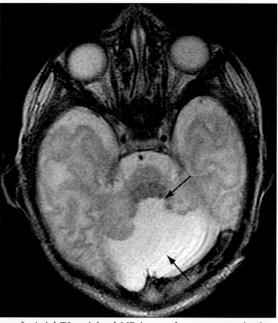

Figure 4. Axial T2-weighted MR image shows communication of fourth ventricle (*white arrow*) with the retrocerebellar cystic collection (*black arrow*) and absence of the inferior vermis.

Case 266

DEMOGRAPHICS/CLINICAL HISTORY

The patient is an infant with prenatal hydrocephalus and spinal abnormality.

FINDINGS

Sagittal T1-weighted magnetic resonance imaging (MRI) of the brain (Fig. 1) shows a towering cerebellum, beaked tectum, low-lying torcular, and cerebellar tonsillar herniation. Axial T2-weighted MRI of the brain (Fig. 2) shows interdigitation of the gyri along the midline. A more caudal axial T2-weighted MR image (Fig. 3) shows finger-like gyri (stenogyria), ventriculomegaly, and a pointed occipital horn. Sagittal T2-weighted MRI through the spine (Fig. 4) shows a thoracolumbar myelomeningocele (with the cord seen along the posterior aspect of the myelomeningocele).

DISCUSSION

Definition/Background
Chiari II malformation consists of many supratentorial and infratentorial abnormalities, and is usually associated with a myelomeningocele.

Characteristic Clinical Features
Prenatal diagnosis of Chiari II malformation is now typical. If patients have not had prenatal care, neonates typically present because of findings of the myelomeningoceles.

Characteristic Radiologic Findings
Findings in the brain include a beaked tectum, downward displacement of the cerebellar tonsils, low-lying torcular, "towering" cerebellum, hydrocephalus, pointing of the occipital horns in patients with mild hydrocephalus, and usually findings of a myelomeningocele.

Less Common Radiologic Manifestations
Other central nervous system abnormalities can be seen in association with Chiari II malformations, including absence of septum pellucidum, gray matter heterotopias, and diastematomyelia. There are reports of patients with coexisting holoprosencephaly and rhombencephalosynapsis.

Differential Diagnosis
- Chiari I malformation
- Chiari III malformation

Discussion
The only radiographic abnormality typically seen in a Chiari I malformation is low-lying tonsils down through the foramen magnum into the upper cervical canal. A Chiari III malformation typically includes findings in Chiari II malformations and high cervical and low occipital encephaloceles.

Diagnosis
Chiari II malformation

Suggested Readings
Ando K, Ishikura R, Ogawa M, et al: MRI tight posterior fossa sign for prenatal diagnosis of Chiari type II malformation. Neuroradiology 49:1033, 2007.

Callen AL, Filly RA: Supratentorial abnormalities in the Chiari II malformation, I: The ventricular "point." J Ultrasound Med 27:33, 2008.

Callen AL, Stengel JW, Filly RA: Supratentorial abnormalities in the Chiari II malformation, II: Tectal morphologic changes. J Ultrasound Med 28:29, 2009.

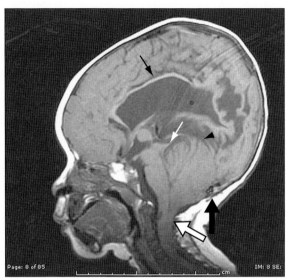

Figure 1. Sagittal T1-weighted MR image of brain shows towering cerebellum (*arrowhead*), beaked tectum (*small white arrow*), low-lying torcular (*large black arrow*), and cerebellar tonsillar herniation (*large white arrow*). The corpus callosum has an abnormal configuration (*small black arrow*).

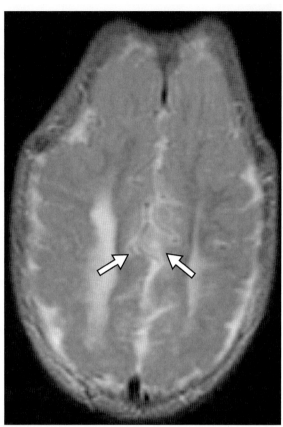

Figure 2. Axial T2-weighted MR image of brain shows interdigitation of gyri along midline (*arrows*).

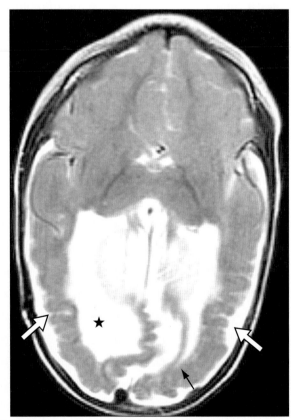

Figure 3. More caudal axial T2-weighted MR image shows finger-like gyri (stenogyria) (*white arrows*), ventriculomegaly (*star*), and pointed occipital horn (*black arrow*).

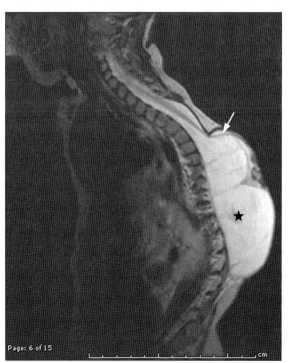

Figure 4. Sagittal T2-weighted MR image through spine shows thoracolumbar myelomeningocele (*star*) with cord seen along posterior aspect of myelomeningocele (*arrow*).

Case 267

DEMOGRAPHICS/CLINICAL HISTORY

The patient is a 3-year-old girl with headaches and enuresis.

FINDINGS

Magnetic resonance imaging (MRI) of the brain through the level of the internal auditory canals (Figs. 1 and 2) reveals bilateral (left larger than right) enhancing masses along the course of the cranial nerve VII and VIII complexes, consistent with bilateral vestibular schwannomas.

DISCUSSION

Definition/Background
Neurofibromatosis type 2 (NF2) is an autosomal dominant condition that affects 1 in 50,000 people. It is characterized by benign tumors of the nerves that transmit sound impulses from the inner ear to the brain (i.e., acoustic neuromas or vestibular schwannomas). NF2 is also called MISME syndrome (i.e., multiple, inherited schwannomas, meningiomas, and ependymomas).

Characteristic Clinical Features
Depending on the location and size of the neuromas or schwannomas, patients may have disturbances of balance and gait; dizziness; headache; facial weakness, numbness, or pain; tinnitus; or progressive hearing loss. Some patients also have juvenile posterior subcapsular opacities, progressive visual impairment, or an increased risk for developing central nervous system tumors.

Characteristic Radiologic Findings
Characteristic MRI findings include bilateral vestibular schwannomas.

Less Common Radiologic Manifestations
NF2 may also manifest as multiple intracranial schwannomas, which are otherwise uncommon in children.

Differential Diagnosis
- Neurofibromatosis type 1 (NF1)

Discussion
NF2, also called von Recklinghausen disease, is a genetic disorder characterized by multiple, benign tumors of nerves and skin (i.e., neurofibromas) and areas of hypopigmentation or hyperpigmentation, which typically include café au lait spots on the trunk and other regions and freckling, particularly in axial and inguinal areas. Patients may also develop Lisch nodules, benign, pigmented, hamartomatous nevi of the iris, or tumors of the cranial nerve.

Diagnosis
Neurofibromatosis type 2

Suggested Readings
Gray J, Swaiman KF: Brain tumors in children with neurofibromatosis: Computed tomography and magnetic resonance imaging. Pediatr Neurol 3:335-341, 1987.
Smirniotopoulos JG, Murphy FM: The phakomatoses. AJNR Am J Neuroradiol 13:725-746, 1992.

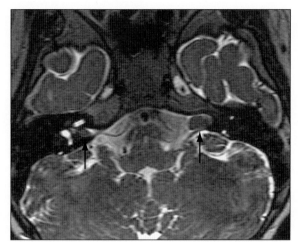

Figure 1. Axial T2-weighted MR image through the levels of the internal auditory canals reveals bilateral (left larger than right) masses along course of cranial nerves VII and VIII (*arrows*).

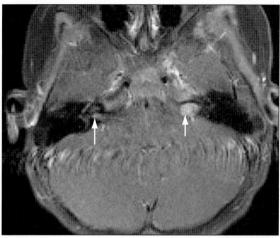

Figure 2. Axial T1-weighted fat-suppressed MR image through the internal auditory canals performed after administration of intravenous contrast agent reveals enhancement of masses (*arrows*).

Case 268

DEMOGRAPHICS/CLINICAL HISTORY

The patient is an 8-month-old infant with a facial birthmark.

FINDINGS

Axial non–contrast-enhanced computed tomography (CT) scan (Fig. 1) shows curvilinear hyperdensities within the cortex and more subtle calcifications at the gray-white junction. Coronal T2-weighted magnetic resonance imaging (MRI) (Fig. 2) shows hemiatrophy of the right cerebral hemisphere. Pial enhancement is seen along the cortex ipsilateral to the hemiatrophy on coronal postcontrast T1-weighted MRI (Fig. 3). In a different patient with Sturge-Weber syndrome, postcontrast fluid attenuated inversion recovery (FLAIR) MRI (Fig. 4) shows pial signal abnormality and enlargement of the ipsilateral choroid plexus.

DISCUSSION

Definition/Background
Sturge-Weber syndrome is also known as encephalotrigeminal angiomatosis, a name that incorporates the leptomeningeal angiomatosis and the port wine stain typically in the distribution of the trigeminal nerve.

Characteristic Clinical Features
Facial port wine stain (i.e., nevus flammeus), typically in the V_1 distribution, is the classic clinical feature for Sturge-Weber syndrome. The leptomeningeal vascular malformation is on the ipsilateral side as the port wine stain.

Characteristic Radiologic Findings
Dystrophic calcifications within the cortex (i.e., "tram track" calcifications) and at the gray-white junction are typical findings and often best seen on CT or gradient-recalled-echo MRI. Cortical atrophy, leptomeningeal enhancement, and enlargement of the ipsilateral choroid plexus are characteristic findings. Thickening of the ipsilateral calvaria and enlargement of the ipsilateral mastoid air cells and sinuses can occur. Single-photon emission computed tomography (SPECT) can show diminished radiotracer localization in the affected hemisphere of the brain.

Less Common Radiologic Manifestations
Although involvement is most commonly unilateral, 8% to 15% of patients can have bilateral involvement, and inspection of the contralateral side for involvement is crucial. Buphthalmos and choroidal angiomas occasionally are seen on imaging. Visceral angiomas have also been described.

Differential Diagnosis
- Meningitis
- Rasmussen encephalitis

Discussion
Leptomeningeal enhancement can be seen in meningitis, but the clinical scenario, absence of other findings, and classic port wine stain can differentiate the two entities. Rasmussen encephalitis may cause hemiatrophy, but the other common radiologic findings in Sturge-Weber syndrome are absent.

Diagnosis
Sturge-Weber syndrome

Suggested Readings
Martí-Bonmatí L, Menor F, Poyatos C, Cortina H: Diagnosis of Sturge-Weber syndrome: Comparison of the efficacy of CT and MR imaging in 14 cases. AJR Am J Roentgenol 158:867-871, 1992.

Wasenko JJ, Rosenbloom SA, Duchesneau PM, et al: The Sturge-Weber syndrome: Comparison of MR and CT characteristics. AJNR Am J Neuroradiol 11:131-134, 1990.

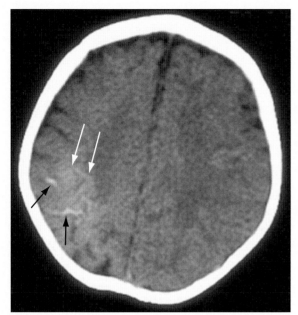

Figure 1. Axial non–contrast-enhanced CT image shows curvilinear hyperdensities (*black arrows*) within cortex and more subtle calcifications at gray-white junction (*white arrows*).

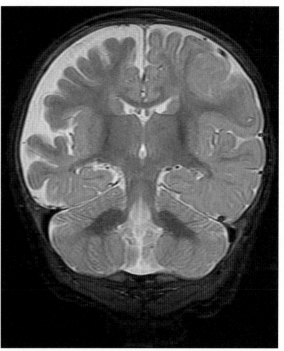

Figure 2. Coronal T2-weighted MR image shows hemiatrophy of right cerebral hemisphere.

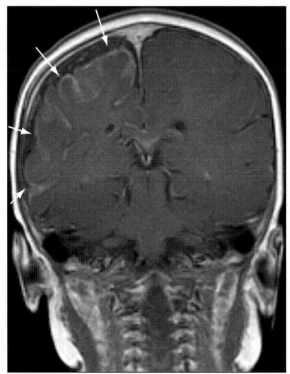

Figure 3. Coronal postcontrast T1-weighted MR image shows pial enhancement (*arrows*) along cortex ipsilateral to hemiatrophy.

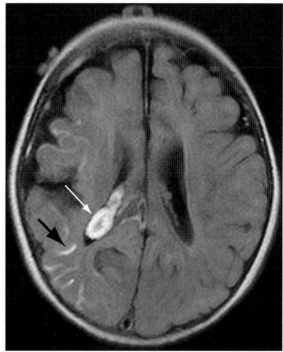

Figure 4. Postcontrast FLAIR MR image in a different patient with Sturge-Weber syndrome shows pial signal abnormality (*black arrow*) and enlargement of the ipsilateral choroid plexus (*white arrow*).

Case 269

DEMOGRAPHICS/CLINICAL HISTORY

The patient is an infant with an abnormality noticed on prenatal screening ultrasound.

FINDINGS

Prenatal ultrasound scan (Fig. 1) shows an echogenic mass within the right ventricle of the heart. Magnetic resonance imaging (MRI) of the infant's brain several weeks after birth reveals abnormal areas of T2 prolongation within the subcortical white matter and subependymal nodules (Fig. 2) that enhance after gadolinium administration (Fig. 3). In a different patient, computed tomography (CT) scan of the abdomen (Fig. 4) shows low attenuation lesions within the left kidney, which is consistent with angiomyolipomas.

DISCUSSION

Definition/Background

Tuberous sclerosis is a hereditary disease characterized by an autosomal dominant inheritance pattern.

Characteristic Clinical Features

The clinical triad consists of seizures, mental retardation, and adenoma sebaceum.

Characteristic Radiologic Findings

MRI of the brain often reveals subependymal and cerebral nodules that are consistent with hamartomas. These nodules are located along the lateral margins of the lateral ventricles.

Less Common Radiologic Manifestations

On brain MRI, the white matter shows foci of abnormal T2-weighted signal that correspond to areas of dysplastic cells.

Diagnosis

Tuberous sclerosis

Suggested Readings

Datta AN, Hahn CD, Sahin M: Clinical presentation and diagnosis of tuberous sclerosis complex in infancy. J Child Neurol 23:268-273, 2008.

Shepherd CW, Houser OW, Gomez MR: MR findings in tuberous sclerosis complex and correlation with seizure development and mental impairment. AJNR Am J Neuroradiol 16:149-155, 1995.

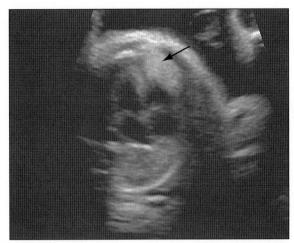

Figure 1. Four-chamber view of the heart from a prenatal ultrasound study reveals large, echogenic mass within right ventricle (*arrow*).

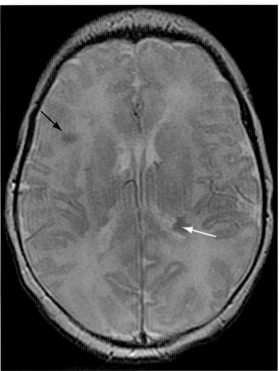

Figure 2. Axial T2-weighted MR image of the brain shows areas of abnormal T2-weighted signal within subcortical white matter (*black arrow*) and subependymal region (*white arrow*).

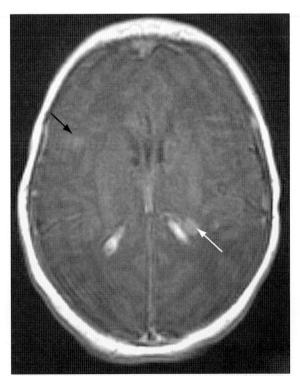

Figure 3. Axial T1-weighted MR image of the brain after administration of intravenous contrast agent shows nodular enhancement in subcortical (*black arrow*) and subependymal (*white arrow*) regions.

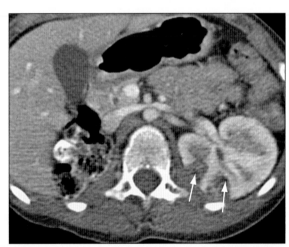

Figure 4. Axial image from contrast-enhanced abdominal CT scan in a different patient shows many low attenuation lesions within left kidney (*arrows*) consistent with angiomyolipomas. The right kidney has been surgically removed.

Case 270

DEMOGRAPHICS/CLINICAL HISTORY

The patient is a 1-month-old girl with poor weight gain, fussiness, and respiratory distress.

FINDINGS

A chest radiograph shows a large cardiac silhouette and pulmonary vascular congestion (Fig. 1) in this patient, who was later found to have aortic coarctation. Renal ultrasound shows both kidneys are fused across midline at the level of the lower poles (Figs. 2 and 3), consistent with a horseshoe kidney.

DISCUSSION

Definition/Background

Turner syndrome is a type of gonadal dysgenesis associated with 45XO karyotype in girls.

Characteristic Clinical Features

This patient was evaluated with echocardiography in light of her respiratory symptoms and was found to have coarctation of the aorta and a bicommissural aortic valve. Patients with Turner syndrome generally are short in stature, have a webbed neck, and have widely spaced nipples.

Characteristic Radiologic Findings

Bone age is often delayed, and patients have short fourth or fifth metacarpals. They often have coarctation of the aorta and renal anomalies, such as horseshoe kidney.

Less Common Radiologic Manifestations

Pleural effusions or ascites at birth may result from lymphedema, which occurs in Turner syndrome.

Differential Diagnosis

- Noonan syndrome
- 46XY gonadal dysgenesis

Discussion

Patients with 46XY gonadal dysgenesis are phenotypically female, but do not have the short stature or physical characteristics of patients with Turner syndrome.

Diagnosis

Turner syndrome

Suggested Readings

Lin AE, Lippe B, Rosenfeld RG: Further delineating or aortic dilation, dissection, and rupture in patients with Turner syndrome. Pediatrics 102:e12, 1998.

Lippe B, Geffner ME, Dietrich RB, et al: Renal malformations in patients with Turner syndrome: Imaging in 141 patients. Pediatrics 82:852-856, 1988.

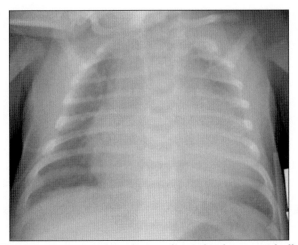

Figure 1. Anteroposterior chest radiograph shows markedly enlarged cardiac silhouette and pulmonary interstitial edema.

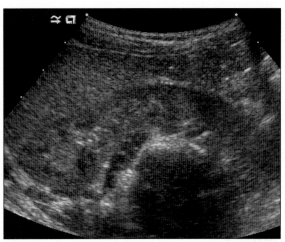

Figure 2. Transverse ultrasound image at the level of the lower pole of the right kidney shows lower pole of kidney crossing midline anterior to vertebral column, consistent with a horseshoe kidney.

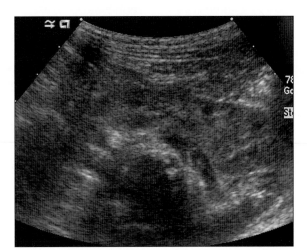

Figure 3. Transverse ultrasound image at the level of the lower pole of the left kidney shows that both lower poles of kidneys are fused across midline, consistent with a horseshoe kidney.

Case 271

DEMOGRAPHICS/CLINICAL HISTORY

The patient is a 3-month-old child with abnormal hands and feet.

FINDINGS

A three-dimensional, reconstructed computed tomography (CT) scan (Fig. 1) shows premature fusion of the right coronal suture. The left coronal suture was also prematurely fused. Axial non–contrast-enhanced CT (Fig. 2) shows a bony protuberance at the coronal sutures from the synostoses. The patient has agenesis of the corpus callosum. A frontal view of the foot (Fig. 3) shows a delta phalanx replacing the normal great toe and soft tissue fusion of the second, third, and fourth phalanges of the foot. A frontal view of the hand (Fig. 4) shows the delta phalanx replacing the normal proximal phalanx of the thumb and soft tissue and osseous fusion of the third and fourth phalanges. Abnormal fusion of the individual proximal and middle phalanges can be seen.

DISCUSSION

Definition/Background
Apert syndrome is an acrocephalosyndactyly (type I), and it is characterized by craniosynostosis and skeletal anomalies, particularly syndactyly of the hands and feet.

Characteristic Clinical Features
Clinical findings include craniofacial suggestion of the underlying synostosis and obvious hand and foot syndactylies of the middle digits.

Characteristic Radiologic Findings
Patients with Apert syndrome have a combination of craniofacial and skeletal anomalies. Abnormalities of the upper and lower limbs typically are symmetric, with various degrees of severity in different patients. Anomalies in the hands and feet include radial deviation of a short thumb or great toe secondary to a delta phalanx and complex or complete syndactylies involving the second, third, and fourth digits. Abnormalities of the shoulders and elbows have been described. Craniosynostosis is typical in patients with Apert syndrome. Intracranial findings associated with Apert syndrome include nonprogressive ventriculomegaly, hydrocephalus, absence of the septum pellucidum, and agenesis or hypogenesis of the corpus callosum. Other common findings seen on CT include abnormal semicircular canals and jugular foraminal stenosis.

Less Common Radiologic Manifestations
Progressive hydrocephalus is less common in Apert syndrome than in other acrocephalosyndactylies, such as Crouzon or Pfeiffer syndrome.

Differential Diagnosis
- Acrocephalosyndactylies

Discussion
Differentiation from other acrocephalosyndactylies typically is based on the characteristic hand and foot findings in Apert syndrome.

Diagnosis
Apert syndrome

Suggested Readings
Prevel CD, Eppley BL, McCarty M: Acrocephalosyndactyly syndromes: A review. J Craniofac Surg 8:279-285, 1997.
Quintero-Rivera F, Robson CD, Reiss RE, et al: Intracranial anomalies detected by imaging studies in 30 patients with Apert syndrome. Am J Med Genet A 140:1337-1338, 2006.

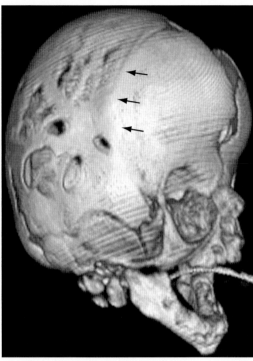

Figure 1. Three-dimensional reconstruction from a CT scan shows premature fusion of right coronal suture (*arrows*). Left coronal suture was also prematurely fused.

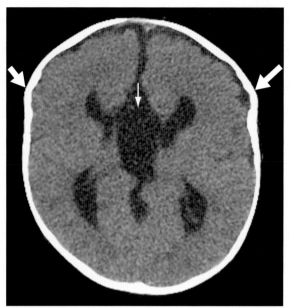

Figure 2. Axial non–contrast-enhanced CT image shows bony protuberance at coronal sutures from synostoses (*large arrows*). The patient also has agenesis of the corpus callosum (*small arrow*).

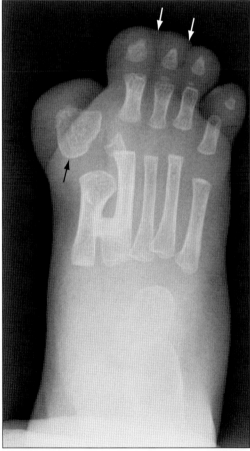

Figure 3. Frontal view of the foot shows delta phalanx (*black arrow*) replacing normal great toe and soft tissue fusion of second, third, and fourth phalanges of the foot (*white arrows*).

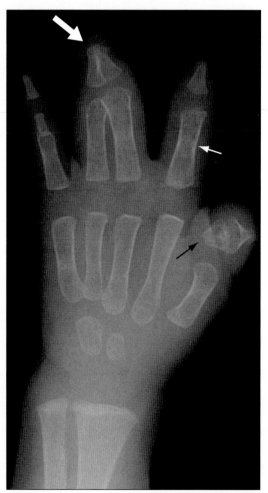

Figure 4. Frontal view of the hand shows delta phalanx (*black arrow*) replacing normal proximal phalanx of thumb and soft tissue and osseous fusion of third and fourth phalanges (*large white arrow*). Abnormal fusion of individual proximal and middle phalanges can be seen; *small white arrow* shows fusion of second digit.

Case 272

DEMOGRAPHICS/CLINICAL HISTORY

The patient is a 14-year-old boy with hepatomegaly and a diagnosis of Niemann-Pick disease.

FINDINGS

A longitudinal ultrasound image of the right kidney (Fig. 1) shows that the right lobe of the liver extends well below the inferior pole of the kidney. A scout image from a chest computed tomography (CT) scan (Fig. 2) shows diffuse, reticular interstitial thickening in both lungs. Moderate cardiomegaly can be seen. Axial, non–contrast-enhanced CT image of the chest through the level of the lower lobes shows diffuse, interlobular septal thickening (Fig. 3).

DISCUSSION

Definition/Background

Niemann-Pick disease refers to a group of congenital lipidoses in which cells and organs in the body abnormally accumulate sphingolipids. The liver, spleen, bone marrow, central nervous system, and lungs are most often affected.

Characteristic Clinical Features

Depending on the specific type of Niemann-Pick disorder, patients may present with psychomotor retardation, hepatosplenomegaly, or respiratory failure. Most patients have thrombocytopenia.

Characteristic Radiologic Findings

Chest radiographs show reticular interstitial thickening, and chest CT shows areas of ground-glass opacities in the upper lobes with interlobular septal thickening in the lower lobes. Abdominal ultrasound or CT reveals hepatosplenomegaly.

Less Common Radiologic Manifestations

Skeletal radiographs may reveal widening of the medullary cavities in the bones, osteopenia, and delayed bone age.

Differential Diagnosis

- Gaucher disease
- Leukemia
- Lymphoma

Discussion

Based on the infiltrative bone marrow replacement process shown on magnetic resonance imaging (MRI), the differential diagnosis includes Gaucher disease, leukemia, and other myelodysplastic syndromes.

Diagnosis

Niemann-Pick disease

Suggested Readings

Mendelson DS, Wasserstein MP, Desnick RJ, et al: Type B Niemann-Pick disease: Findings at chest radiography, thin-section CT, and pulmonary function testing. Radiology 238:339-345, 2006.

Muntaner L, Galmes A, Chabas A, et al: Imaging features of type-B Niemann-Pick disease. Eur Radiol 7:361-364, 1997.

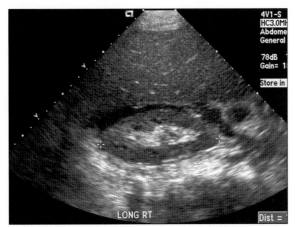

Figure 1. Longitudinal ultrasound image of right kidney shows that right lobe of liver extends well below inferior pole of kidney.

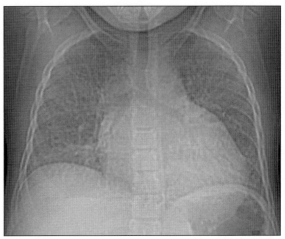

Figure 2. Scout image from chest CT shows diffuse, reticular interstitial thickening in both lungs. Moderate cardiomegaly can be seen.

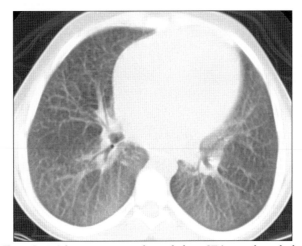

Figure 3. Axial non–contrast-enhanced chest CT image through the level of the lower lobes shows diffuse, interlobular septal thickening.

Case 273

DEMOGRAPHICS/CLINICAL HISTORY

The patient is a 13-year-old girl with a diagnosis of Noonan syndrome since early childhood.

FINDINGS

Posteroanterior (Fig. 1) and lateral (Fig. 2) radiographs of the chest show stents overlying the left and right pulmonary arteries and a vascular closure device overlying the heart. A posteroanterior radiograph of the entire spine (Fig. 3) shows moderate dextroscoliosis of the thoracic spine and compensatory levoscoliosis of the lumbar spine.

DISCUSSION

Definition/Background

Noonan syndrome is an autosomal dominant condition characterized by short stature, dysmorphic features, and congenital heart defects.

Characteristic Clinical Features

Patients with Noonan syndrome have characteristic facial features, including hypertelorism, down-slanting palpebral fissures, low-set ears, low hairline, ptosis, and neck pterygia. Patients also have short stature and psychomotor retardation.

Characteristic Radiologic Findings

The diagnosis of Noonan syndrome is rarely a radiographic one. Many of these patients have pulmonic stenosis. Chest radiographs reveal decreased pulmonary blood flow, although patients usually are treated early in life, and radiographs show stents in the pulmonary arteries.

Differential Diagnosis

- Turner syndrome
- Neurofibromatosis–Noonan syndrome
- LEOPARD syndrome

Discussion

Neurofibromatosis–Noonan syndrome is a disorder similar to Noonan syndrome that has features of both diseases. Patients with LEOPARD syndrome have lentigenes, electrocardiographic conduction defects, ocular hypertelorism, pulmonic stenosis, abnormal genitalia, retardation of growth, and sensorineural deafness. It is an autosomal recessive condition.

Diagnosis

Noonan syndrome

Suggested Readings

Mendez HM, Opitz JM: Noonan syndrome: A review. Am J Med Genet 21:493-506, 1985.

Sznajer Y, Keren B, Baumann C, et al: The spectrum of cardiac anomalies in Noonan syndrome as a result of mutations in the PTPN11 gene. Pediatrics 119:e1325-e1331, 2007.

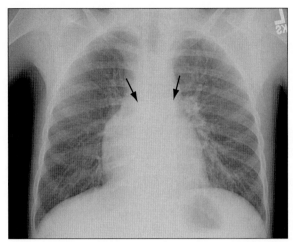

Figure 1. Posteroanterior chest radiograph shows stents overlying left and right pulmonary arteries (*arrows*) and vascular closure device overlying the heart.

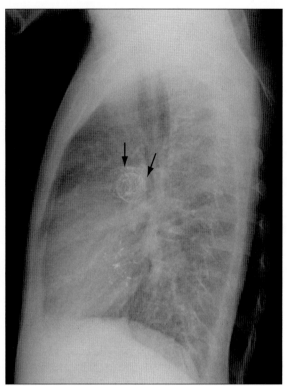

Figure 2. Lateral chest radiograph shows stents overlying left and right pulmonary arteries (*arrows*) and vascular closure device overlying the heart.

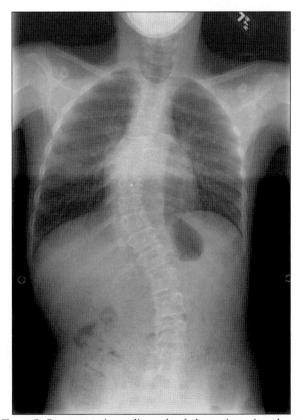

Figure 3. Posteroanterior radiograph of the entire spine shows moderate dextroscoliosis of thoracic spine and compensatory levoscoliosis of lumbar spine.

Case 274

DEMOGRAPHICS/CLINICAL HISTORY

The patient is a 3-year-old girl with hepatomegaly.

FINDINGS

Axial (Fig. 1) and coronal (Fig. 2) T1-weighted images from magnetic resonance imaging (MRI) of the abdomen show hepatomegaly and splenomegaly. An anteroposterior radiograph of the knee (Fig. 3) shows the characteristic "Erlenmeyer flask" deformity of the distal femoral metaphysis related to undertubulation of long bones.

DISCUSSION

Definition/Background

Gaucher disease is a hereditary lysosomal storage disease that leads to the accumulation of glucosylceramide in the reticuloendothelial system (liver, spleen, lymph nodes, and bone marrow).

Characteristic Clinical Features

Patients may be entirely asymptomatic. Symptoms include painful bone crises related to bone involvement with development of avascular necrosis; hepatomegaly and liver dysfunction, which may lead to liver failure; and splenomegaly.

Characteristic Radiologic Findings

Ultrasound, computed tomography (CT), and MRI of the abdomen reveal hepatomegaly. Skeletal radiographs demonstrate osteopenia, cortical thinning, and "Erlenmeyer flask" deformity of the lower legs.

Less Common Radiologic Manifestations

Radiographs and CT of the chest reveal a diffuse reticulonodular pattern in the lungs.

Differential Diagnosis

- Peliosis hepatis
- Sarcoidosis
- Tyrosinemia

Discussion

Peliosis hepatis of the liver is characterized by hepatosplenomegaly. In contrast to Gaucher disease, there are multiple blood-filled cavities within the liver and spleen. Sarcoidosis may involve the liver in a child and is characterized by hepatosplenomegaly with granulomas and lymphadenopathy. Tyrosinemia is characterized by hepatomegaly, enlarged echogenic kidneys, and rickets.

Diagnosis

Gaucher disease

Suggested Readings

Hainaux B, Christophe C, Hanquinet S, et al: Gaucher's disease: Plain radiography, US, CT and MR diagnosis of lungs, bone, and liver lesions. Pediatr Radiol 22:78-79, 1992.

Terk MR, Esplin J, Lee K, et al: MR imaging of patients with type 1 Gaucher's disease: Relationship between bone and visceral changes. AJR Am J Roentgenol 165:599-604, 1995.

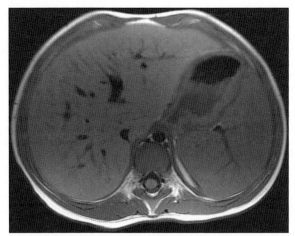

Figure 1. Axial T1-weighted MR image of the abdomen shows hepatomegaly and splenomegaly.

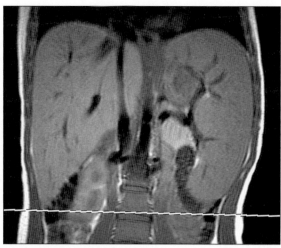

Figure 2. Coronal T1-weighted MR image of the abdomen shows hepatomegaly and splenomegaly.

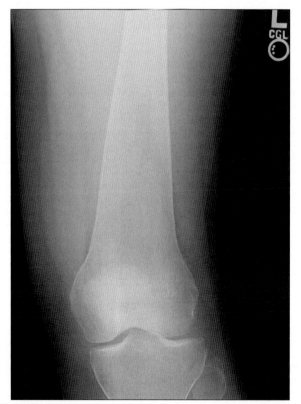

Figure 3. Anteroposterior radiograph of the knee shows characteristic "Erlenmeyer flask" deformity of distal femoral metaphysis, related to undertubulation of long bones.

Case 275

DEMOGRAPHICS/CLINICAL HISTORY

The patient is an 8-year-old child with Goldenhar syndrome.

FINDINGS

A three-dimensional craniofacial computed tomography (CT) reconstruction (Fig. 1) shows left facial microsomia, with a hypoplastic left orbit, left maxilla, and left mandible. Right lateral view of the CT reconstruction (Fig. 2) shows the normal osseous external auditory canal, normal body of the ramus of the mandible, and normal zygomatic arch on the right. Left lateral view of the CT reconstruction (Fig. 3) shows absence of a normal osseous external auditory canal in expected location and ipsilateral mandibular and zygomatic arch hypoplasia.

DISCUSSION

Definition/Background

Goldenhar syndrome, also known as oculoauriculovertebral dysplasia, is a severe form of hemifacial microsomia.

Characteristic Clinical Features

Goldenhar syndrome is characterized by asymmetric facial features, in particular, abnormal position or appearance of the ipsilateral ear.

Characteristic Radiologic Findings

Hemifacial microsomia is seen, with mandibular hypoplasia, deformity of the ipsilateral ear, ocular abnormalities, and vertebral and skull base abnormalities. Associated ipsilateral facial musculature is hypoplastic.

Less Common Radiologic Manifestations

Brain and vascular anomalies have rarely been reported.

Differential Diagnosis

- Other craniofacial syndromes (e.g., Treacher Collins syndrome)

Discussion

Goldenhar syndrome affects only one side of the face, whereas other craniofacial syndromes may be bilateral.

Diagnosis

Goldenhar syndrome

Suggested Readings

Binaghi S, Gudinchet F, Rilliet B: Three-dimensional spiral CT of craniofacial malformations in children. Pediatr Radiol 30:856-860, 2000.

Santos DT, Miyazaki O, Cavalcanti MG: Clinical-embryological and radiological correlations of oculo-auriculo-vertebral spectrum using 3D-CT. Dentomaxillofac Radiol 32:8-14, 2003.

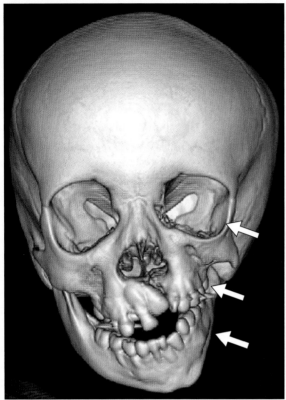

Figure 1. Three-dimensional craniofacial CT reconstruction shows left facial microsomia, with hypoplastic left orbit, left maxilla, and left mandible (*arrows*).

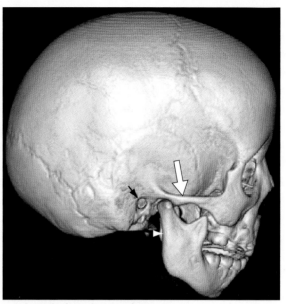

Figure 2. Right lateral view of CT reconstruction shows normal osseous external auditory canal (*black arrow*), normal body of ramus of mandible (*arrowhead*), and normal zygomatic arch (*white arrow*) on right.

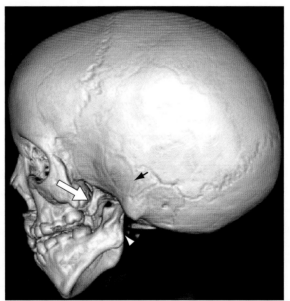

Figure 3. Left lateral view of CT reconstruction shows absence of normal osseous external auditory canal (*black arrow*) in expected location and ipsilateral mandibular (*arrowhead*) and zygomatic arch (*white arrow*) hypoplasia.

Case 276

DEMOGRAPHICS/CLINICAL HISTORY

The patient is a 2-year-old boy with bowing deformity of the lower leg.

FINDINGS

Anteroposterior (Fig. 1) and lateral (Fig. 2) radiographs of the lower leg show lateral bowing of the tibia and fibula with evidence of a pseudarthrosis at the midshaft of the tibia.

DISCUSSION

Definition/Background

Neurofibromatosis 1 is also known as von Recklinghausen disease. It is a hereditary phakomatosis that affects the skin, nervous system, bones, endocrine glands, and other organs.

Characteristic Clinical Features

Patients often have multiple areas of skin pigmentation accompanied by dermal and neural tumors of various types. Peripheral manifestations of the disease include limb hemihypertrophy, pseudarthrosis, and peripheral nerve neurofibromas.

Characteristic Radiologic Findings

Pseudarthrosis of the tibia is characteristic of neurofibromatosis. It is believed to be secondary to mesodermal defects that result in bowing deformities leading to pathologic fracture, poor healing, and subsequent pseudarthrosis.

Less Common Radiologic Manifestations

Cortically based lucencies in the tibia around the knee are characteristic of neurofibromatosis. These lesions resemble nonossifying fibromas on plain radiographs, although they are usually greater in size and number.

Differential Diagnosis

- Post-traumatic pseudarthrosis
- Nonossifying fibroma

Discussion

Pseudarthrosis of the tibia may occur after traumatic fracture of the tibia with abnormal healing. The characteristic bowing deformity of neurofibromatosis lesions is rarely present in this situation. The cortically based cystic lesions of the tibia that occur in patients with neurofibromatosis resemble nonossifying fibromas, although nonossifying fibromas tend to be smaller and fewer in number.

Diagnosis

Neurofibromatosis 1

Suggested Readings

Fortman BJ, Kuszyk BS, Urban BA, et al: Neurofibromatosis type 1: A diagnostic mimicker at CT. RadioGraphics 21:601-612, 2001.

Levine SM, Lambiase RE, Petchprapa CN: Cortical lesions of the tibia: Characteristic appearance at conventional radiography. RadioGraphics 23:157-177, 2003.

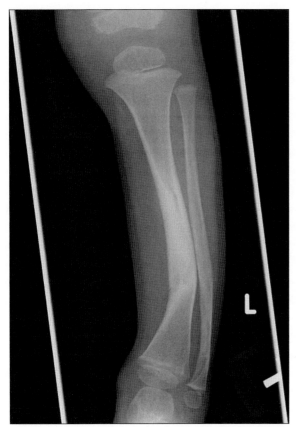

Figure 1. Anteroposterior radiograph of lower leg shows lateral bowing of tibia and fibula with evidence of pseudarthrosis at mid-shaft of tibia.

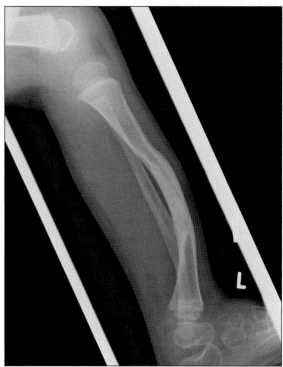

Figure 2. Lateral radiograph of lower leg shows anterior bowing of tibia and fibula.

Case 277

DEMOGRAPHICS/CLINICAL HISTORY

The patient is a 1-month-old girl with inability to pass a nasogastric tube through the right nares.

FINDINGS

Fig. 1 shows enlargement of the midline vomer and membranous connection causing right-sided choanal atresia. Lesions can be bilateral, as in the patient shown in Fig. 2 with CHARGE syndrome and combination bony and membranous anomalies causing bilateral choanal atresia.

DISCUSSION

Definition/Background
Approximately half of patients with choanal atresia have other major anomalies (e.g., CHARGE syndrome) or brain anomalies. Choanal atresia can be composed of bony or membranous abnormalities, or a combination (most common).

Characteristic Clinical Features
When choanal atresia is bilateral (approximately 50% of cases), newborns present at birth with respiratory distress. If choanal atresia is unilateral, patients may go undiagnosed until attempted passage of a nasogastric tube or obstructive pathology on the contralateral side elicits respiratory difficulty.

Characteristic Radiologic Findings
Bony atresia (approximately 30% of cases) is shown by fusion of an enlarged vomer with the medially bowed palatine bone. Purely membranous atresia is rarer, with normal vomer and palatine bones. Most commonly, atresia has bony and membranous components.

Differential Diagnosis
- Piriform aperture stenosis
- Mid-nose stenosis
- Choanal stenosis

Discussion
Piriform aperture stenosis is the most anterior obstruction of the nasal passage. Mid-nose stenosis is less common and often associated with other craniofacial abnormalities. Choanal stenosis is narrowing of the choana, but with incomplete obstruction.

Diagnosis
Choanal atresia

Suggested Readings
Keller JL, Kacker A: Choanal atresia, CHARGE association, and congenital nasal stenosis. Otolaryngol Clin North Am 33:1343, 2000.

Slovis TL, Renfro B, Watts FB, et al: Choanal atresia: Precise CT evaluation. Radiology 155:345, 1985.

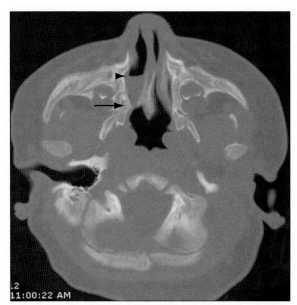

Figure 1. Computed tomography (CT) scan shows enlargement of vomer to the right with medial bowing of right palatine bone (*arrow*) and membranous connection causing right-sided choanal atresia. Air-fluid level is seen in right nasal passage, consistent with obstruction (*arrowhead*).

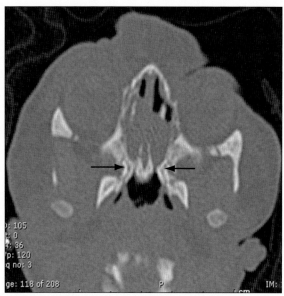

Figure 2. In a different patient, a newborn with CHARGE syndrome and respiratory distress, CT scan shows combination bony and membranous anomalies causing bilateral choanal atresia (*arrows*).

Case 278

DEMOGRAPHICS/CLINICAL HISTORY

The patient is a child with an incidental finding on a computed tomography (CT) scan performed for trauma.

FINDINGS

Magnetic resonance imaging (MRI) shows a small T2-weighted hyperintense lesion (Fig. 1) in the right cerebellopontine angle, causing mild mass effect. The lesion shows suppression of signal on fluid attenuated inversion recovery (FLAIR) MRI (Fig. 2). Mild signal intensity is seen in the lesion on diffusion-weighted MRI (Fig. 3). Apparent diffusion coefficient mapping shows hyperintensity of the lesion, which indicates that the lesion does not have true restricted diffusion (Fig. 4). Postcontrast imaging (not shown) did not show any enhancement.

DISCUSSION

Definition/Background
Arachnoid cysts are thought to be congenital in origin, with the etiology still controversial. When located in a supratentorial location, they are most commonly found in the middle cranial fossa; when located infratentorially, they are often found in the cerebellopontine angle.

Characteristic Clinical Features
No clinical findings are particular to arachnoid cysts because they are typically found incidentally; however, headaches can be found with complications such as hemorrhage or symptoms related to the location of the cyst (including obstructive hydrocephalus) secondary to mass effect from cyst expansion.

Characteristic Radiologic Findings
Arachnoid cysts typically are similar to cerebrospinal fluid (CSF) density or intensity on imaging. No enhancement or restricted diffusion is seen in arachnoid cysts.

Less Common Radiologic Manifestations
Occasionally, septations can be seen. Any non-CSF density or intensity characteristics may be due to hemorrhage, but are atypical.

Differential Diagnosis
- Epidermoid
- Subdural fluid
- Astrocytoma

Discussion
Epidermoids often have similar locations and T2 characteristics as arachnoid cysts; however, they typically display restricted diffusion and incomplete suppression on FLAIR MRI. Subdural fluid collections tend to have slightly different T2 and FLAIR characteristics than CSF. Astrocytomas typically have slightly different FLAIR signal than CSF and have an adjacent enhancing component.

Diagnosis
Arachnoid cyst

Suggested Readings
Cincu R, Agrawal A, Eiras J: Intracranial arachnoid cysts: Current concepts and treatment alternatives. Clin Neurol Neurosurg 109:837-843, 2007.

Gosalakkal JA: Intracranial arachnoid cysts in children: A review of pathogenesis, clinical features, and management. Pediatr Neurol 26:93-98, 2002.

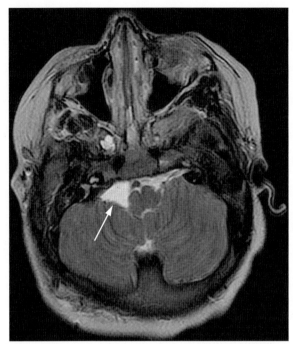

Figure 1. Axial T2-weighted MR image shows small hyperintense lesion in right cerebellopontine angle (*arrow*), causing mild mass effect.

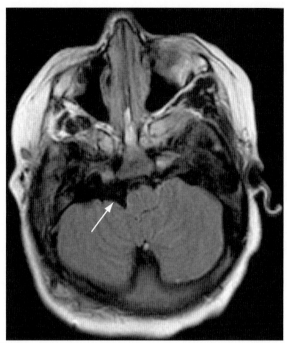

Figure 2. On axial FLAIR MRI, lesion (*arrow*) shows suppression of signal, similar to CSF.

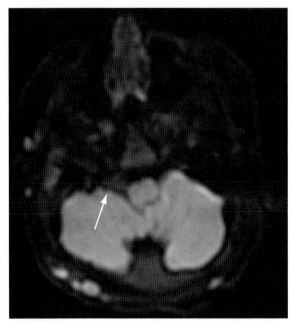

Figure 3. On diffusion-weighted MRI, minimal signal is seen in lesion (*arrow*).

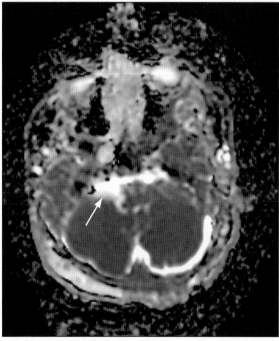

Figure 4. Apparent diffusion coefficient mapping shows hyperintensity of lesion (*arrow*), which indicates that the lesion does not have true restricted diffusion.

Case 279

DEMOGRAPHICS/CLINICAL HISTORY

The patient is a 16-year-old child with von Hippel-Lindau (VHL) disease

FINDINGS

A posterior fossa mass with multiple flow voids within and around the mass is seen on axial T2-weighted fluid attenuated inversion recovery (FLAIR) magnetic resonance imaging (MRI) (Fig. 1). Postcontrast sagittal T1-weighted MRI (Fig. 2) shows the intensely enhancing mass. Axial computed tomography (CT) scan of the patient's abdomen with intravenous contrast (Fig. 3) shows many cysts within the pancreas. Sagittal T1-weighted postcontrast MRI (Fig. 4) in another child with VHL disease shows a hemangioblastoma with a nonenhancing cystic component and a solid, enhancing mural nodule.

DISCUSSION

Definition/Background

Hemangioblastomas typically occur in young and middle-aged adults, and when seen in children, they are often associated with syndromes, typically VHL disease. Multiple hemangioblastomas suggest the presence of a syndrome.

Characteristic Clinical Features

Many patients who have the diagnosis of VHL disease are screened for hemangioblastomas. Patients who present with de novo hemangioblastomas may have symptoms from mass effect or hemorrhage, including ataxia, nausea, vomiting, and headache.

Characteristic Radiologic Findings

Hemangioblastomas are typically found in the posterior fossa or within the spinal cord. The most common appearance is a cystic mass with an enhancing mural nodule adjacent to a pial surface. Solid, enhancing masses without cysts also are common. MRI often can show flow voids, reflecting the vascularity of the tumor.

Less Common Radiologic Manifestations

Occasionally, hemangioblastomas have little or no solid components, which can make them difficult to distinguish from an arachnoid cyst.

Differential Diagnosis

- Arachnoid cyst
- Pilocytic astrocytoma
- Medulloblastoma
- Ependymoma

Discussion

Depending on the particular composition of the hemangioblastoma, the imaging appearance can mimic several other entities. The clinical history of VHL disease should suggest the diagnosis. The presence of flow voids can suggest hemangioblastoma over other entities.

Diagnosis

Posterior fossa hemangioblastoma

Suggested Readings

Richard S, Campello C, Taillandier L, et al: Haemangioblastoma of the central nervous system in von Hippel-Lindau disease. French VHL Study Group. J Intern Med 243:547-553, 1998.

Richard S, David P, Marsot-Dupuch K, et al: Central nervous system hemangioblastomas, endolymphatic sac tumors, and von Hippel-Lindau disease. Neurosurg Rev 23:1-22, 2000.

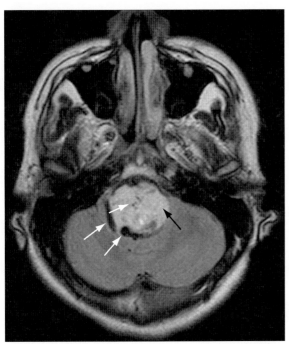

Figure 1. Axial T2-weighted FLAIR MR image shows posterior fossa mass (*black arrow*) with multiple flow voids (*white arrows*) within and around mass.

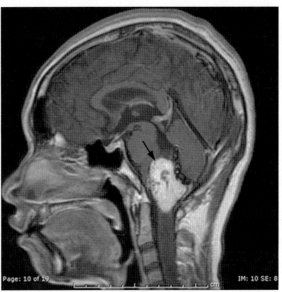

Figure 2. Postcontrast sagittal T1-weighted MR image shows intense enhancement of mass (*arrow*).

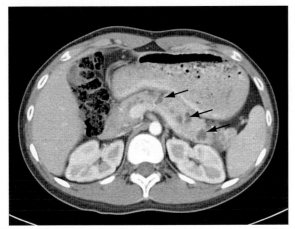

Figure 3. Axial CT scan of abdomen with contrast agent shows multiple cysts within pancreas (*arrows*).

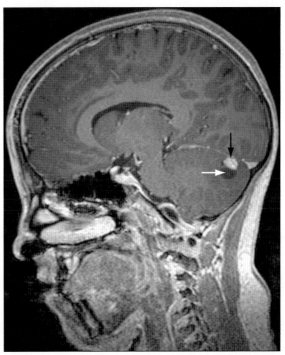

Figure 4. In a different patient, sagittal T1-weighted postcontrast MR image shows hemangioblastoma with nonenhancing cystic component (*white arrow*) and enhancing solid mural nodule (*black arrow*).

Case 280

DEMOGRAPHICS/CLINICAL HISTORY

The patient is an 8-year-old child with morning emesis for 5 days.

FINDINGS

Axial computed tomography (CT) scan (Fig. 1) shows a suprasellar mass with hypodense and hyperdense components. Sagittal CT reconstruction (Fig. 2) shows calcifications within the inferior aspect of the suprasellar mass. Coronal T1 weighted magnetic resonance imaging (MRI) (Fig. 3) shows hypointense and hyperintense cystic components. Rim enhancement of the hypointense cyst and enhancement of an inferior solid component are seen on postcontrast T1-weighted MRI (Fig. 4).

DISCUSSION

Definition/Background
Craniopharyngiomas are the most common type of pediatric suprasellar tumor.

Characteristic Clinical Features
Patients can present with symptoms from the mass effect on the adjacent structures (e.g., visual defects, abnormalities in hypothalamic-pituitary axis) or with signs of increased intracranial pressure (e.g., nausea, vomiting, headaches).

Characteristic Radiologic Findings
Craniopharyngiomas typically have cystic and solid components, often with areas of calcification. CT delineates the calcification best. MRI shows the different cystic components and the solid enhancing components. Cystic components can have various densities (CT) and intensities (MRI), depending on the amount of proteinaceous fluid within them. MRI better delineates tumor extent and involvement of adjacent structures.

Differential Diagnosis
- Pituitary adenoma
- Rathke cleft cyst
- Astrocytoma

Discussion
Craniopharyngiomas may extend into the sella, but the pituitary is typically normal in appearance, which differentiates it from a pituitary adenoma. Rathke cleft cysts usually are small and do not have solid, enhancing components. When astrocytomas are located in the hypothalamus, they can extend into the suprasellar cistern and mimic craniopharyngiomas. Differentiating the two can be difficult, but if the center of the solid enhancing portion is within the hypothalamus, the diagnosis of astrocytoma should be considered.

Diagnosis
Craniopharyngioma

Suggested Readings

Choi SH, Kwon BJ, Na DG, et al: Pituitary adenoma, craniopharyngioma, and Rathke cleft cyst involving both intrasellar and suprasellar regions: differentiation using MRI. Clin Radiol 62:453-462, 2007.

Tsuda M, Takahashi S, Higano S, et al: CT and MR imaging of craniopharyngioma. Eur Radiol 7:464-469, 1997.

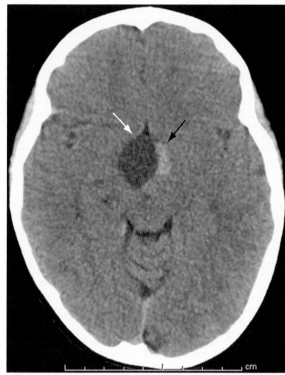

Figure 1. Axial CT scan shows suprasellar mass with hypodense (*white arrow*) and hyperdense (*black arrow*) components.

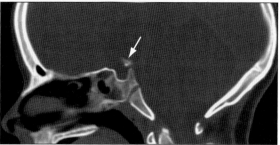

Figure 2. Sagittal CT reconstruction shows calcifications within inferior aspect of suprasellar mass (*arrow*).

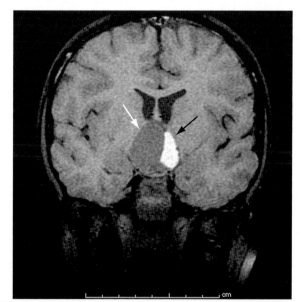

Figure 3. Coronal T1-weighted MR image shows hypointense (*white arrow*) and hyperintense (*black arrow*) cystic components.

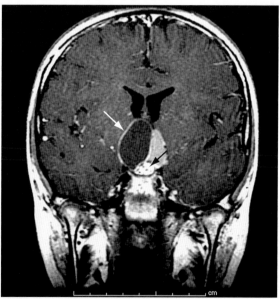

Figure 4. Postcontrast T1-weighted MR image shows rim enhancement of hypointense cyst (*white arrow*) and enhancement of inferior solid component (*black arrow*).

Case 281

DEMOGRAPHICS/CLINICAL HISTORY

The patient is a 2-year-old child with headaches and vomiting.

FINDINGS

Axial non–contrast-enhanced computed tomography (CT) scan of the head (Fig. 1) shows an isodense mass in the fourth ventricle. Axial T2-weighted magnetic resonance imaging (MRI) (Fig. 2) shows extension of the mass through the left foramen of Luschka into the cerebellopontine angle. Diffusion weighted imaging (DWI) demonstrates intermediate signal within the mass. Postcontrast sagittal T1-weighted MRI (Fig. 4) shows the hydrocephalus resulting from obstruction of the fourth ventricle by the enhancing mass.

DISCUSSION

Definition/Background
Ependymomas most commonly occur in the posterior fossa, but they can occur in the supratentorial brain and within the spine.

Characteristic Clinical Features
Presenting symptoms, such as nausea, vomiting, and headaches, reflect increased intracranial pressure from hydrocephalus.

Characteristic Radiologic Findings
Ependymomas often spread through the foramina of Luschka and Magendie and into the upper cervical canal. Ependymomas can have fine calcifications or hemorrhage. Rarely, ependymomas spread through the cerebrospinal fluid, and imaging of the spine should be performed to look for metastases.

Less Common Radiologic Manifestations
Metastatic spread to bone, liver, or lung is rare.

Differential Diagnosis
- Medulloblastoma
- Pilocytic astrocytoma

Discussion
Medulloblastomas can have an appearance similar to an ependymoma, but are more likely to be hyperdense on CT, to have restricted diffusion on MRI, to have leptomeningeal metastatic spread, and are less likely to spread through the foramina. Pilocytic astrocytomas are more likely to have cystic components, are less cellular than ependymomas, and are less likely to spread through the foramina.

Diagnosis
Ependymoma

Suggested Readings
Fitz CR: Neuroradiology of posterior fossa tumors in children. Clin Neurosurg 30:189-202, 1983.
Schneider JF, Viola A, Confort-Gouny S, et al: Infratentorial pediatric brain tumors: The value of new imaging modalities. J Neuroradiol 34:49-58, 2007.

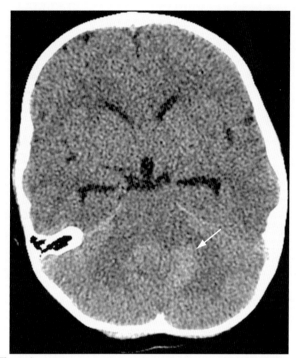

Figure 1. Axial non–contrast-enhanced CT scan of the head shows isodense mass in fourth ventricle (*arrow*).

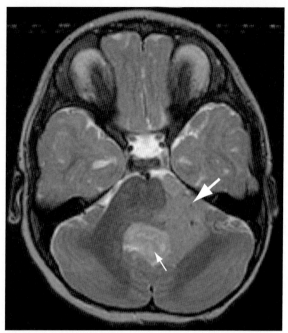

Figure 2. Axial T2-weighted MR image shows extension of mass (*small arrow*) through left foramen of Luschka into cerebellopontine angle (*large arrow*).

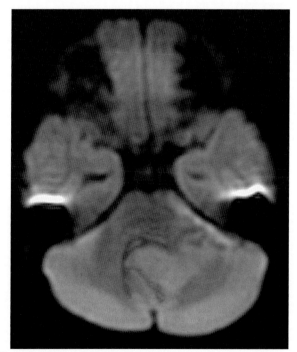

Figure 3. Diffusion weighted imaging (DWI) demonstrates intermediate signal within the mass.

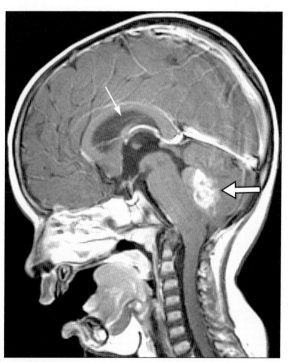

Figure 4. Postcontrast sagittal T1-weighted MR image shows hydrocephalus (*small arrow*) resulting from obstruction of fourth ventricle by enhancing mass (*large arrow*).

Case 282

DEMOGRAPHICS/CLINICAL HISTORY

The patient is a 2-year-old child with vomiting.

FINDINGS

Axial non–contrast-enhanced computed tomography (CT) (Fig. 1) shows a large, hyperdense mass in the fourth ventricle, causing hydrocephalus. Sagittal T1-weighted magnetic resonance imaging (MRI) with contrast agent (Fig. 2) shows enhancement of the mass and abnormal enhancement of the leptomeninges along the brainstem and cerebellum. Increased signal intensity on diffusion-weighted imaging (Fig. 3) and restricted diffusion on apparent diffusion coefficient map (Fig. 4) show the hypercellularity of the tumor.

DISCUSSION

Definition/Background

Medulloblastomas are aggressive tumors of the posterior fossa. Approximately one third of patients presenting with medulloblastoma already have leptomeningeal metastases.

Characteristic Clinical Features

Most patients present with signs of increased intracranial pressure, such as nausea, vomiting, and headaches, caused by obstructive hydrocephalus.

Characteristic Radiologic Findings

Medulloblastomas are highly cellular tumors and are typically hyperdense on CT. Obstructive hydrocephalus is a typical finding. On MRI, the mass can be located in the midline along the fourth ventricle or vermis, but an eccentric intracerebellar location also can be seen. Intense enhancement is typical within the tumor. Leptomeningeal enhancement representing metastatic disease is common. Restricted diffusion is a characteristic finding of medulloblastomas.

Less Common Radiologic Manifestations

Rarely, medulloblastomas can have cysts and calcification.

Differential Diagnosis

- Ependymoma
- Pilocytic astrocytoma

Discussion

Posterior fossa ependymomas can have an appearance similar to medulloblastomas, but ependymomas are more likely to extend into the foramina of Magendie and Luschka and are less likely to have restricted diffusion and leptomeningeal metastases. Pilocytic astrocytomas typically have prominent cystic components and do not have restricted diffusion or leptomeningeal metastases.

Diagnosis

Medulloblastoma

Suggested Readings

Fitz C: Neuroradiology of posterior fossa tumors in children. Clin Neurosurg 30:189-202, 1983.

Schneider JF, Viola A, Confort-Gouny S, et al: Infratentorial pediatric brain tumors: The value of new imaging modalities. J Neuroradiol 34:49-58, 2007.

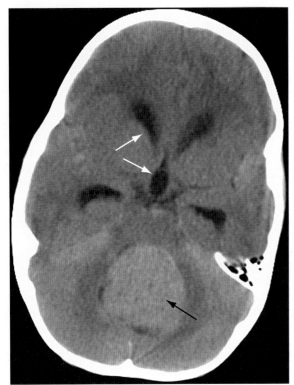

Figure 1. Axial non–contrast-enhanced CT scan shows large hyperdense mass (*black arrow*) in fourth ventricle, causing hydrocephalus (*white arrows*).

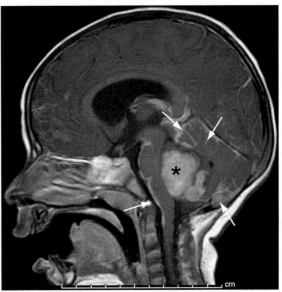

Figure 2. Sagittal T1-weighted MRI with contrast agent shows enhancement of mass (*asterisk*) and abnormal enhancement of leptomeninges along brainstem and cerebellum (*white arrows*).

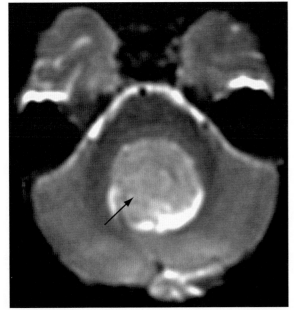

Figure 3. Diffusion-weighted imaging shows increased signal intensity (*arrow*).

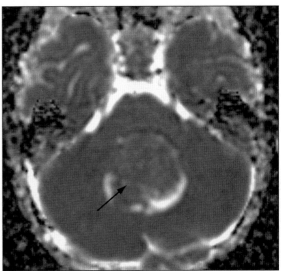

Figure 4. Apparent diffusion coefficient map confirms restricted diffusion (*arrow*), representing hypercellularity of tumor.

Case 283

DEMOGRAPHICS/CLINICAL HISTORY

The patient is a 5-year-old child with vomiting.

FINDINGS

An axial non–contrast-enhanced computed tomography (CT) scan (Fig. 1) shows a mass in the cerebellum with a large cystic component and a hypodense solid component. Axial T2-weighted magnetic resonance imaging (MRI) (Fig. 2) better delineates the cystic components and hyperintense solid component. Intense enhancement of the solid component is seen on postcontrast T1-weighted MRI (Fig. 3). Diffusion-weighted imaging (Fig. 4) does not show hyperintensity or restricted diffusion (apparent diffusion coefficient map not shown) of the cystic or solid portions.

DISCUSSION

Definition/Background

After medulloblastoma, astrocytoma is the second most common posterior fossa tumor in children. Pilocytic astrocytomas are the most common subtype of astrocytoma in children, and they have an excellent prognosis.

Characteristic Clinical Features

Patients typically present with symptoms including nausea, vomiting, headaches, and ataxia, caused by the mass effect in the cerebellum and obstruction of the fourth ventricle.

Characteristic Radiologic Findings

Pilocytic astrocytomas typically have cystic components that are seen as hypodense areas on CT and hyperintense areas on T2-weighted MRI. They can occasionally have hemorrhage or contain proteinaceous material, which can make the cysts hyperintense on T1-weighted MRI. The solid components are not hypercellular and typically show high signal intensity on T2-weighted MRI. Solid portions usually show homogeneous enhancement, and the cystic components sometimes have wall enhancement. Diffusion-weighted imaging usually does not show restricted diffusion of the mass.

Less Common Radiologic Manifestations

Some low-grade astrocytomas do not show significant enhancement. Calcifications are rare in pilocytic astrocytomas. Leptomeningeal metastases are extremely rare.

Differential Diagnosis

- Ependymoma
- Medulloblastoma

Discussion

Ependymomas and medulloblastomas usually do not have large cystic components. Ependymomas often spread through the foramina, and medulloblastoma typically spreads through the cerebrospinal fluid, seeding the leptomeninges. Medulloblastomas typically have restricted diffusion on diffusion-weighted imaging.

Diagnosis

Pilocytic astrocytoma

Suggested Readings

Fitz CR: Neuroradiology of posterior fossa tumors in children. Clin Neurosurg 30:189-202, 1983.

Schneider JF, Viola A, Confort-Gouny S, et al: Infratentorial pediatric brain tumors: The value of new imaging modalities. J Neuroradiol 34:49-58, 2007.

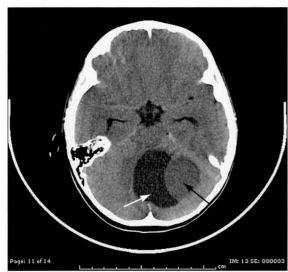

Figure 1. Axial non–contrast-enhanced CT scan shows mass in cerebellum with large cystic component (*white arrow*) and a hypodense solid component (*black arrow*).

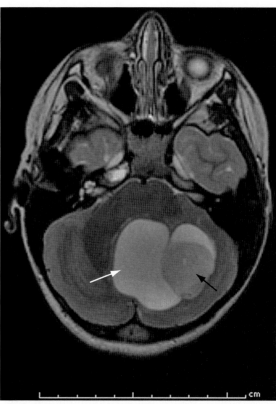

Figure 2. Axial T2-weighted MR image better delineates cystic components (*white arrow*) and hyperintense solid component (*black arrow*).

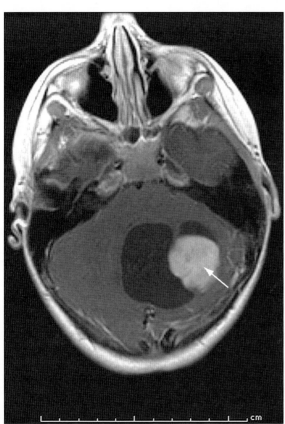

Figure 3. Postcontrast T1-weighted MR image shows intense enhancement of solid component (*arrow*).

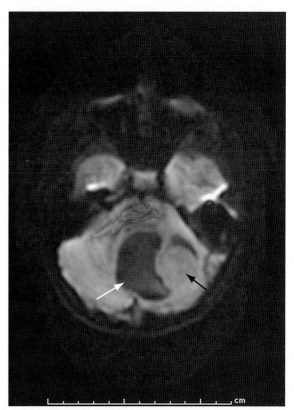

Figure 4. Diffusion-weighted imaging does not show hyperintensity or restricted diffusion of cystic (*white arrow*) or solid (*black arrow*) portions.

Case 284

DEMOGRAPHICS/CLINICAL HISTORY

The patient is a 4-year-old girl presenting for preoperative evaluation for atrial septal defect closure.

FINDINGS

A frontal radiograph (Fig. 1) of the chest shows a right-sided mass that does not obscure the diaphragm or right heart border. Congenital vertebral anomalies in the lower cervical and upper thoracic spine were incidentally found. Lateral radiograph (Fig. 2) confirms the location of the mass within the posterior mediastinum. Axial contrast-enhanced computed tomography (CT) scan (Fig. 3) of the mass shows a low-density (30 HU) posterior mediastinal mass, without calcifications or involvement within the neural foramina. Coronal postcontrast T1-weighted magnetic resonance imaging (MRI) (Fig. 4) shows heterogeneous enhancement of the mass and confirms an intrathoracic location, with the mass sitting atop the dark diaphragm on the T1-weighted image.

DISCUSSION

Definition/Background
Ganglioneuromas are benign, well-differentiated neural neoplasms.

Characteristic Clinical Features
Ganglioneuromas often are found incidentally in asymptomatic patients during imaging. Pain and other symptoms can occur if the tumor involves the neural foramina, nerve roots, or a mass effect on the cord. The average age of patients with ganglioneuroma is slightly older than the average age of patients with neuroblastoma.

Characteristic Radiologic Findings
Ganglioneuromas typically are located in the posterior mediastinum, and they seldom occur in the abdomen, involving the adrenal gland. Although there is no specific imaging difference between neuroblastomas and ganglioneuromas, the latter is less likely to have calcifications or intraspinal involvement. In some patients, the imaging appearance is identical to neuroblastoma, with a heterogeneous appearance; calcifications, encasement, and displacement of vessels; involvement of neural foramina; and a mass effect on the spinal cord.

Less Common Radiologic Manifestations
Ganglioneuromas are typically surgically resected because there are many case reports of malignant peripheral nerve sheath tumors occurring within conservatively treated ganglioneuromas. Ganglioneuromas that are incompletely resected or not resected should be followed radiographically for any changes.

Differential Diagnosis
- Neuroblastoma (pediatric)
- Ganglioneuroblastoma

Discussion
The appearances of neuroblastoma, ganglioneuroblastoma, and ganglioneuroma can be identical, and the diagnosis must be based on examination of a pathologic specimen.

Diagnosis
Ganglioneuroma

Suggested Readings
Lonergan GJ, Schwab CM, Suarez ES, Carlson CL: Neuroblastoma, ganglioneuroblastoma, and ganglioneuroma: Radiologic-pathologic correlation. RadioGraphics 22:911-934, 2002.
Schulman H, Laufer L, Barki Y, et al: Ganglioneuroma: An 'incidentaloma' of childhood. Eur Radiol 8:582-584, 1998.

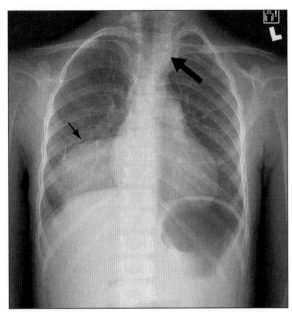

Figure 1. Frontal radiograph of chest shows right-sided mass (*small arrow*) that does not obscure diaphragm or right heart border. Incidentally identified are congenital vertebral anomalies in lower cervical and upper thoracic spine (*large arrow*).

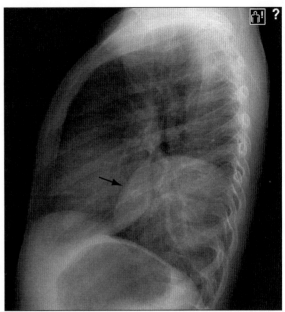

Figure 2. Lateral radiograph confirms location of mass (*arrow*) within posterior mediastinum.

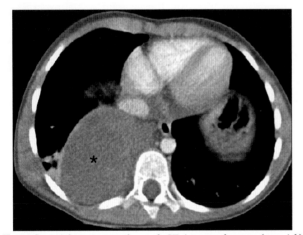

Figure 3. Axial contrast-enhanced CT image of mass (*asterisk*) shows low-density (30 HU) posterior mediastinal mass, without calcifications or involvement within neural foramina.

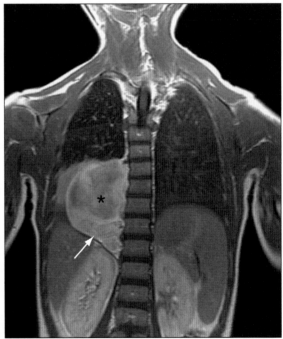

Figure 4. Coronal postcontrast T1-weighted MR image shows heterogeneous enhancement of mass (*asterisk*) and confirms intrathoracic location, with mass sitting atop dark diaphragm (*arrow*). Axial images confirmed no extension into neural foramina, and pathologic examination confirmed lesion to be a ganglioneuroma.

Case 285

DEMOGRAPHICS/CLINICAL HISTORY

The patient is a 1-year-old child with leukocoria.

FINDINGS

Axial fluid attenuated inversion recovery (FLAIR) magnetic resonance imaging (MRI) (Fig. 1) shows isointense masses along the retina in the left and right globes. Hyperintensity in the left subretinal space represents subretinal hemorrhage. Axial T2-weighted MRI (Fig. 2) in a slightly more superior plane shows additional retinal lesions. Surgical pathologic examination determined that this patient had bilateral retinoblastomas.

DISCUSSION

Definition/Background

Retinoblastoma is the most common pediatric intraocular tumor.

Characteristic Clinical Features

Leukocoria is the typical clinical feature.

Characteristic Radiologic Findings

On computed tomography (CT), calcifications typically are seen within the retinoblastoma mass; approximately 95% of patients may have calcifications. MRI is used to detect bilateral disease and to look for extension or involvement of the optic nerve. The tumor shows enhancement on MRI.

Less Common Radiologic Manifestations

Intracranial extension can occur with leptomeningeal seeding. So-called trilateral retinoblastoma refers to the rare occurrence of bilateral retinoblastomas and a pineal mass, typically a pineoblastoma.

Differential Diagnosis

- Coats disease
- *Toxocara* endophthalmitis
- Persistent hyperplastic primary vitreous, pediatric orbit
- Retinal astrocytic hamartomas

Discussion

Coats disease, also known as exudative retinitis or retinal telangiectasia, causes hemorrhage of retinal capillaries, retinal detachment, and microphthalmos. *Toxocara* endophthalmitis, a granulomatous reaction in the vitreous or uvea due to the dead or dying larvae of *Toxocara canis* or *Toxocara cati*, has an appearance similar to Coats disease, and patients have serologic results that suggest the diagnosis. Calcifications are rare in Coats disease and *Toxocara* endophthalmitis. Persistent hyperplastic primary vitreous has a typical "trumpet horn" appearance of the subretinal fluid outlining the persistent hyaloid artery and fibrous connection, and the proliferation lacks calcification. Retinal astrocytic hamartomas can have calcifications, but they are confined to the sensory retina or optic disk and usually do not cause hemorrhage.

Diagnosis

Retinoblastoma

Suggested Readings

Chung EM, Specht CS, Schroeder JW: From the archives of the AFIP: Pediatric orbit tumors and tumorlike lesions: Neuroepithelial lesions of the ocular globe and optic nerve. RadioGraphics 27:1159-1186, 2007.

Kaufman LM, Mafee MF, Song CD: Retinoblastoma and simulating lesions: Role of CT, MR imaging and use of Gd-DTPA contrast enhancement. Radiol Clin North Am 36:1101-1117, 1998.

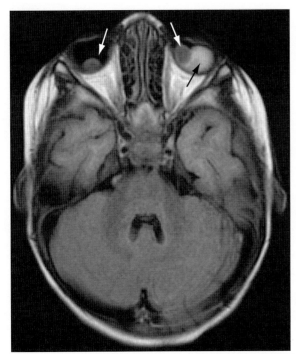

Figure 1. Axial FLAIR MR image shows isointense masses (*white arrows*) along retina in left and right globes. Hyperintensity in left subretinal space (*black arrow*) represents subretinal hemorrhage.

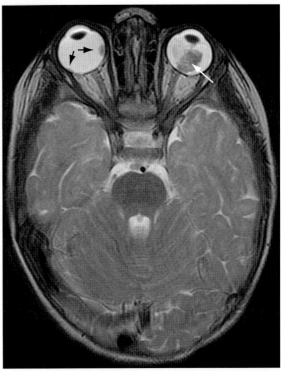

Figure 2. Axial T2-weighted MR image in slightly more superior plane shows additional retinal lesions (*arrows*). Surgical pathologic examination confirmed that the patient had bilateral retinoblastomas.

Case 286

DEMOGRAPHICS/CLINICAL HISTORY

The patient is a 13-year-old child with epistaxis and a suspected nasal mass.

FINDINGS

A nasopharyngeal mass is seen extending posteriorly to the sella on sagittal T1-weighted magnetic resonance imaging (MRI) (Fig. 1). Postcontrast sagittal T1-weighted MRI (Fig. 2) shows avid enhancement of the mass extending up to the tuberculum sellae. Axial postcontrast T1-weighted MRI (Fig. 3) shows the enhancing mass and central nonenhancement, suggesting necrosis. No invasion of the pterygopalatine fossa is seen. Coronal contrast-enhanced T1-weighted MRI (Fig. 4) shows low signal intensity curvilinear structures, representing the many flow voids within the hypervascular mass.

DISCUSSION

Definition/Background

Although juvenile nasopharyngeal angiofibromas are benign tumors, they are locally aggressive.

Characteristic Clinical Features

The typical presentation is a young boy with epistaxis.

Characteristic Radiologic Findings

The mass typically originates in and fills the nasal cavity, often invading the pterygopalatine fossa. The mass is hypervascular and shows avid postcontrast enhancement. When invasion of the skull base occurs, recurrence and residual disease are common.

Differential Diagnosis

- Nasopharyngeal carcinoma

Discussion

Nasopharyngeal carcinomas can have a similar imaging appearance, but are much less common than juvenile nasopharyngeal angiofibromas.

Diagnosis

Juvenile nasopharyngeal angiofibroma

Suggested Readings

Kania RE, Sauvaget E, Guichard JP, et al: Early postoperative CT scanning for juvenile nasopharyngeal angiofibroma: Detection of residual disease. AJNR Am J Neuroradiol 26:82-88, 2005.

Momeni AK, Roberts CC, Chew FS: Imaging of chronic and exotic sinonasal disease: Review. AJR Am J Roentgenol 189(Suppl):S35-S45, 2007.

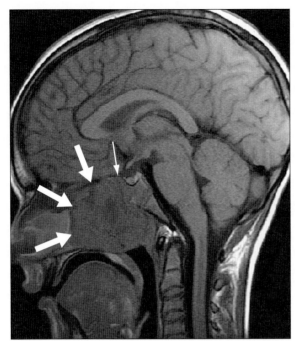

Figure 1. Sagittal T1-weighted MR image shows nasopharyngeal mass (*large arrows*) extending posteriorly to sella (*small arrow*).

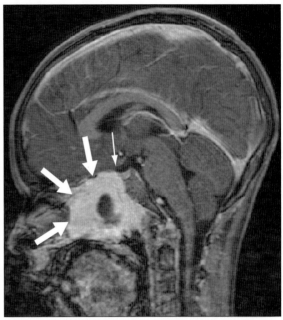

Figure 2. Postcontrast sagittal T1-weighted MR image shows avid enhancement of mass (*large arrows*) extending up to the tuberculum sellae (*small arrow*).

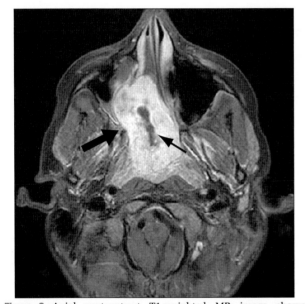

Figure 3. Axial postcontrast T1-weighted MR image shows enhancing mass and central nonenhancement (*small arrow*), suggesting necrosis. No invasion of pterygopalatine fossa is seen (*large arrow*).

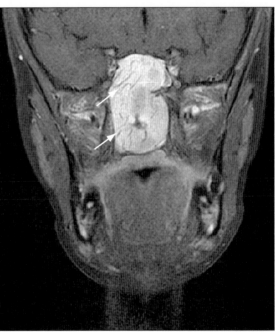

Figure 4. Coronal postcontrast T1-weighted MR image shows low signal intensity curvilinear structures (*arrows*), representing many flow voids within hypervascular mass.

Case 287

DEMOGRAPHICS/CLINICAL HISTORY

The patient is an 18-year-old young adult with increasing nasal congestion.

FINDINGS

Proptosis of the right orbit is seen on a contrast-enhanced computed tomography (CT) scan of the sinuses (Fig. 1). A heterogeneous mass is expanding the right ethmoid air cells. Osseous windowing of the CT scan (Fig. 2) shows destruction of the right lamina papyracea with minimal residual calcifications within the mass. Coronal T1-weighted postcontrast magnetic resonance imaging (MRI) (Fig. 3) shows the heterogeneously enhancing mass with intracranial extension, dural enhancement, and secondary obstruction of the right maxillary sinus. Sagittal T1-weighted postcontrast MRI (Fig. 4) shows the extension of the mass within the nasal cavity, ethmoid air cells, and frontal sinus, with intracranial extension and dural enhancement.

DISCUSSION

Definition/Background
Rhabdomyosarcoma is the most common pediatric soft tissue sarcoma.

Characteristic Clinical Features
Although no specific features are characteristic, rhabdomyosarcoma symptoms reflect the location of the mass. Pain, swelling, nasal obstruction, and proptosis can be symptoms of a head and neck rhabdomyosarcoma.

Characteristic Radiologic Findings
Rhabdomyosarcomas have an aggressive radiologic appearance. Destruction of adjacent bones, enhancement, and intracranial involvement all can be seen on imaging of head and neck rhabdomyosarcomas.

Differential Diagnosis
- Lymphoma
- Carcinoma
- Neuroblastoma

Discussion
The differential diagnosis depends on the exact location of the soft tissue mass. There may not be specific radiologic findings to suggest rhabdomyosarcoma as the diagnosis, and a biopsy typically is needed.

Diagnosis
Rhabdomyosarcoma of the sinus

Suggested Readings
Callender TA, Weber RS, Janjan N, et al: Rhabdomyosarcoma of the nose and paranasal sinuses in adults and children. Otolaryngol Head Neck Surg 112:252-257, 1995.

Latack JT, Hutchinson RJ, Heyn RM: Imaging of rhabdomyosarcomas of the head and neck. AJNR Am J Neuroradiol 8:353-359, 1987.

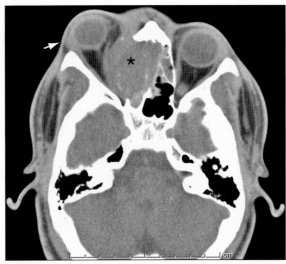

Figure 1. Contrast-enhanced CT scan of sinuses shows proptosis of right orbit (*arrow*). Heterogeneous mass is seen within and expanding right ethmoid air cells (*asterisk*).

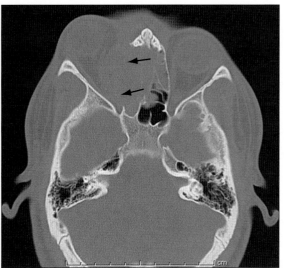

Figure 2. Osseous windowing of CT image shows destruction of right lamina papyracea, with minimal residual calcifications within mass (*arrows*).

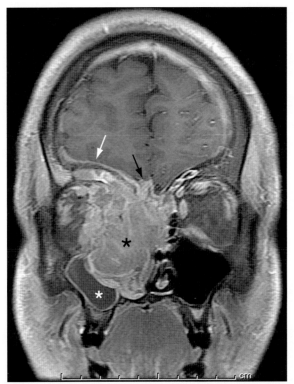

Figure 3. Coronal T1-weighted postcontrast MR image shows heterogeneously enhancing mass (*black asterisk*), with intracranial extension (*black arrow*), dural enhancement (*white arrow*), and secondary obstruction of right maxillary sinus (*white asterisk*).

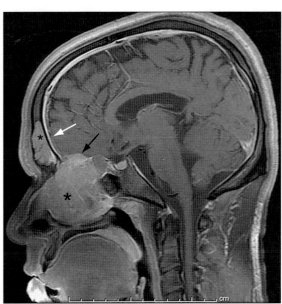

Figure 4. Sagittal T1-weighted postcontrast MR image shows extension of mass within nasal cavity, ethmoid air cells, and frontal sinus (*asterisks*), with intracranial extension (*black arrow*) and dural enhancement (*white arrow*).

Case 288

DEMOGRAPHICS/CLINICAL HISTORY

The patient is a 19-year-old young adult with neurofibromatosis 1.

FINDINGS

Axial T2-weighted magnetic resonance imaging (MRI) (Fig. 1) shows many hyperintense nodules and masses in the psoas and dorsal paraspinal muscles. Many of these nodules show central hypointensity in a target pattern on T2-weighted MRI. Enlargement of exiting nerve roots can be seen. Axial T2-weighted MRI (Fig. 2) shows fusiform enlargement of the exiting nerve roots and widening of the neural foramina, and smaller nodules can be seen in the paraspinal muscles. Axial T2-weighted MRI (Fig. 3) through the sacrum shows innumerable targetoid lesions within and anterior to the sacrum, representing an extensive plexiform neurofibroma. Coronal postcontrast T1-weighted MRI (Fig. 4) shows enhancement of the enlarged exiting nerve roots.

DISCUSSION

Definition/Background
Neurofibromas can occur as an isolated mass, but plexiform neurofibromas are associated with neurofibromatosis 1.

Characteristic Clinical Features
Patients often present with cutaneous and subcutaneous nodules, café au lait spots, and abnormal pigmenting of the iris. They can present with symptoms caused by neural and neurofibromatosis-associated tumors.

Characteristic Radiologic Findings
On computed tomography (CT), neurofibromas appear as soft tissue masses with enhancement. The MRI appearance is characteristic, with hyperintensity on T2-weighted MR images that has a ringlike pattern. Enhancement of the neurofibromas can be homogeneous or ringlike. Plexiform neurofibromas have a ropelike and serpiginous appearance in the nerve roots and branching nerves, with a target appearance on cross-sectional imaging of the nerve. Rapid growth of lesions or heterogeneous enhancement requires attention because these lesions can degenerate into malignant peripheral nerve sheath tumors.

Differential Diagnosis
- Neuroblastoma, pediatric

Discussion
Although neuroblastomas can occur in the paraspinal region with intraspinal extension, the imaging appearance should differentiate them from neurofibromas. Neuroblastomas often have calcification on CT and do not usually have the targetoid or serpiginous appearance that plexiform neurofibromas have.

Diagnosis
Plexiform neurofibroma

Suggested Readings
Levy AD, Patel N, Dow N, et al: From the archives of the AFIP: Abdominal neoplasms in patients with neurofibromatosis type 1: Radiologic-pathologic correlation. RadioGraphics 25:455-480, 2005.

Tucker T, Wolkenstein P, Revuz J, et al: Association between benign and malignant peripheral nerve sheath tumors in NF1. Neurology 65:205-211, 2005.

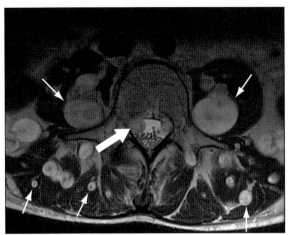

Figure 1. Axial T2-weighted MR image shows many hyperintense nodules and masses in psoas and dorsal paraspinal muscles (*small arrows*). Many nodules show central T2-weighted hypointensity in a target pattern. Enlargement of exiting nerve roots also can be seen (*large arrow*).

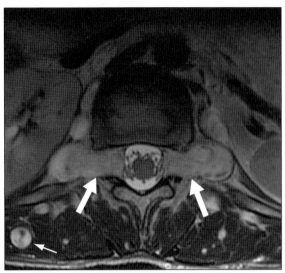

Figure 2. Axial T2-weighted MR image shows fusiform enlargement of exiting nerve roots (*large arrows*) and widening of neural foramina. Smaller nodules can be seen in paraspinal muscles (*small arrow*).

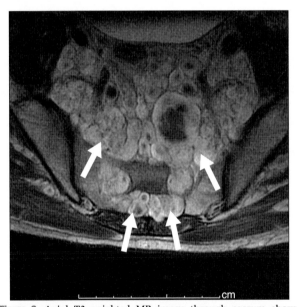

Figure 3. Axial T2-weighted MR image through sacrum shows many targetoid lesions (*arrows*) within and anterior to sacrum, representing extensive plexiform neurofibroma.

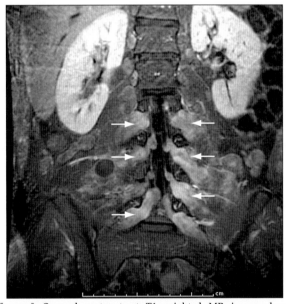

Figure 4. Coronal postcontrast T1-weighted MR image shows enhancement of enlarged exiting nerve roots (*arrows*).

Case 289

DEMOGRAPHICS/CLINICAL HISTORY

The patient is a 4-year-old child with a 1-year history of limp and back pain.

FINDINGS

Bony erosion of the pedicles and canal expansion are seen in a frontal radiograph of the thoracic spine (Fig. 1), reflecting a long-standing intraspinal process. Sagittal T2-weighted magnetic resonance imaging (MRI) (Fig. 2) of the cervicothoracic cord shows an intramedullary mass in the upper thoracic cord with an associated cyst. Cord edema extends up to the craniocervical junction. Sagittal T1-weighted MRI (Fig. 3) shows the isointense mass and T1-weighted hypointense associated cyst. Sagittal T1-weighted postcontrast MRI (Fig. 4) shows enhancement within the mass, but no enhancement of the superior cystic collection is seen.

DISCUSSION

Definition/Background

Astrocytomas, gangliogliomas, and ependymomas constitute most intramedullary spinal tumors in children.

Characteristic Clinical Features

Children can present with back pain, radiculopathy, scoliosis, gait disturbance, or bowel and bladder dysfunction.

Characteristic Radiologic Findings

Intramedullary spinal tumors can vary in the amount of solid and cystic composition and in the degree of tumoral enhancement. Some tumors are poorly defined and infiltrate the cord, whereas others may be well demarcated.

Differential Diagnosis

- Acute disseminated encephalomyelitis
- Multiple sclerosis

Discussion

Because demyelinating processes can have cord edema and variable enhancement, they can mimic a tumor. Brain imaging findings and a clinical history of acute onset may suggest the diagnosis of a demyelinating process, as can follow-up imaging.

Diagnosis

Intramedullary spinal tumor—astrocytoma

Suggested Readings

Auguste KI, Gupta N: Pediatric intramedullary spinal cord tumors. Neurosurg Clin N Am 17:51-61, 2006.

Rossi A, Gandolfo C, Morana G, Tortori-Donati P: Tumors of the spine in children. Neuroimaging Clin N Am 17:17-35, 2007.

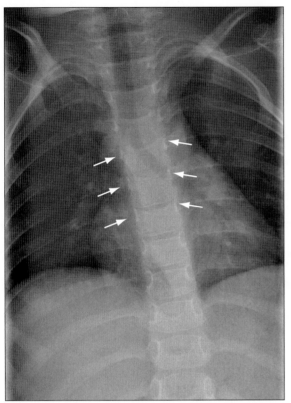

Figure 1. Frontal radiograph of thoracic spine shows bony erosion of pedicles and canal expansion (*arrows*), reflecting long-standing intraspinal process.

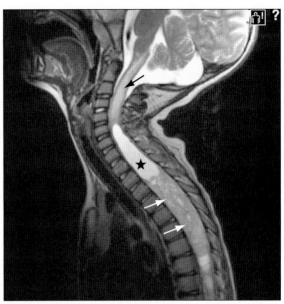

Figure 2. Sagittal T2-weighted MR image of cervicothoracic cord shows intramedullary mass (*white arrows*) in upper thoracic cord, with associated cyst (*asterisk*). Cord edema (*black arrow*) extends up to craniocervical junction.

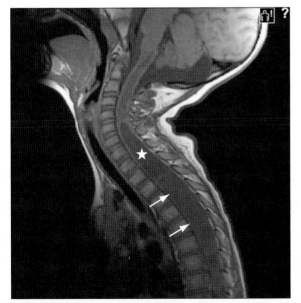

Figure 3. Sagittal T1-weighted MR image shows isointense mass (*arrows*) and T1-weighted hypointense cyst (*asterisk*).

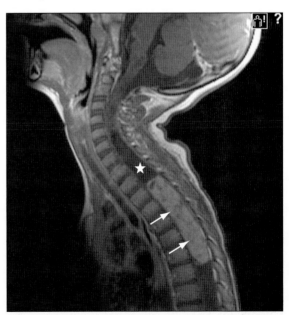

Figure 4. Sagittal T1-weighted postcontrast MR image shows enhancement within mass (*arrows*). There is no enhancement of superior cystic collection (*asterisk*).

Case 290

DEMOGRAPHICS/CLINICAL HISTORY

The patient is a 5-year-old boy with microcephaly and seizures.

FINDINGS

Agenesis of the corpus callosum is seen on sagittal T1-weighted magnetic resonance imaging (MRI) (Fig. 1). Coronal T2-weighted MRI (Fig. 2) shows the absence of crossing callosal fibers, the typical "longhorn" appearance of the frontal horns of the lateral ventricles, the white matter that would have formed the corpus callosum (i.e., Probst bundles), and prominence of the temporal horns. Parallel configuration of the lateral ventricles is shown on the axial fluid attenuated inversion recovery (FLAIR) sequence (Fig. 3). Sagittal T1-weighted MRI in a different patient with hypogenesis of the corpus callosum (Fig. 4) shows the presence of the genu and body of the corpus callosum, with absence of the splenium and rostrum. An associated midline lipoma and a portion of the cingulate gyrus can be seen anteriorly.

DISCUSSION

Definition/Background
The corpus callosum consists of tightly packed white matter fibers that connect the two cerebral hemispheres. The corpus callosum forms from anterior to posterior (genu, body, and splenium), with the anteroinferior portion (rostrum) forming last.

Characteristic Clinical Features
Patients with callosal abnormalities can present with seizures or developmental delay. With improved prenatal care, many patients with agenesis of the corpus callosum are diagnosed prenatally.

Characteristic Radiologic Findings
Abnormalities of the corpus callosum include complete agenesis, hypogenesis (i.e., incomplete formation in proper order), and dysgenesis (i.e., incomplete formation in an abnormal order). In complete agenesis, the lateral ventricles take a parallel configuration in the axial plane with dilation of the occipital horns (colpocephaly). The frontal horns have a "longhorn" appearance in the coronal plane. In the sagittal plane, because the corpus callosum is not present and the cingulate gyrus is not seen, radial appearance of the sulcal-gyral pattern is seen. Abnormalities of the corpus callosum are associated with other midline anomalies, particularly the presence of a midline lipoma, which appears hyperechoic on ultrasound, hypodense on computed tomography (CT), and hyperintense with suppression on fat saturation on T1-weighted MRI. Interhemispheric cysts can be present.

Less Common Radiologic Manifestations
Associated abnormalities include gray matter heterotopias, encephaloceles, and Dandy-Walker malformations.

Differential Diagnosis
- Postoperative and ischemic defects of the corpus callosum

Discussion
The clinical history and postoperative changes can suggest a surgical cause for interruption of the corpus callosum. Gliosis, ex vacuo dilation, and white matter volume loss can suggest prior ischemic injury as the cause for thinning or loss of a portion of the corpus callosum.

Diagnosis
Agenesis of the corpus callosum

Suggested Readings

Rubinstein D, Cajade-Law AG, Youngman V, et al: The development of the corpus callosum in semilobar and lobar holoprosencephaly. Pediatr Radiol 26:839-844, 1996.

Sztriha L: Spectrum of corpus callosum agenesis. Pediatr Neurol 32: 94-101, 2005.

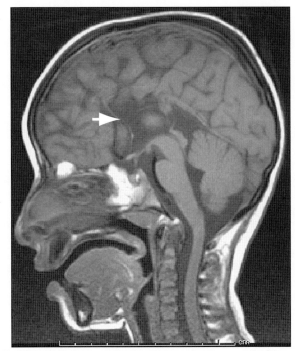

Figure 1. Sagittal T1-weighted MR image shows agenesis of corpus callosum (*arrow*).

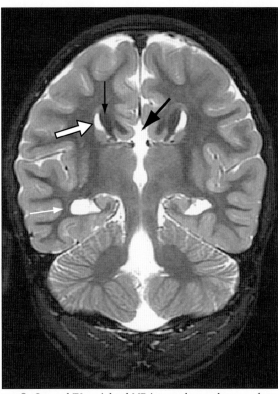

Figure 2. Coronal T2-weighted MR image shows absence of crossing callosal fibers (*large black arrow*), typical "longhorn" appearance of frontal horns of lateral ventricles (*large white arrow*), white matter that would have formed corpus callosum (i.e., Probst bundles) (*small black arrow*), and prominence of temporal horns (*small white arrow*).

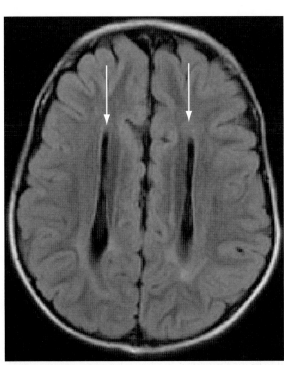

Figure 3. Axial FLAIR MRI sequence shows parallel configuration of lateral ventricles (*arrows*).

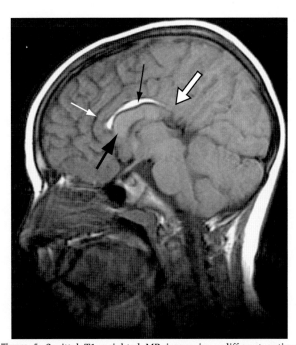

Figure 4. Sagittal T1-weighted MR image in a different patient with hypogenesis of the corpus callosum shows presence of genu and body of corpus callosum (*large black arrow*), with absence of splenium (*large white arrow*) and rostrum. Associated midline lipoma (*small black arrow*) can be seen, and a portion of cingulate gyrus can be seen anteriorly (*small white arrow*).

Case 291

DEMOGRAPHICS/CLINICAL HISTORY

The patient is a 12-year-old girl with a known congenital brain anomaly.

FINDINGS

Axial computed tomography (CT) scan (Fig. 1) shows alobar holoprosencephaly with a lack of cleavage of the frontal lobes and a large monoventricle. In a different patient with semilobar holoprosencephaly, sagittal T1-weighted magnetic resonance imaging (MRI) (Fig. 2) shows dysgenesis of the corpus callosum, with formation of only the splenium. Coronal T2-weighted MRI in the same patient in as Fig. 2 shows a midline cleft palate (Fig. 3).

DISCUSSION

Definition/Background

Holoprosencephaly is caused by a failure of cleavage of the prosencephalon. There are different degrees of severity, identified as alobar (most severe), semilobar, and lobar (less severe) subtypes. A middle interhemispheric variant, or syntelencephaly, has been described as a subtype of holoprosencephaly.

Characteristic Clinical Features

"The face predicts the brain" is commonly said about holoprosencephaly. Often, patients have facial anomalies, particularly along the midline, including cyclopism, a single nostril, or cleft lip or palate.

Characteristic Radiologic Findings

In alobar holoprosencephaly, there is a large single ventricle and absence of the septum, corpus callosum, falx, and interhemispheric fissure (IHF). The thalami and basal ganglia are typically fused. Semilobar holoprosencephaly also has a single ventricle and absence of the septum, but the IHF and falx are partially formed posteriorly, and the only portion of the corpus callosum that is typically well formed is the splenium. Fusion of the thalami and basal ganglia varies. In lobar holoprosencephaly, the septum is absent, but the remainder of the brain is relatively well formed, with a normal-appearing posterior and partial formation of the anterior IHF and falx. The frontal horns may be small and dysplastic, the genu of the corpus callosum may be aplastic or hypoplastic, and there may be minimal frontal lobe fusion.

Less Common Radiologic Manifestations

The interhemispheric variant is rare and typically has connection of the sylvian fissures across the midline over the vertex and often has cortical dysplasias and heterotopias.

Differential Diagnosis

- Septo-optic dysplasia

Discussion

Differentiation of septo-optic dysplasia from lobar holoprosencephaly can be difficult. Subtleties of frontal lobe fusion and anomalies of the anterior falx and IHF can suggest lobar holoprosencephaly.

Diagnosis

Holoprosencephaly

Suggested Readings

Dubourg C, Bendavid C, Pasquier L, et al: Holoprosencephaly. Orphanet J Rare Dis 2:8, 2007.
Hahn JS, Pinter JD: Holoprosencephaly: Genetic, neuroradiological, and clinical advances. Semin Pediatr Neurol 9:309-319, 2002.

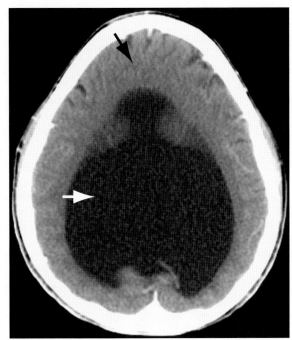

Figure 1. Axial CT image shows lack of cleavage of frontal lobes (*black arrow*) and single ventricle (*white arrow*).

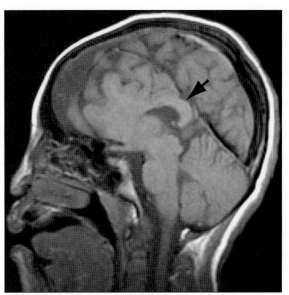

Figure 2. Sagittal T1-weighted MR image in a different patient with semilobar holoprosencephaly shows dysgenesis of corpus callosum, with formation of splenium only (*arrow*).

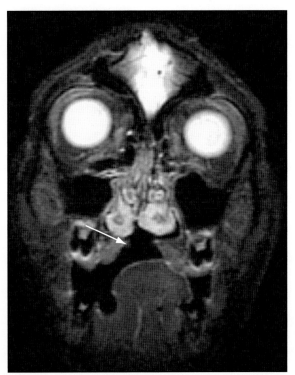

Figure 3. Coronal T2-weighted MR image in the same patient as in Fig. 2 shows midline cleft palate (*arrow*).

Case 292

DEMOGRAPHICS/CLINICAL HISTORY

The patient is a 4-year-old child with seizures.

FINDINGS

Axial T1-weighted magnetic resonance imaging (MRI) (Fig. 1) shows a focus of gray matter heterotopia adjacent to the left lateral ventricle. Coronal T1-weighted MRI (Fig. 2) shows the subependymal heterotopia (and an abnormal cortex superior to the heterotopic gray matter). In a different patient, coronal T2-weighted MRI (Fig. 3) shows the band type of heterotopia. The band heterotopia is isointense to cortex. A thin layer of white matter is seen between the cortex and band heterotopia.

DISCUSSION

Definition/Background

Gray matter heterotopia is the result of failure of migration of the cortical fibers from the germinal matrix (along the lateral ventricle) to the cortical mantle. Heterotopia can be categorized as subependymal, subcortical, and band subtypes.

Characteristic Clinical Features

Seizures are the typical presentation. If both hemispheres are affected, mental retardation and developmental delay are associated features.

Characteristic Radiologic Findings

Heterotopic gray matter is isointense with gray matter on all sequences. Heterotopia can be located anywhere from the subependymal location to the subcortical position. Band heterotopia has an appearance of a double cortex, with a thin band of white matter between the heterotopic band and the cortex. Heterotopia can be associated with other malformations of the brain, such as agenesis of the corpus callosum and cephaloceles.

Less Common Radiologic Manifestations

The cortex seen near the heterotopia can be abnormal, particularly deficient, because of the abnormal migration.

Differential Diagnosis

- Tuberous sclerosis

Discussion

Subependymal nodules associated with tuberous sclerosis do not follow gray matter signal intensity on all sequences. Other stigmata of tuberous sclerosis are typically present, such as cortical or subcortical tubers.

Diagnosis

Gray matter heterotopia

Suggested Readings

Barkovich AJ, Kuzniecky RI: Gray matter heterotopia. Neurology 55:1603-1608, 2000.
Guerrini R, Carrozzo R: Epilepsy and genetic malformations of the cerebral cortex. Am J Med Genet 106:160-173, 2001.

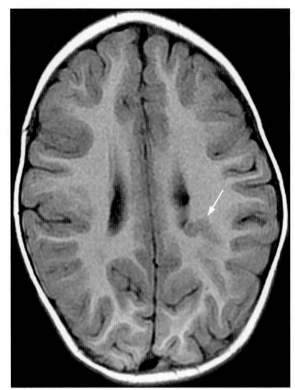

Figure 1. Axial T1-weighted MR image shows focus of gray matter heterotopia (*arrow*) adjacent to left lateral ventricle.

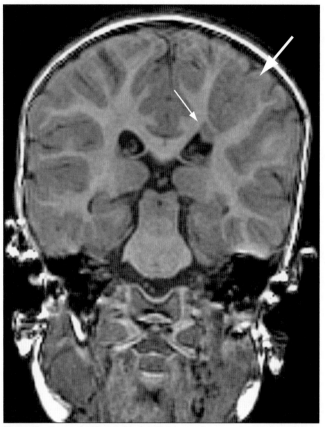

Figure 2. Coronal T1-weighted MR image shows subependymal heterotopia (*small arrow*) and abnormal cortex superior to heterotopic gray matter (*large arrow*).

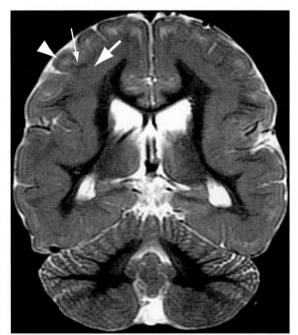

Figure 3. Coronal T2-weighted MR image in a different patient with band-type heterotopia. Band heterotopia (*large arrow*) is isointense to cortex (*arrowhead*). Thin layer of white matter (*small arrow*) is seen between cortex and band heterotopia.

Case 293

DEMOGRAPHICS/CLINICAL HISTORY

The patient is a 5-week-old infant with Down syndrome with seizures and an apparent life-threatening event (ALTE).

FINDINGS

A cleft is seen in the right frontal lobe, shown on axial T1-weighted magnetic resonance imaging (MRI) (Fig. 1). The cleft is lined by gray matter. Dimpling along the right lateral ventricle is a subtle indicator of closed-lip schizencephaly. The gray matter lining of the cleft is more prominent on axial T2-weighted MRI (Fig. 2). Dimpling is seen along the lateral ventricle. Coronal MRI (Fig. 3) shows the gray matter–lined cleft extending from the pial surface to the lateral ventricle. A more anterior coronal view (Fig. 4) shows absence of the septum pellucidum.

DISCUSSION

Definition/Background

The presence of gray matter–lined clefts extending from the cortex to the ventricular surface is called *schizencephaly*. The closed-lip subtype shows apposition of the two "lips" of the cleft, whereas the lips in an open-lip subtype do not come in close contact.

Characteristic Clinical Features

Typically, patients present with seizures, hemiparesis, developmental delay, and often blindness.

Characteristic Radiologic Findings

Gray matter–lined clefts extending from the cortex to the lateral ventricles is the defining characteristic of schizencephaly. Slightly more than half of patients have unilateral schizencephaly; the remaining patients have bilateral clefts. Most clefts are open-lipped. Approximately 70% of patients with schizencephaly have no septum pellucidum.

Less Common Radiologic Manifestations

Optic nerve hypoplasia can be seen in one third of patients with schizencephaly. Thinning and expansion of the calvaria can sometimes be seen adjacent to areas of open-lip schizencephaly.

Differential Diagnosis

- Infarction
- Porencephaly
- Transmantle cortical dysplasia

Discussion

An area of infarction and porencephaly does not have gray matter lining the clefts. Transmantle cortical dysplasia can look similar to closed-lip schizencephaly. One subtle clue to differentiate the two is the presence of the dimple in the lateral ventricle, which suggests closed-lip schizencephaly.

Diagnosis

Closed-lip schizencephaly

Suggested Readings

Oh KY, Kennedy AM, Frias AE Jr, Byrne JL: Fetal schizencephaly: Pre- and postnatal imaging with a review of the clinical manifestations. RadioGraphics 25:647-657, 2005.

Packard AM, Miller VS, Delgado MR: Schizencephaly: Correlations of clinical and radiologic features. Neurology 48:1427-1434, 1997.

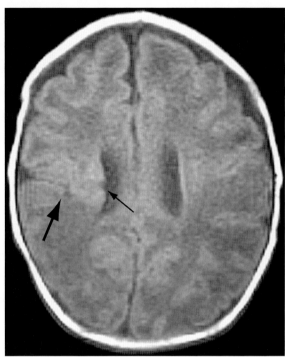

Figure 1. Axial T1-weighted MR image shows cleft in right frontal lobe that connects subarachnoid space with right lateral ventricle, consistent with closed-lip schizencephaly. Schizencephaly is lined by gray matter from cortex to ventricular surface (*large arrow*). Dimpling along right lateral ventricle (*small arrow*) is a subtle indicator of closed-lip schizencephaly.

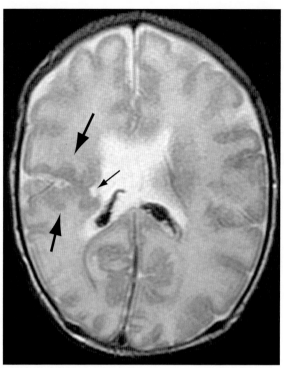

Figure 2. Axial T2-weighted MR image accentuates gray matter lining of schizencephaly (*large arrows*). Dimpling is seen along lateral ventricle (*small arrow*).

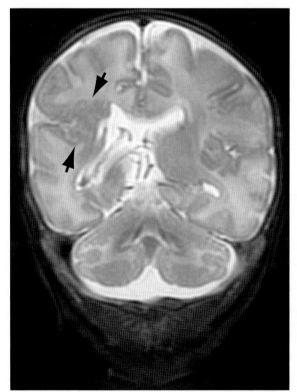

Figure 3. Coronal T2-weighted MR image shows gray matter lining of closed lip schizencephaly (*arrows*).

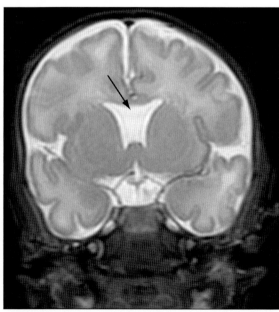

Figure 4. More anterior coronal image reveals absence of septum pellucidum (*arrow*).

Case 294

DEMOGRAPHICS/CLINICAL HISTORY

The patient is a 4-year-old adopted child who is asymptomatic but with a small scar on the lower back and unknown back surgery.

FINDINGS

A bony septum is seen bridging the canal from the posterior vertebral body to the abnormally shaped posterior element on sagittal T1-weighted (Fig. 1) and sagittal T2-weighted (Fig. 2) magnetic resonance imaging (MRI). A fatty filum is shown best in Fig. 1. On axial T1-weighted (Fig. 3) and axial T2-weighted (Fig. 4) MRI, the bony septum is identified with two hemicords.

DISCUSSION

Definition/Background

Diastematomyelia is a congenital condition in which the spinal cord is split into two symmetric hemicords. The two hemicords can be encased in separate dural tubes by an osseous or osteocartilaginous septum (type 1) or encased in a single dural tube (type 2), often separated by a fibrous septum and occasionally without a septum.

Characteristic Clinical Features

Clinical features include scoliosis; hairy tuft; and symptoms of tethered cord syndrome, including motor and sensory dysfunction, muscle atrophy, abnormal reflexes, urinary incontinence, and foot and hip deformities.

Characteristic Radiologic Findings

Conventional radiographic abnormalities include vertebral anomalies, scoliosis, and widening of the interpedicular distance with a bony septum. Classic computed tomography (CT) and MRI findings include division of the spinal cord into two hemicords typically by an osteocartilaginous or fibrous septum. The hemicords can reform a single cord distal to the septum or remain split down to the filum. Hydromyelia can be seen in the normal cord or within the hemicords. Myelomeningoceles (or hemimyelomeningoceles), filar lipomas, and tight fila can be associated.

Less Common Radiologic Manifestations

Occasionally, no septum is identified. Also, two separate septa can occur, causing asymmetry of the hemicords.

Differential Diagnosis

- Cord atrophy

Discussion

Central cord atrophy could simulate the appearance of a hemicord, at least partially. This condition is typically accompanied by a history of trauma, infection, or tumor, and the bony or fibrous septum is absent.

Diagnosis

Diastematomyelia with bony septum

Suggested Readings

Chopra S, Gulati MS, Paul SB, et al: MR spectrum in spinal dysraphism. Eur Radiol 11:497, 2001.

Rossi A, Gandolfo C, Morana G, et al: Current classification and imaging of congenital spinal abnormalities. Semin Roentgenol 41:250, 2006.

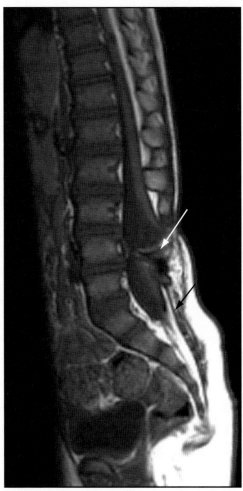

Figure 1. Sagittal T1-weighted MR image shows bony septum (*black arrow*) bridging canal from posterior vertebral body to abnormally shaped posterior element. A fatty filum is shown (*white arrow*).

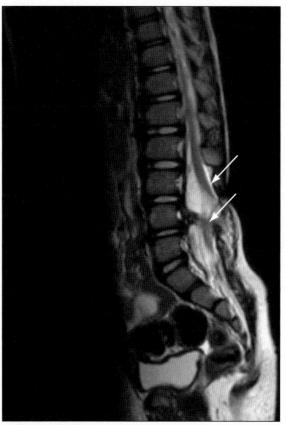

Figure 2. T2-weighted MR image shows bony septum better delineated by hyperintensity from cerebrospinal fluid within spinal canal. Posteriorly positioned portion of spinal cord appears partially tethered (*white arrow*).

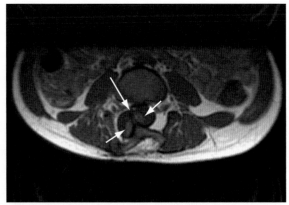

Figure 3. Axial T1-weighted MR image identifies bony septum (*long arrow*) separating two hemicords (*short arrows*).

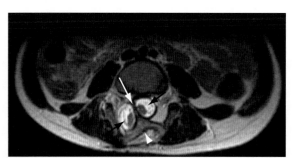

Figure 4. T2-weighted MR image shows septum (*white arrow*) and hemicords (*black arrows*) against cerebrospinal fluid hyperintensity. Note abnormal shape of posterior ring (*arrowhead*).

Case 295

DEMOGRAPHICS/CLINICAL HISTORY

The patient is a 7-year-old child with a left intranasal mass.

FINDINGS

A contrast-enhanced computed tomography (CT) scan (Fig. 1) shows a round nonenhancing hypodense mass within the left nasal cavity. The mass is also seen more superiorly along the anterior ethmoid air cells (Fig. 2). At surgery, there was a fibrous stalk connecting the mass to the intracranial contents through a patent foramen cecum.

DISCUSSION

Definition/Background
Nasal glial heterotopia (nasal gliomas) are non-neoplastic and caused by failure of the closure of the foramen cecum with migration of neural tissue through the defect and subsequent involution of the intracranial connection.

Characteristic Clinical Features
A reddish, firm, lobular mass is seen typically located along the nasal dorsum, particularly the glabella; 30% are intranasal and can cause nasal obstruction.

Characteristic Radiologic Findings
Nasal glial heterotopia are well-circumscribed masses that show similar density (on CT) and signal intensity (on magnetic resonance imaging [MRI]) as gray matter. Heterotopia do not show enhancement, but adjacent compressed nasal tissue can enhance. A patent foramen cecum may be visualized.

Differential Diagnosis
- Hemangioma
- Nasal dermoid/epidermoid
- Nasolacrimal duct cyst

Discussion
Hemangiomas can be differentiated on imaging because they are vascular masses that show avid enhancement. Dermoids often have a sinus tract, pit, or hair along the nasal dorsum; they typically show high T2 signal intensity on MRI and restricted diffusion on diffusion-weighted imaging. Nasolacrimal duct cysts can be seen into the nasal cavity, but are fluid density and intensity and can be traced from the nasal cavity back to the nasolacrimal duct along the medial orbit.

Diagnosis
Nasal glial heterotopion

Suggested Readings
Hedlund G: Congenital frontonasal masses: Developmental anatomy, malformations, and MR imaging. Pediatr Radiol 36:647, 2006.
Huisman TA, Schneider JF, Kellenberger CJ, et al: Developmental nasal midline masses in children: Neuroradiological evaluation. Eur Radiol 14:243, 2004.

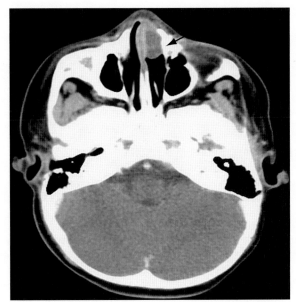

Figure 1. Contrast-enhanced axial CT scan shows round nonenhancing hypodense mass within left nasal cavity (*arrow*).

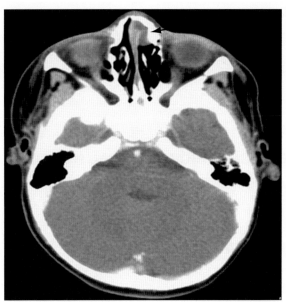

Figure 2. Contrast-enhanced axial CT scan shows nonenhancing mass (*arrow*) more superiorly along anterior ethmoid air cells.

Case 296

DEMOGRAPHICS/CLINICAL HISTORY

The patient is a 3-day-old infant with hypotonia and born to a diabetic mother.

FINDINGS

Absence of the sacrum is shown on an anteroposterior radiograph of the spine (Fig. 1) along with a vertebral anomaly in the cervicothoracic region. The lateral view of the spine (Fig. 2) shows the complete absence of the sacrum. T1-weighted magnetic resonance imaging (MRI) (Fig. 3) shows a small amount of fat within the filum and a terminal lipoma. Blunting of the conus and lumbosacral hypoplasia are seen on T2-weighted MRI (Fig. 4).

DISCUSSION

Definition/Background

Caudal regression syndrome includes a spectrum of abnormalities, but the milder lumbosacral hypogenesis and anal atresia are the most common forms. Maternal diabetes is present in approximately one sixth of cases.

Characteristic Clinical Features

Lumbosacral hypogenesis is often associated with genitourinary anomalies, and any anomalies noticed at birth should prompt a spinal evaluation. If the child has isolated lumbosacral hypogenesis, he or she may also have motor defects, such as leg weakness and neurogenic bladder.

Characteristic Radiologic Findings

Lumbosacral hypogenesis or agenesis is typical and can vary in severity. There often is some combination of a blunted conus, cord tethering, and a thick or fatty filum.

Less Common Radiologic Manifestations

Terminal myelocystoceles, lipomas, lipomyeloceles, and hydromyelia are less common findings. VACTERL (vertebral anomalies, anorectal malformations, cardiac malformations, tracheoesophageal fistulas, renal anomalies, and limb anomalies) and OEIS (omphalocele, cloacal exstrophy, imperforate anus, and spinal deformities) associations have mild associations with lumbosacral hypogenesis.

Differential Diagnosis

- VACTERL association

Discussion

Caudal regression is not always present with VACTERL association; radiography and MRI can help evaluate vertebral and cord anomalies.

Diagnosis

Caudal regression

Suggested Readings

Estin D, Cohen AR: Caudal agenesis and associated caudal spinal cord malformations. Neurosurg Clin North Am 6:377-391, 1995.
Singh SK, Singh RD, Sharma A: Caudal regression syndrome: Case report and review of the literature. Pediatr Surg Int 21:578-581, 2005.

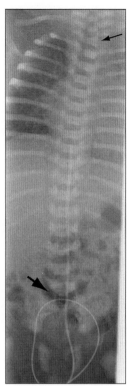

Figure 1. Anteroposterior radiograph of spine shows absence of sacrum (*large arrow*) with vertebral anomaly in cervicothoracic region (*small arrow*).

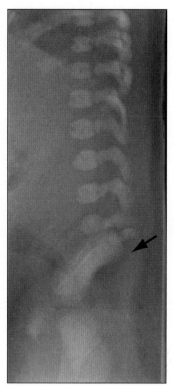

Figure 2. Lateral radiograph of spine shows complete absence of sacrum (*arrow*).

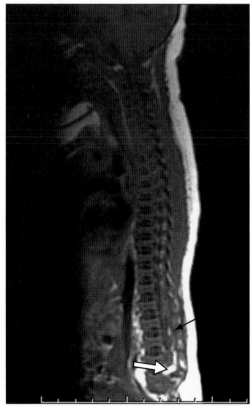

Figure 3. Sagittal T1-weighted MR image shows small amount of fat within filum (*black arrow*) and terminal lipoma (*white arrow*).

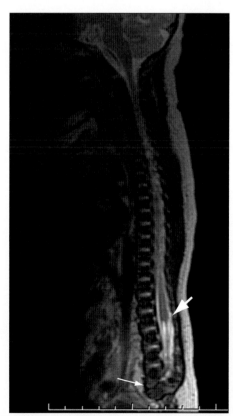

Figure 4. Sagittal T2-weighted MR image shows blunting of conus (*large arrow*) and lumbosacral hypoplasia (*small arrow*).

Case 297

DEMOGRAPHICS/CLINICAL HISTORY

The patient is a newborn with a sacral dimple.

FINDINGS

Longitudinal ultrasound of the spine (Fig. 1) shows the tip of the conus medullaris and a hypoechoic ovoid structure along the filum terminale. Transverse ultrasound of the spine (Fig. 2) shows the hypoechoic structure.

DISCUSSION

Definition/Background

Small fluid collections occurring in the conus medullaris (ventriculus terminale) and filum terminale (filar cyst) in a neonate are thought to be normal developmental variants.

Characteristic Clinical Features

No specific clinical features suggest ventricular or filar cysts; however, these are incidentally found in patients being imaged for sacral dimples. Development of neurologic symptoms requires repeat imaging.

Characteristic Radiologic Findings

Typically imaged by ultrasonography, these cysts appear as ovoid hypoechoic collections at the tip of the conus medullaris or within the filum. These are occasionally seen on neonatal magnetic resonance imaging (MRI) as simple nonenhancing cysts.

Differential Diagnosis
- Syringomyelia
- Tumor

Discussion

Syringomyelia is dilation of the central canal of the spinal cord and typically extends superiorly. The neonatal age of the patient and classic description of the cysts make tumor unlikely.

Diagnosis

Filar cyst

Suggested Readings

Coleman LT, Zimmerman RA, Rorke LB: Ventriculus terminalis of the conus medullaris: MR findings in children. AJNR Am J Neuroradiol 16:1421-1426, 1995.

Irani N, Goud AR, Lowe LH: Isolated filar cyst on lumbar spine sonography in infants: A case-control study. Pediatr Radiol 36:1283-1288, 2006.

Kriss VM, Kriss TC, Coleman RC: Sonographic appearance of the ventriculus terminalis cyst in the neonatal spinal cord. J Ultrasound Med 19:207-209, 2000.

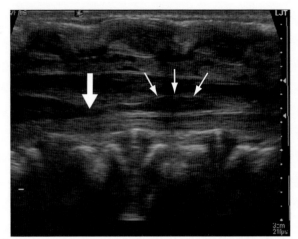

Figure 1. Longitudinal ultrasound of spine shows tip of conus medullaris (*large arrow*) and hypoechoic ovoid structure (*small arrows*) along filum terminale.

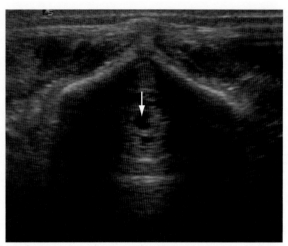

Figure 2. Transverse ultrasound of spine shows hypoechoic structure (*arrow*).

Case 298

DEMOGRAPHICS/CLINICAL HISTORY

The patient is a 12-week-old infant with a sacral dimple.

FINDINGS

Sagittal T1-weighted magnetic resonance imaging (MRI) of the spine (Fig. 1) shows a low-lying conus and tethered cord terminating in a large T1-weighted hyperintense mass, representing a lipoma. A dermal sinus tract and sacral osseous abnormalities are suggested. Sagittal T2-weighted MRI (Fig. 2) shows a syrinx, low-lying conus, and dermal sinus tract. The large lipoma is well seen on axial T1-weighted MRI (Fig. 3). The syrinx is seen within the distal cord on axial T2-weighted MRI (Fig. 4).

DISCUSSION

Definition/Background

Tethered cords are often associated with lipomatous malformations. Other associated abnormalities include segmentation and fusion anomalies, split-cord malformations, and dermal sinus tracts.

Characteristic Clinical Features

On physical examination, children can have a deep sacral dimple, hemangioma, or tuft of hair at the base of the spine. Symptoms of a tethered cord include bowel or bladder dysfunction and toe walking.

Characteristic Radiologic Findings

The normal conus should not terminate below L2. Tethered cords often are associated with a thickened or fatty filum or spinal lipoma. Patients may have an associated cord syrinx or dermal sinus tract.

Less Common Radiologic Manifestations

The cord can be tethered to a lipomyelomeningocele or myelomeningocele.

Diagnosis

Tethered cord

Suggested Readings

Lew SM, Kothbauer KF: Tethered cord syndrome: An updated review. Pediatr Neurosurg 43:236-248, 2007.

Michelson DJ, Ashwal S: Tethered cord syndrome in childhood: Diagnostic features and relationship to congenital anomalies. Neurol Res 26:745-753, 2004.

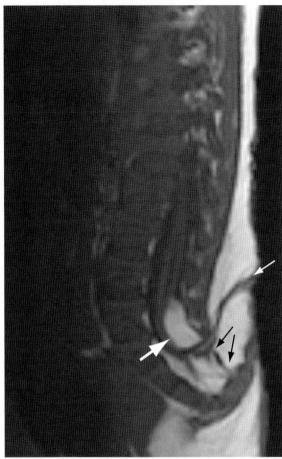

Figure 1. Sagittal T1-weighted MR image of the spine shows low-lying conus and tethered cord terminating in large, T1-weighted hyperintense mass, representing a lipoma (*large arrow*). Low signal intensity extending from filum to dorsal cutaneous surface suggests dermal sinus tract (*small white arrow*). Sacral osseous abnormalities are also seen (*small black arrows*).

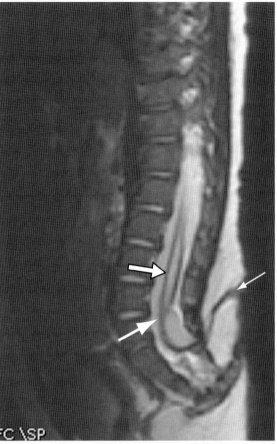

Figure 2. Sagittal T2-weighted MR image shows syrinx (*black-outlined arrow*), low-lying conus (*large white arrow*), and dermal sinus tract (*small white arrow*).

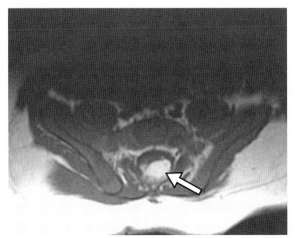

Figure 3. Axial T1-weighted MR image shows large lipoma (*arrow*).

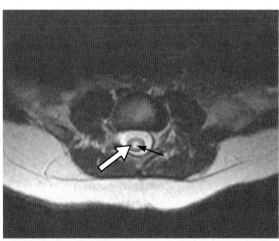

Figure 4. Axial T2-weighted MR image shows syrinx (*white arrow*) within distal cord (*black arrow*).

Case 299

DEMOGRAPHICS/CLINICAL HISTORY

The patient is a 9-year-old boy with progressive visual and intellectual decline, ataxia, and corticospinal tract signs.

FINDINGS

Axial fluid attenuated inversion recovery (FLAIR) image from magnetic resonance imaging (MRI) of the brain shows a pattern of symmetric, posterior white matter signal abnormality in the parietooccipital lobes, also involving the splenium of the corpus callosum (Fig. 1). Axial T1-weighted MRI acquired after administration of intravenous contrast agent shows peripheral enhancement in the areas of signal abnormality on the FLAIR image (Fig. 2).

DISCUSSION

Definition/Background
X-linked adrenoleukodystrophy refers to a group of inherited disorders characterized by disruption of the breakdown of long-chain fatty acids.

Characteristic Clinical Features
This disease is hereditary (X-linked) and affects mainly boys. Patients present with adrenal problems, muscle spasticity, strabismus, declining communication and writing skills, and progressive nervous system deterioration.

Characteristic Radiologic Findings
MRI of the brain shows marked increased signal intensity within the white matter around the atria of the lateral ventricles on T2-weighted images. The T2 signal abnormality also involves the posterior aspect of the corpus callosum.

Differential Diagnosis
- Multiple sclerosis
- Acute disseminated encephalomyelitis

Discussion
Multiple sclerosis is an autoimmune condition leading to demyelination of the white matter tracts in the central nervous system that most often affects young women. Acute disseminated encephalomyelitis is a condition characterized by inflammation of the brain and spinal cord, secondary to damage to myelin, that occurs in young children. Both of these conditions tend to have focal areas of demyelination rather than large confluent areas.

Diagnosis
X-linked adrenoleukodystrophy

Suggested Readings
Suda S, Komaba Y, Kumagai T, et al: Progression of the olivopontocerebellar form of adrenoleukodystrophy as shown by MRI. Neurology 66:144-145, 2006.
Volkow ND, Patchell L, Kulkarni MV, et al: Adrenoleukodystrophy: Imaging with CT, MRI and PET. J Nucl Med 28:524-527, 1987.

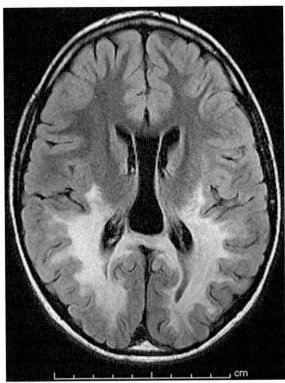

Figure 1. Axial FLAIR image from MRI of the brain shows pattern of symmetric, posterior white matter signal abnormality in parietooccipital lobes, also involving splenium of corpus callosum.

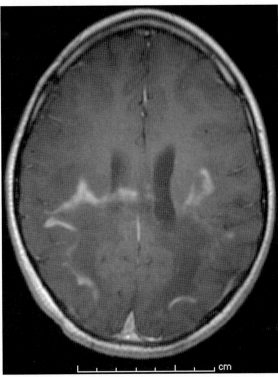

Figure 2. Axial T1-weighted MR image acquired after intravenous contrast agent administration shows peripheral enhancement in areas of signal abnormality on FLAIR image.

Case 300

DEMOGRAPHICS/CLINICAL HISTORY

The patient is a 2-year-old child with a firm orbital mass, undergoing magnetic resonance imaging (MRI).

FINDINGS

A small, homogeneous, T1-weighted, isointense to slightly hyperintense mass is seen at the left zygomaticofrontal suture (Fig. 1). The mass shows high signal intensity on T2-weighted MRI (Fig. 2). Axial, T1-weighted, postcontrast, fat-saturated MRI (Fig. 3) shows thin, peripheral enhancement around the mass, without internal enhancement of the mass.

DISCUSSION

Definition/Background
Dermoid cysts are the most common orbital mass in children. They are slow growing and are caused by sequestration of ectoderm that is typically located within the sutures of the skull, particularly the zygomaticofrontal and frontoethmoidal sutures.

Characteristic Clinical Features
Dermoid and epidermoid cysts of the orbit typically manifest in the first decade of life as firm, subcutaneous masses and often are located at the zygomaticofrontal suture.

Characteristic Radiologic Findings
Dermoid cysts are hypodense on computed tomography (CT). MRI of dermoids often shows hyperintensity on T1-weighted images due to their proteinaceous and sebaceous lipid content. If the cyst ruptured or infected, inflammatory changes can be seen around the mass. Diffusion weighted images (DWI) may demonstrate decreased diffusion within the dermoid-epidermoid cysts.

Less Common Radiologic Manifestations
Rarely, orbital dermoids can have intracranial extension or minimal wall calcifications.

Differential Diagnosis
- Metastatic neuroblastoma
- Langerhans cell histiocytosis
- Cellulitis

Discussion
When inflammatory changes are present, differentiating dermoids from other entities can be challenging. Dermoids are slow growing and can cause benign erosive changes of the bone. A periosteal reaction or other evidence of aggressive changes suggests an alternative diagnosis.

Diagnosis
Orbital dermoid

Suggested Readings
Abou-Rayyah Y, Rose GE, Konrad H, et al: Clinical, radiological and pathological examination of periocular dermoid cysts: Evidence of inflammation from an early age. Eye 16:507-512, 2002.

Pryor SG, Lewis JE, Weaver AL, Orvidas LJ: Pediatric dermoid cysts of the head and neck. Otolaryngol Head Neck Surg 132:938-942, 2005.

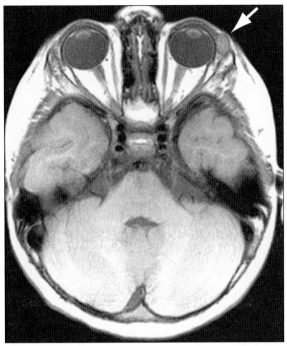

Figure 1. Axial T1-weighted MR image shows small, homogeneous, isointense to slightly hyperintense mass at left zygomaticofrontal suture (*arrow*).

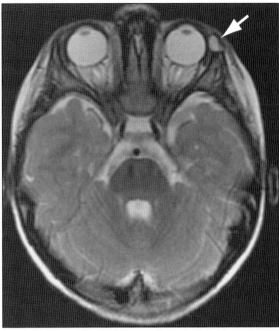

Figure 2. On T2-weighted MRI, mass (*arrow*) shows hyperintensity.

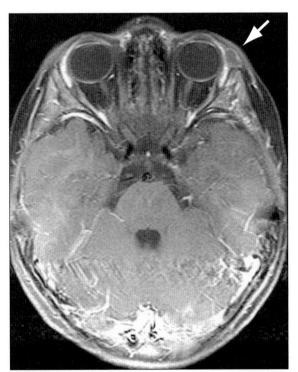

Figure 3. Axial T1-weighted postcontrast fat-saturated MR image shows thin peripheral enhancement around mass, without internal enhancement of mass (*arrow*).

Case 301

DEMOGRAPHICS/CLINICAL HISTORY

The patient is a 2-year-old girl with a large orbital mass and proptosis.

FINDINGS

Axial T2-weighted magnetic resonance imaging (MRI) (Fig. 1) shows a large hyperintense left orbital mass with numerous flow voids and prominent vessels in and adjacent to the mass. The mass shows homogeneous enhancement and peritumoral prominent vessels on coronal postcontrast T1-weighted fat-saturated MRI (Fig. 2). In another patient with proptosis, axial computed tomography (CT) scan with contrast agent (Fig. 3) shows a homogeneously enhancing right orbital mass with extraconal and intraconal compartments. The mass causes displacement of the globe anteriorly (see Fig. 3) and laterally, with lateral displacement of the inferior rectus muscle, as seen on the coronal reformatted CT image (Fig. 4).

DISCUSSION

Definition/Background

Hemangiomas are benign endothelial tumors that typically manifest within the first few months of life, undergo a phase of proliferation, usually lasting 1 to 2 years, and then regress over the next few years. Orbital hemangiomas are the most common orbital vascular tumor in infants.

Characteristic Clinical Features

Orbital hemangiomas often cause proptosis and globe displacement, and they can cause amblyopia.

Characteristic Radiologic Findings

Because of the vascular nature of the tumors, hemangiomas show homogeneous enhancement after administration of contrast medium on CT and MRI. MRI often shows flow voids within and around the tumor, particularly on T2-weighted MRI.

Less Common Radiologic Manifestations

During the involuting phase, hemangiomas can have fibrous and fatty components, causing slight heterogeneity after contrast enhancement.

Differential Diagnosis

- Rhabdomyosarcoma
- Vascular malformation
- Metastatic neuroblastoma
- Orbital dermoid

Discussion

The clinical history and appearance often help in differentiating hemangiomas from other entities in the differential diagnosis. Evidence of heterogeneous enhancement or osseous involvement on imaging can represent a more ominous condition, such as rhabdomyosarcoma or metastatic neuroblastoma. Vascular malformations are not tumors and typically do not have the same homogeneous avid arterial enhancement. Orbital dermoids typically are located at the zygomaticofrontal suture and can shows calcifications on CT and hyperintensity on T1-weighted MRI.

Diagnosis

Orbital hemangioma

Suggested Readings

Chung EM, Smirniotopoulos JG, Specht CS, et al: From the archives of the AFIP: Pediatric orbit tumors and tumorlike lesions: Nonosseous lesions of the extraocular orbit. RadioGraphics 27:1777-1799, 2007.

Smoker WR, Gentry LR, Yee NK, et al: Vascular lesions of the orbit: More than meets the eye. RadioGraphics 28:185-204, 2008.

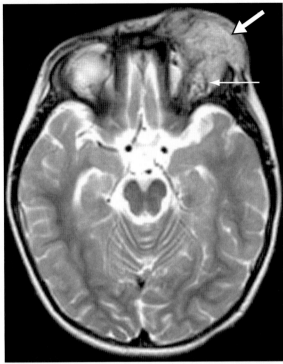

Figure 1. Axial T2-weighted MR image shows large left hyperintense orbital mass (*thick arrow*), with numerous flow voids and prominent vessels in and adjacent to mass (*thin arrow*).

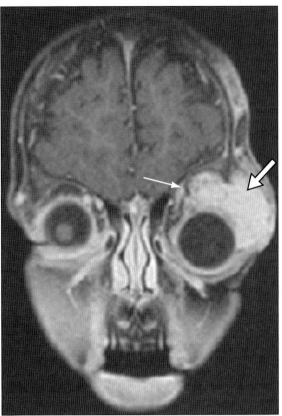

Figure 2. Coronal postcontrast T1-weighted fat-saturated MR image shows homogeneous enhancement of mass (*thick arrow*) and peritumoral prominent vessels (*thin arrow*).

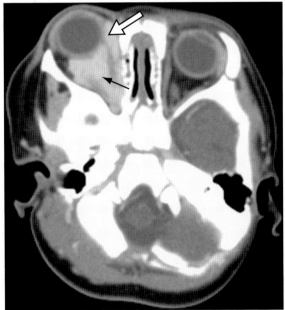

Figure 3. Axial CT scan with contrast agent in another patient with proptosis shows homogeneously enhancing right orbital mass with extraconal (*white arrow*) and intraconal compartments (*black arrow*).

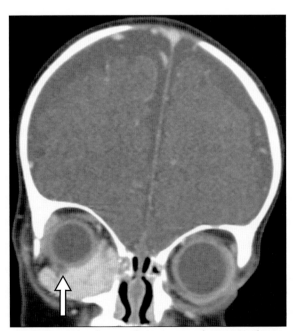

Figure 4. Coronal reformatted CT image of mass in the same patient as in Fig. 3 shows displacement of globe with lateral displacement of inferior rectus muscle (*arrow*).

Case 302

DEMOGRAPHICS/CLINICAL HISTORY

The patient is a 7-year-old child with developmental delay and abnormal eye examination results.

FINDINGS

T2-weighted magnetic resonance imaging (MRI) (Fig. 1) shows an abnormal lens and retrolental mass. A left middle cranial fossa arachnoid cyst is incidentally noted. Subretinal fluid is hyperintense on T2-weighted fluid attenuated inversion recovery (FLAIR) MRI (Fig. 2). The fibrovascular stalk representing the persistent hyaloid vascular system (i.e., Cloquet canal) can be seen. Sagittal oblique T1-weighted MRI (Fig. 3) through the right orbit shows the hyperintense subretinal fluid.

DISCUSSION

Definition/Background
Persistent hyperplastic primary vitreous (PHPV) represents the lack of regression of the embryonic hyaloid vascular system.

Characteristic Clinical Features
Patients with PHPV can present with leukocoria, lens opacification, microphthalmos, and vitreous hemorrhage. Findings are typically unilateral, but can be bilateral in conditions such as Norrie disease or Warburg syndrome.

Characteristic Radiologic Findings
Findings of an abnormally small lens, microphthalmos, cone-shaped retrolental mass, and persistent hyaloid fibrovascular stalk are seen on computed tomography (CT), but are more easily discernible on MRI. Postcontrast imaging shows enhancement of the retrolental mass. A small, ipsilateral optic nerve and fluid-fluid levels in the vitreous can be seen.

Differential Diagnosis
- Coats disease
- Retinopathy of prematurity
- Retinoblastoma
- Retinal detachment

Discussion
Microphthalmos, seen in PHPV, is not typically present in early Coats disease. Calcifications are absent in PHPV, which separates the findings from those of retinoblastoma. Absence of a history of prolonged oxygen therapy in a premature infant precludes the diagnosis of retinopathy of prematurity.

Diagnosis
Persistent hyperplastic primary vitreous

Suggested Readings
Edward DP, Mafee MF, Garcia-Valenzuela E, Weiss RA: Coats' disease and persistent hyperplastic primary vitreous: Role of MR imaging and CT. Radiol Clin North Am 36:1119-1131, 1998.

Magill HL, Hanna SL, Brooks MT, et al: Persistent hyperplastic primary vitreous (PHPV). RadioGraphics 10:515-518, 1990.

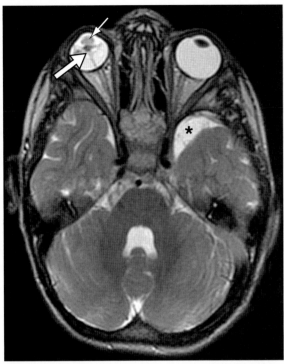

Figure 1. T2-weighted MR image shows small, misshapen, hyperintense lens (*thin arrow*) and retrolental mass (*thick arrow*). Incidentally noticed is a left middle cranial fossa arachnoid cyst (*asterisk*).

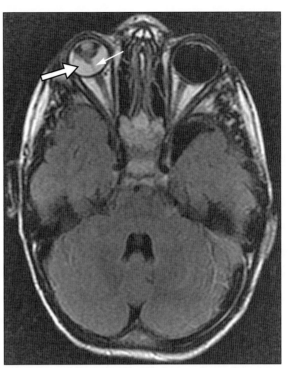

Figure 2. T2-weighted FLAIR MR image shows hyperintense subretinal fluid (*thick arrow*). Fibrovascular stalk representing persistent hyaloid vascular system can be seen (*thin arrow*).

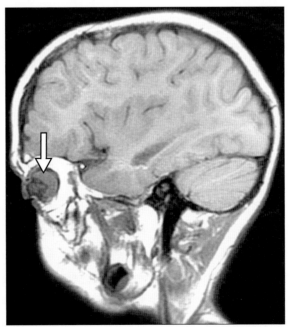

Figure 3. Sagittal oblique T1-weighted MR image through right orbit shows hyperintense subretinal fluid (*arrow*).

Case 303

DEMOGRAPHICS/CLINICAL HISTORY

The patient is a 2-year-old child with sensorineural hearing loss.

FINDINGS

Enlargement of the vestibular aqueduct is seen on axial thin-section computed tomography (CT) scanning (Fig. 1). The cochlea in this patient is dysplastic, with a decreased number of turns and an abnormal modiolus. The enlarged aqueduct is seen at a slightly different level (Fig. 2) joining the vestibule. The vestibular aqueduct should not be wider than the adjacent posterior semicircular canal.

DISCUSSION

Definition/Background

The vestibular aqueduct is considered to be enlarged when the diameter is greater than 1.5 mm or is wider than the adjacent posterior semicircular canal.

Characteristic Clinical Features

Patients present with sensorineural (typically) or mixed hearing loss.

Characteristic Radiologic Findings

Enlargement of the vestibular aqueduct typically is characterized on CT scanning by a diameter greater than 1.5 mm. Magnetic resonance imaging (MRI) often shows an enlarged endolymphatic duct and sac. Anomalies of the cochlea may be associated and can be seen on CT and MRI.

Diagnosis

Vestibular aqueduct syndrome

Suggested Readings

Mafee MF, Charletta D, Kumar A, Belmont H: Large vestibular aqueduct and congenital sensorineural hearing loss. AJNR Am J Neuroradiol 13:805-819, 1992.

Rodriguez K, Shah RK, Kenna M: Anomalies of the middle and inner ear. Otolaryngol Clin North Am 40:81-96, 2007.

Swartz JD: An overview of congenital/developmental sensorineural hearing loss with emphasis on the vestibular aqueduct syndrome. Semin Ultrasound CT MR 25:353-368, 2004.

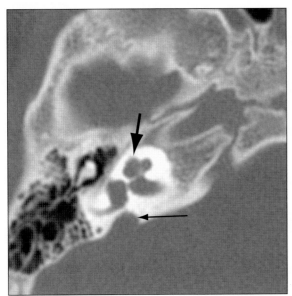

Figure 1. Axial thin-section CT image shows enlargement of vestibular aqueduct (*small arrow*). Cochlea (*large arrow*) is also dysplastic, with decreased number of turns and abnormal modiolus.

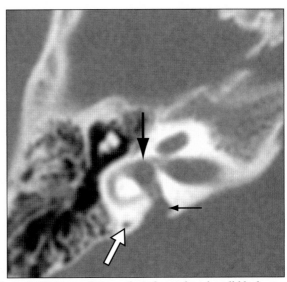

Figure 2. CT image shows enlarged aqueduct (*small black arrow*) at slightly different level joining vestibule (*large black arrow*). Vestibular aqueduct should not be wider than adjacent posterior semicircular canal (*white arrow*).

Case 304

DEMOGRAPHICS/CLINICAL HISTORY

The patient is a child with an abnormality seen on prenatal ultrasound.

FINDINGS

A prenatal sonogram with Doppler (Fig. 1) shows a dilated midline vascular structure. Postnatal T2-weighted magnetic resonance imaging (MRI) shows multiple arterial flow voids (Fig. 2). The arterial flow voids drain into the enlarged and dilated vein of Galen (Fig. 3). A persistent falcine sinus drains the vein of Galen into the superior sagittal sinus. Magnetic resonance venography (MRV) (Fig. 4) shows the vein of Galen malformation and the superiorly oriented, persistent falcine sinus, which is present instead of the normal straight sinus.

DISCUSSION

Definition/Background

Vein of Galen malformation is an arteriovenous malformation, with multiple feeding arteries originating from the choroidal, anterior cerebral, and transmesencephalic arteries and draining into the vein of Galen or into the veins that drain into the vein of Galen.

Characteristic Clinical Features

The diagnosis can be suggested prenatally by ultrasound. If patients are not diagnosed prenatally, they typically present as neonates or infants with heart failure or hydrocephalus, which is thought to result from obstruction of the aqueduct by a mass effect or decreased absorption of cerebrospinal fluid because of high venous pressures.

Characteristic Radiologic Findings

Ultrasound shows the dilated vein of Galen, but does not delineate the feeding arterial vessels well. Angiography can be used for diagnostic and therapeutic purposes and can show the feeding vessels from the choroidal arteries and any additional arterial suppliers. MRI can show evidence of parenchymal ischemia and atrophy. Other venous anomalies are common, particularly the presence of a persistent falcine sinus, a fetal remnant, and absence of the straight sinus.

Differential Diagnosis
- Vein of Galen varix
- Enlarged vein of Galen from nearby arteriovenous malformation

Discussion

MRI and arteriography can distinguish true vein of Galen malformations from other causes of vein of Galen dilation because the arterial feeders can be seen draining into the vein of Galen.

Diagnosis

Vein of Galen malformation

Suggested Readings

Alvarez H, Garcia Monaco R, Rodesch G, et al: Vein of Galen aneurysmal malformations. Neuroimaging Clin N Am 17:189-206, 2007.

Jones BV, Ball WS, Tomsick TA, et al: Vein of Galen aneurysmal malformation: Diagnosis and treatment of 13 children with extended clinical follow-up. AJNR Am J Neuroradiol 23:1717-1724, 2002.

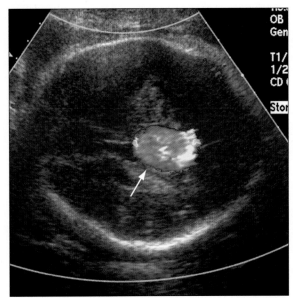

Figure 1. Prenatal sonogram with Doppler shows dilated midline vascular structure (*arrow*).

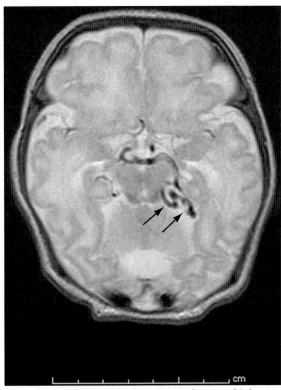

Figure 2. Postnatal T2-weighted MR image shows multiple arterial flow voids (*arrows*).

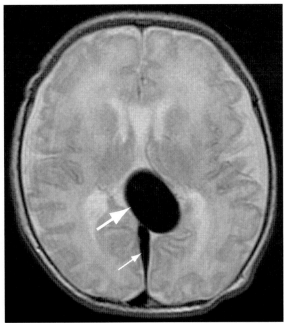

Figure 3. MR image shows arterial flow voids draining into enlarged and dilated vein of Galen (*large arrow*). Persistent falcine sinus (*small arrow*) drains vein of Galen into deep sinuses.

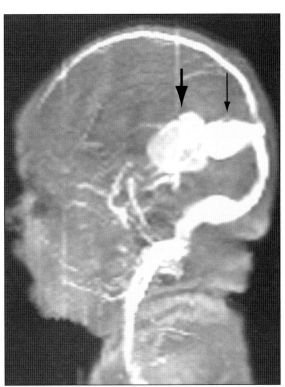

Figure 4. MRV shows vein of Galen malformation (*large arrow*) and superiorly oriented, persistent falcine sinus (*small arrow*), which is present instead of normal straight sinus.

Case 305

DEMOGRAPHICS/CLINICAL HISTORY

The patient is a 5-week-old infant, born prematurely at 29 weeks' gestation.

FINDINGS

Coronal ultrasound through the anterior fontanelle (Fig. 1) shows cystic changes in the periventricular and deep white matter. A more posterior angulation (Fig. 2) shows significant white matter cystic changes and an area of mixed echogenicity in the right periventricular white matter, representing an area of parenchymal hemorrhage. Sagittal T1-weighted magnetic resonance imaging (MRI) (Fig. 3) shows the cystic changes in the white matter, not only in a periventricular distribution. An axial diffusion B-zero image (Fig. 4) shows a cavity with a low intensity rim, representing hemosiderin deposition from a parenchymal hemorrhage.

DISCUSSION

Definition/Background

The term *periventricular leukomalacia* (PVL) is often used. However, injury to the white matter may occur in many areas, not just the periventricular regions. Other descriptors for this appearance such as *focal necrosis in the white matter* or *white matter injury of prematurity*, are also used.

Characteristic Clinical Features

Premature infants are often screened by cranial ultrasound because there are few distinctive signs of injury in these infants. Common reasons for additional imaging include a history of prolonged resuscitation, birth asphyxia, poor Apgar scores, hemorrhage, and any neurologic sign.

Characteristic Radiologic Findings

On ultrasound, early white matter injury can appear as echogenic areas that are typically as bright or brighter than the echogenic choroid plexus. In the weeks after injury, the echogenic areas may transform into cystic areas. Although ultrasonography is a good screening tool, MRI is more sensitive in detecting areas of white matter injury. On T1-weighted MRI, foci of hyperintensity can reflect areas of coagulation necrosis. The cystic areas of white matter injury also are shown. Diffusion-weighted imaging can show acute changes in the white matter.

Diagnosis

White matter injury of prematurity (also known as periventricular leukomalacia)

Suggested Readings

Inder TE, Anderson NJ, Spencer C, et al: White matter injury in the premature infant: A comparison between serial cranial sonographic and MR findings at term. AJNR Am J Neuroradiol 24:805-809, 2003.

Miller SP, Cozzio CC, Goldstein RB, et al: Comparing the diagnosis of white matter injury in premature newborns with serial MR imaging and transfontanel ultrasonography findings. AJNR Am J Neuroradiol 24:1661-1669, 2003.

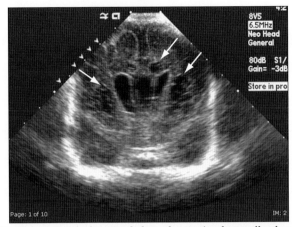

Figure 1. Coronal ultrasound through anterior fontanelle shows cystic changes in periventricular and deep white matter (*arrows*).

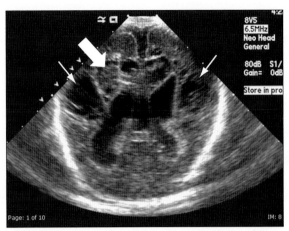

Figure 2. More posterior angulation shows significant white matter cystic changes (*small arrows*) and area of mixed echogenicity in right periventricular white matter that represents parenchymal hemorrhage (*large arrow*).

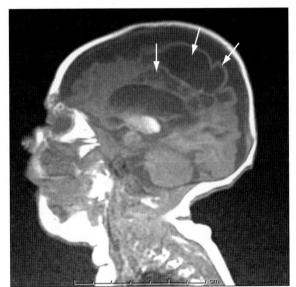

Figure 3. Sagittal T1-weighted MR image shows extensive cystic changes in white matter (*arrows*).

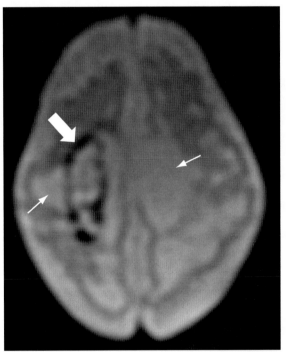

Figure 4. Axial, diffusion B-zero image shows cavity with a low signal intensity rim (*large arrow*), representing hemosiderin deposition from parenchymal hemorrhage. Areas of cystic white matter change are indicated (*small arrows*).

Case 306

DEMOGRAPHICS/CLINICAL HISTORY

The patient is a 6-month-old girl with a head circumference 95% of normal, poor head control, and nystagmus.

FINDINGS

Axial T2-weighted magnetic resonance imaging (MRI) (Fig. 1) shows increased signal intensity throughout the white matter and abnormal high signal intensity within the globi pallidi. Axial T1-weighted MRI (Fig. 2) shows low signal intensity within the white matter. Magnetic resonance spectroscopy (MRS) (Fig. 3) shows a significantly elevated *N*-acetyl aspartate (NAA) peak.

DISCUSSION

Definition/Background

Canavan disease is a white matter disease (i.e., leukodystrophy) with buildup of NAA because of a lack of the enzyme aspartoacylase. Patients are typically of Ashkenazi Jewish descent.

Characteristic Clinical Features

Patients with Canavan disease usually present between 3 and 9 months with some combination of macrocephaly, gross motor delay, poor head control, and reduced visual response.

Characteristic Radiologic Findings

Diffuse low density is seen on computed tomography (CT) in the cerebellar and cerebral white matter. MRI shows low signal intensity on T1-weighted and high signal intensity on T2-weighted images within the white matter. Subcortical white matter is affected early, and the globi pallidi are almost always affected, with sparing of putamen. The thalami are often affected. No contrast enhancement is seen. MRS characteristically shows a significantly elevated NAA peak.

Differential Diagnosis
- Leukodystrophy

Discussion

Other leukodystrophies can have similar white matter abnormalities late in their courses, but the characteristic spectroscopic finding of increased NAA levels is distinctive to Canavan disease.

Diagnosis

Canavan disease

Suggested Readings

Cheon JE, Kim IO, Hwang YS, et al: Leukodystrophy in children: a pictorial review of MR imaging features. RadioGraphics 22:461-476, 2002.

Marks HG, Caro PA, Wang ZY, et al: Use of computed tomography, magnetic resonance imaging, and localized 1H magnetic resonance spectroscopy in Canavan's disease: A case report. Ann Neurol 30:106-110, 1991.

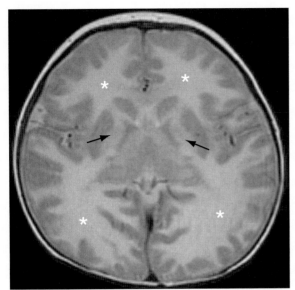

Figure 1. Axial T2-weighted MR image shows increased signal intensity throughout white matter (*asterisks*) and abnormal high signal intensity within globi pallidi (*arrows*).

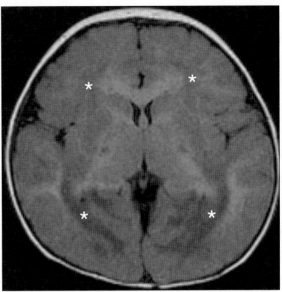

Figure 2. Axial T1-weighted MR image shows low signal intensity within white matter (*asterisks*).

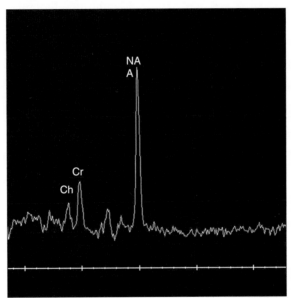

Figure 3. MRS shows significantly elevated NAA peak.

Case 307

DEMOGRAPHICS/CLINICAL HISTORY

The patient is a 2-year-old child with precocious puberty.

FINDINGS

Sagittal T1-weighted magnetic resonance imaging (MRI) (Fig. 1) shows a mass isointense to gray matter that is posterior to the optic chiasm and anterior to the midbrain. The pituitary has a normal appearance. Axial T2-weighted MRI (Fig. 2) better delineates the slightly hyperintense mass as separate from the optic chiasm. The mass does not enhance, as seen on postcontrast sagittal T1-weighted MRI (Fig. 3).

DISCUSSION

Definition/Background

Hypothalamic hamartomas are congenital non-neoplastic masses.

Characteristic Clinical Features

Patients typically present with precocious puberty or seizures, or both. Gelastic seizures are a particularly unusual feature that suggests a hypothalamic hamartoma.

Characteristic Radiologic Findings

Depending on the size, the masses may be difficult to diagnose on computed tomography (CT). Masses can be sessile or pedunculated, coming from the hypothalamus, mammillary bodies, or the tuber cinereum proper. The signal intensity profile of hamartomas is isodense to hypodense (to gray matter) on T1-weighted MRI and isodense to hyperdense on T2-weighted MRI, and there is no contrast enhancement.

Less Common Radiologic Manifestations

Arachnoid cysts have been associated with hamartomas. Pallister-Hall syndrome includes a hypothalamic hamartoma and has many other associated findings, including polydactyly, kidney and lung abnormalities, and imperforate anus. Rarely, other congenital cortical malformations or migrational anomalies may be present, which are important to document if the patient has presenting symptoms of seizures.

Differential Diagnosis

- Hypothalamic gliomas
- Duplicated pituitary gland

Discussion

Hypothalamic gliomas are more commonly heterogeneous and typically show some enhancement after administration of contrast agent. Duplicated pituitary glands can have a precontrast appearance similar to that of a pedunculated small hypothalamic hamartoma, but postcontrast imaging should show avid enhancement of the pituitary tissue.

Diagnosis

Hypothalamic hamartoma

Suggested Readings

Boyko OB, Curnes JT, Oakes WJ, Burger PC: Hamartomas of the tuber cinereum: CT, MR, and pathologic findings. AJNR Am J Neuroradiol 12:309-314, 1991.

Freeman JL, Coleman LT, Wellard RM, et al: MR imaging and spectroscopic study of epileptogenic hypothalamic hamartomas: Analysis of 72 cases. AJNR Am J Neuroradiol 25:450-462, 2004.

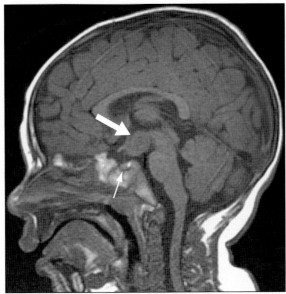

Figure 1. Sagittal T1-weighted MR image shows mass (*large arrow*) isointense to gray matter that is posterior to optic chiasm and anterior to midbrain. The pituitary (*small arrow*) has a normal appearance.

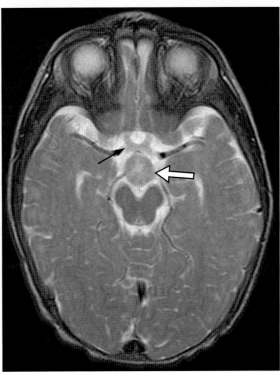

Figure 2. Axial T2-weighted MR image better delineates slightly hyperintense mass (*white arrow*) as separate from optic chiasm (*black arrow*).

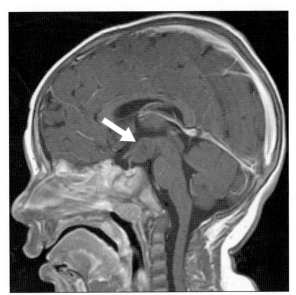

Figure 3. Mass (*arrow*) does not enhance on postcontrast sagittal T1-weighted MRI.

Case 308

DEMOGRAPHICS/CLINICAL HISTORY

The patient is a 22-month-old girl with abnormal gait.

FINDINGS

Magnetic resonance imaging (MRI) of the lumbar spine (Figs. 1 and 2) shows abnormal signal at the L3-L4 intervertebral disk that extends to involve the superior aspect of L4 and the inferior aspect of L3. There is associated narrowing of the intervertebral disk space and posterior protrusion into the spinal canal (see Fig. 2). An anterior projection image from a radiolabeled bone scan (Fig. 3) shows increased radiotracer uptake at the L3-L4 level.

DISCUSSION

Definition/Background

Diskitis is infection of an intervertebral disk space that tends to be caused by hematogenous spread. Diskitis typically occurs in children 4 to 10 years old.

Characteristic Clinical Features

Patients present with back pain and lack of mobility. Affected children are usually afebrile.

Characteristic Radiologic Findings

Early on, plain radiographs are normal, with changes developing later in the course of infection, including disk space narrowing and irregularity of the vertebral end plates. MRI shows decreased signal on T1-weighted images and increased signal on fluid sensitive sequences within the intervertebral disk space, which may be abnormally narrow. Surrounding enhancement may be seen. Adjacent osteomyelitis or abscess may be present.

Differential Diagnosis

- Vertebral osteomyelitis
- Tuberculous spondylitis

Discussion

Vertebral osteomyelitis is an infection of the vertebral body, usually by *Staphylococcus aureus*, that is more common in older patients with diabetes as a risk factor. Tuberculous spondylitis is an infection of the spine caused by *Mycobacterium tuberculosis*. Tuberculosis may involve the vertebral bodies more than the disk, but often biopsy and serology are necessary.

Diagnosis

Diskitis

Suggested Readings

Brown R, Hussain M, McHugh K, et al: Discitis in young children. J Bone Joint Surg Br 83:106-111, 2001.

Kocher MS, Lee B, Dolan M, et al: Pediatric orthopedic infections: Early detection and treatment. Pediatr Ann 35:112-122, 2006.

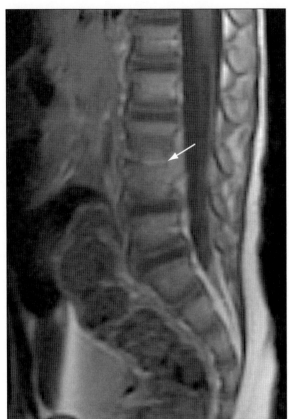

Figure 1. Sagittal T1-weighted MR image of the lumbar spine shows abnormal decreased signal at L3-L4 intervertebral disk that extends to involve superior aspect of L4 and inferior aspect of L3. There is associated narrowing of intervertebral disk space and posterior protrusion into spinal canal (*arrow*).

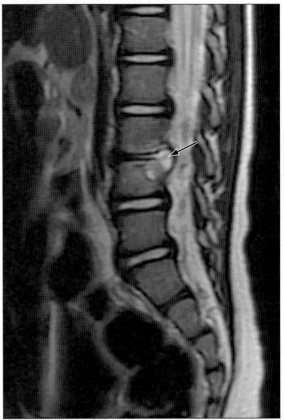

Figure 2. Sagittal T2-weighted MR image of the lumbar spine shows abnormal signal at L3-L4 intervertebral disk that extends to involve superior aspect of L4 and inferior aspect of L3. There is associated narrowing of intervertebral disk space and posterior protrusion into spinal canal (*arrow*).

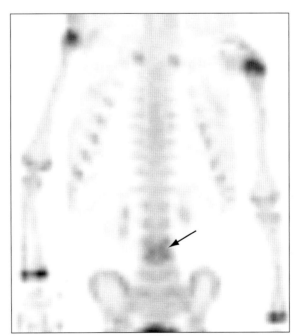

Figure 3. Anterior projection image from radiolabeled bone scan shows increased radiotracer uptake at L3-L4 level (*arrow*).

Case 309

DEMOGRAPHICS/CLINICAL HISTORY

The patient is a 2-year-old child with seizures and recent symptoms of upper respiratory infection.

FINDINGS

Axial fluid attenuated inversion recovery (FLAIR) magnetic resonance imaging (MRI) through the posterior fossa (Fig. 1) shows an abnormal increased signal within the middle cerebellar peduncles. Axial FLAIR MRI (Fig. 2) shows increased signal intensity in the subcortical and deep white matter, the thalami, the left genu and splenium of the corpus callosum, and the posterior limb of the right internal capsule.

DISCUSSION

Definition/Background

Acute disseminated encephalomyelitis (ADEM) typically affects children and adolescents. Patients often have a history of recent viral infection or immunization.

Characteristic Clinical Features

Clinical presentations include headaches, vomiting, fever, and more significant neurologic signs such as seizures or coma.

Characteristic Radiologic Findings

On computed tomography (CT), hypodense areas often can be seen in involved areas. MRI is the most sensitive modality for localizing lesions, typically demonstrating many ill-defined, hyperintense areas on T2-weighted and FLAIR images. Lesions often are located in white and gray matter. Lesions in the basal ganglia and thalami are often symmetric, whereas white matter lesions are often asymmetric. The posterior fossa often is involved. Contrast enhancement varies, and lack of enhancement is common. Diffusion-weighted imaging may show restricted diffusion in the acute phase, but this does not necessarily reflect permanent damage. Concomitant spinal lesions are seen in many patients. Follow-up imaging usually shows near-complete resolution of signal abnormalities, and minimal residual gliosis can be seen.

Less Common Radiologic Manifestations

Involvement of the cord usually affects smaller segments, but involvement of the entire cord has been described.

Differential Diagnosis

- Multiple sclerosis

Discussion

Multiple sclerosis is the primary differential diagnosis. Although findings can be similar, the predominance of periventricular lesions, absence of gray matter lesions, and radial involvement of the corpus callosum suggest multiple sclerosis. Follow-up imaging and clinical follow-up usually distinguish the two because multiple sclerosis is a chronic condition, and acute disseminated encephalomyelitis typically occurs as a single episode.

Diagnosis

Acute disseminated encephalomyelitis (ADEM)

Suggested Readings

Rossi A: Imaging of acute disseminated encephalomyelitis. Neuroimaging Clin N Am 18:149-161, 2008.

Tenembaum S, Chitnis T, Ness J, Hahn JS: International Pediatric MS Study Group: Acute disseminated encephalomyelitis. Neurology 68(Suppl 2):S23-S36, 2007.

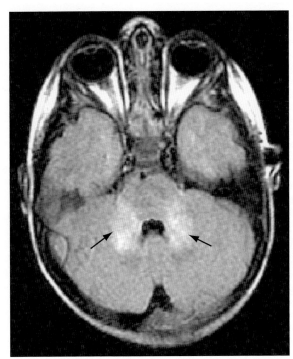

Figure 1. Axial FLAIR MR image through posterior fossa shows abnormal increased signal within middle cerebellar peduncles (*arrows*).

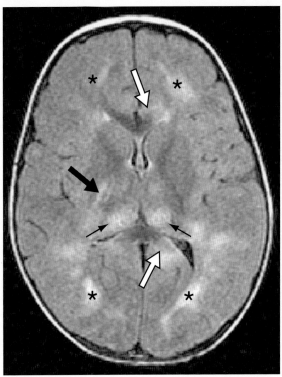

Figure 2. Axial FLAIR MR image shows increased signal in subcortical and deep white matter (*asterisks*), thalami (*small black arrows*), left genu and splenium of the corpus callosum (*white arrows*), and posterior limb of right internal capsule (*large black arrow*).

Case 310

DEMOGRAPHICS/CLINICAL HISTORY

The patient is a 34-week gestational age newborn with microcephaly.

FINDINGS

Coronal transcranial ultrasound through the anterior fontanelle (Fig. 1) shows ventriculomegaly and multiple echogenic foci along the ventricles and within the basal ganglia. A non–contrast-enhanced axial computed tomography (CT) scan at the level of the third ventricle (Fig. 2) shows multiple periventricular calcifications. Parenchymal and periventricular calcifications are seen at a more cranial level of the non–contrast-enhanced CT scan (Fig. 3). T2-weighted fluid attenuated inversion recovery (FLAIR) magnetic resonance imaging (MRI) obtained at 14 months of age (Fig. 4) shows thickened nodular gray matter representing polymicrogyria and abnormal hyperintensity within the visualized white matter. The patient was diagnosed after birth with congenital cytomegalovirus (CMV) infection.

DISCUSSION

Definition/Background
TORCH is an acronym referring to specific perinatal infections (*t*oxoplasmosis, *o*ther [e.g., syphilis, human immunodeficiency virus], *r*ubella, *c*ytomegalovirus, and *h*erpes). These infections can have skeletal and central nervous system (CNS) manifestations.

Characteristic Clinical Features
Fever and poor feeding can be early clinical manifestations of TORCH infections. Seizures can be present in patients with CNS manifestations.

Characteristic Radiologic Findings
Radiographic manifestations vary depending on which infection is present. Intraparenchymal and periventricular calcifications are classic CNS manifestations and can be the initial finding to suggest a TORCH infection. Hydrocephalus and cortical malformations (particularly polymicrogyria secondary to CMV) are other CNS manifestations. Skeletal changes in rubella and CMV infection include metaphyseal striations ("celery stalk" appearance). Delayed ossification of the knee epiphyses has been associated with congenital rubella.

Differential Diagnosis
■ Aicardi-Goutières syndrome

Discussion
Aicardi-Goutières syndrome is an early-onset encephalopathy caused by genetic mutations and can have similar CNS manifestations as TORCH infections, with negative serology.

Diagnosis
TORCH infection (cytomegalovirus)

Suggested Readings
Altman NR: Intracranial infection in children. Top Magn Reson Imaging 5:143, 1993.
Baskin HJ, Hedlund G: Neuroimaging of herpesvirus infections in children. Pediatr Radiol 37:949, 2007.
Hedlund GL, Boyer RS: Neuroimaging of postnatal pediatric central nervous system infections. Semin Pediatr Neurol 6:299, 1999.

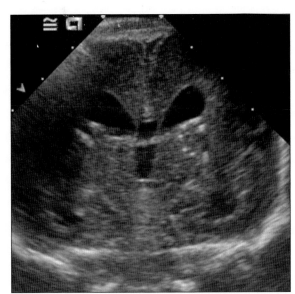

Figure 1. Coronal transcranial ultrasound through anterior fontanelle shows ventriculomegaly and multiple echogenic foci along ventricles and within basal ganglia.

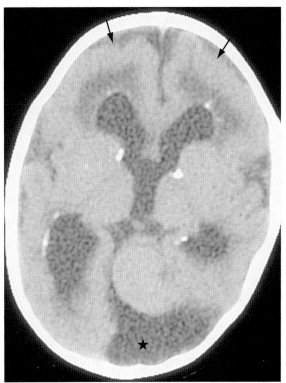

Figure 2. Non–contrast-enhanced axial CT scan at level of third ventricle shows multiple periventricular calcifications. There is abnormal configuration of frontal gray matter (*arrows*) and ventriculomegaly. Large posterior fossa cyst (*star*) and cerebellar hypoplasia (not shown) are also present.

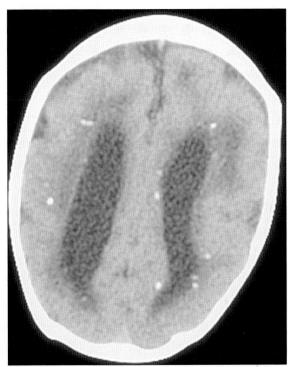

Figure 3. Non–contrast-enhanced axial CT scan at more cranial level shows parenchymal and periventricular calcifications.

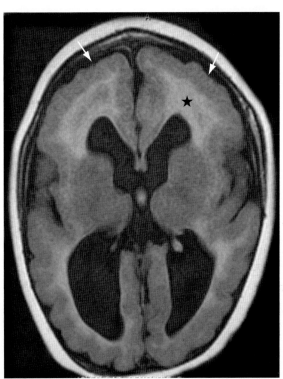

Figure 4. T2-weighted FLAIR MR image at 14 months of age shows thickened nodular gray matter representing polymicrogyria (*arrows*) and abnormal hyperintensity within visualized white matter (*star*).

Case 311

DEMOGRAPHICS/CLINICAL HISTORY

The patient is a 3-year-old child with a possible right cholesteatoma.

FINDINGS

Axial computed tomography (CT) scan through the temporal bones (Fig. 1) shows a soft tissue mass within the medial aspect of the right anterior epitympanum medial to the neck of the malleus. Axial CT scan of the normal contralateral side (Fig. 2) shows the normal aeration of this region. Coronal reformatted CT scan (Fig. 3) shows the soft tissue lies under the anterior tegmen tympani without dehiscence. Coronal reformatted CT scan (Fig. 4) through the intact scutum also identifies normal aeration of Prussak space and intact ossicles.

DISCUSSION

Definition/Background
Cholesteatomas are collections of keratin within an epithelial sac. They are typically acquired and less often congenital.

Characteristic Clinical Features
Patients often have a whitish mass behind the tympanic membrane that is found on otoscopic examination.

Characteristic Radiologic Findings
CT is the primary imaging modality for evaluation of the osseous temporal bone and for the diagnosis of cholesteatoma. Acquired cholesteatomas often manifest as a soft tissue mass centered in Prussak space. Erosion of the scutum, tegmen tympani, and ossicles is commonly

seen in progressive disease. Cholesteatomas can become superinfected and cause intracranial complications, such as meningitis. Congenital cholesteatomas are less common and can occur in several locations, including the middle ear, external auditory canal, mastoid, squamous portion of the temporal bone, and the petrous apex. Intact tympanic membrane without a history of otitis media suggests a congenital cause.

Less Common Radiologic Manifestations
If erosion into the lateral semicircular canal occurs, a fistula can form.

Differential Diagnosis
- Thickening of the tympanic membrane
- Persistent stapedial artery
- Temporal bone and middle ear tumors

Discussion
Chronic infections can cause thickening of the tympanic membrane, but they usually do not have a masslike appearance and do not cause erosion of the ossicles or scutum. The course of a persistent stapedial artery can be followed, and the absence of the foramen spinosum suggests the diagnosis. Tumors within the temporal bone and middle ear are rare in children; they may be suggested by clinical history and presentation.

Diagnosis
Cholesteatoma

Suggested Readings
El-Bitar MA, Choi SS, Emamian SA, Vezina LG: Congenital middle ear cholesteatoma: Need for early recognition—role of computed tomography scan. Int J Pediatr Otorhinolaryngol 67:231-235, 2003.
Phelps PD, Wright A: Imaging cholesteatoma. Clin Radiol 41:156-162, 1990.

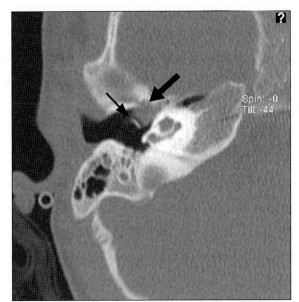

Figure 1. Axial CT image through the temporal bones shows soft tissue mass within medial aspect of right anterior epitympanum (*large arrow*) that is medial to neck of malleus (*small arrow*).

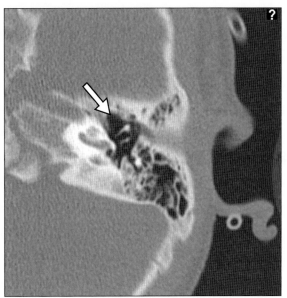

Figure 2. Axial CT image of normal contralateral side shows normal aerated appearance of this region (*arrow*).

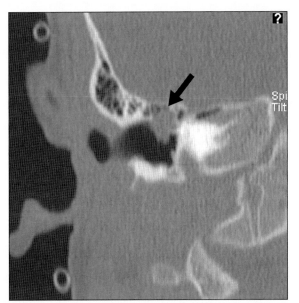

Figure 3. Coronal reformatted CT image shows soft tissue mass lies under anterior tegmen tympani (*arrow*) without dehiscence.

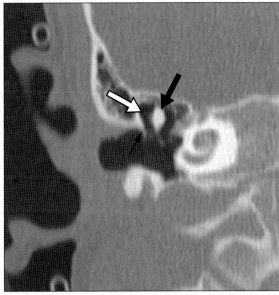

Figure 4. Coronal reformatted CT image through intact scutum (*small arrow*) identifies normal aeration of Prussak space (*white arrow*) and intact ossicles (*large arrow*).

Case 312

DEMOGRAPHICS/CLINICAL HISTORY

The patient is a 2-year-old girl receiving antibiotics for otitis media who presented with otalgia.

FINDINGS

Axial fluid attenuated inversion recovery (FLAIR) magnetic resonance imaging (MRI) (Fig. 1) shows abnormal collections adjacent to and within the left mastoid air cells. Contrast-enhanced, axial T1-weighted MRI (Fig. 2) shows rim enhancement around the subperiosteal collection, within the infected mastoid cells, and surrounding the epidural abscess. Contrast-enhanced coronal T1-weighted MRI (Fig. 3) shows the intracranial extension and the extracranial subperiosteal collection. Diffusion-weighted MRI (Fig. 4) shows restricted diffusion within the epidural abscess, mastoid air cells, and subperiosteal abscess.

DISCUSSION

Definition/Background

Epidural abscesses often result from direct extension from sinusitis, instrumentation, or meningitis.

Characteristic Clinical Features

Patients with epidural abscesses can present with persistent fevers, headaches, and seizures.

Characteristic Radiologic Findings

Computed tomography (CT) can show rim enhancement around a low density lentiform collection. MRI shows hypointensity on T1-weighted images, hyperintensity on T2-weighted images, rim enhancement on postcontrast images, and restricted diffusion on diffusion-weighted images. Adjacent dural enhancement is typically seen. If infections are adjacent to a venous sinus, thrombosis is a dangerous complication. If caused by meningitis or instrumentation, leptomeningeal and ventricular enhancement and intraparenchymal abscesses can be seen.

Differential Diagnosis
- Epidural hematoma

Discussion

Epidural hematomas follow the density (on CT) and signal (on MRI) characteristics of blood products. Fractures typically are seen adjacent to epidural hematomas, and the clinical history can help to differentiate the two.

Diagnosis

Epidural abscess from mastoiditis

Suggested Readings

Germiller JA, Monin DL, Sparano AM, Tom LW: Intracranial complications of sinusitis in children and adolescents and their outcomes. Arch Otolaryngol Head Neck Surg 132:969-976, 2006.

Tsai YD, Chang WN, Shen CC, et al: Intracranial suppuration: A clinical comparison of subdural empyemas and epidural abscesses. Surg Neurol 59:191-196, 2003.

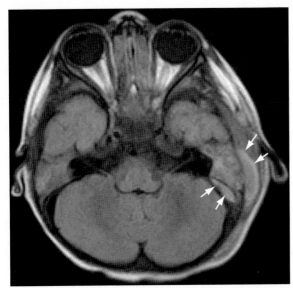

Figure 1. Axial FLAIR MR image shows abnormal collections adjacent to and within left mastoid air cells (*arrows*).

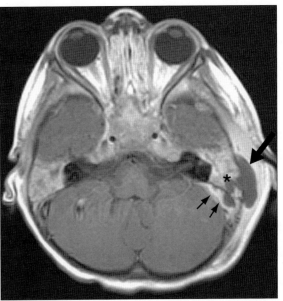

Figure 2. Postcontrast axial T1-weighted MR image shows rim enhancement around subperiosteal collection (*large arrow*), within infected mastoid cells (*asterisk*), and surrounding epidural abscess (*small arrows*). No adjacent venous sinus thrombosis was seen (*not shown*).

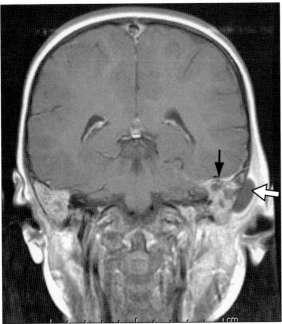

Figure 3. Postcontrast coronal T1-weighted MR image shows intracranial extension (*black arrow*) and extracranial subperiosteal collection (*white arrow*).

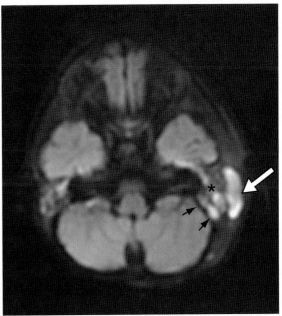

Figure 4. Diffusion-weighted MR image shows restricted diffusion within epidural abscess (*black arrows*), mastoid air cells (*asterisk*), and subperiosteal abscess (*white arrow*).

Case 313

DEMOGRAPHICS/CLINICAL HISTORY

The patient is a 2-week-old infant with a skull fracture.

FINDINGS

A frontal radiograph of the skull (Fig. 1) shows a thin elevation of bone along the right parietal bone. Axial computed tomography (CT) scan through soft tissue windows (Fig. 2) shows the thin shell of calcification, representing the elevated periosteum. Axial CT scan through bone windows (Fig. 3) shows the thin shell of calcification and a fracture line.

DISCUSSION

Definition/Background

Cephalhematomas (also known as cephalohematomas) are caused by a subperiosteal hematoma and are most common along the parietal or occipital bones.

Characteristic Clinical Features

Most cephalhematomas are detected at birth or within the first few weeks of life. A focal area of swelling is detected, and the shell of bone can be felt as the cephalhematoma resorbs. Resorption can take 2 months, and residual thickening of the calvaria may remain.

Characteristic Radiologic Findings

The early imaging appearance shows a focal hematoma, which is limited by the presence of the periosteal attachments at the sutures. As the cephalhematoma evolves, the shell of periosteum surrounding the hematoma matures and thickens. The hematoma slowly resorbs, and the outer table can remain thickened after resorption. Cephalhematomas are sometimes associated with skull fractures.

Less Common Radiologic Manifestations

Occasionally, a small cystic pocket between the mature periosteum and the outer table can remain after the hematoma resorbs. Early cephalhematomas can become superinfected, as reflected by clinical and radiologic signs of inflammation. If a craniosynostosis is present, cephalhematomas can cross the fused suture.

Differential Diagnosis

- Subgaleal and subcutaneous collections

Discussion

Subgaleal and subcutaneous collections can clinically simulate cephalhematomas. Imaging findings suggest the alternate spatial locations.

Diagnosis

Cephalhematoma cephalohematoma

Suggested Readings

Gupta PK, Mathew GS, Malik AK, Al Derazi T: Ossified cephalhematoma. Pediatr Neurosurg 43:492-497, 2007.

Wong CH, Foo CL, Seow WT: Calcified cephalohematoma: Classification, indications for surgery and techniques. J Craniofac Surg 17:970-979, 2006.

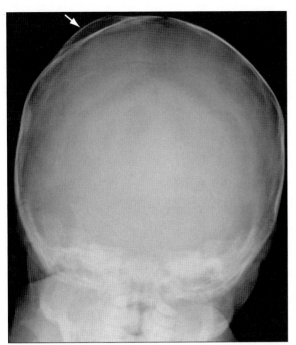

Figure 1. Frontal radiograph of skull shows cephalhematoma (*arrow*) along right parietal bone.

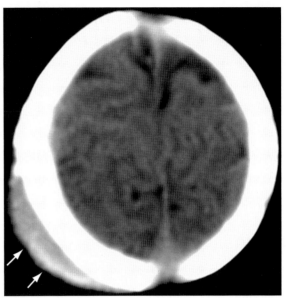

Figure 2. Axial CT image through soft tissue windows shows thin shell of calcification (*arrow*), representing elevated periosteum.

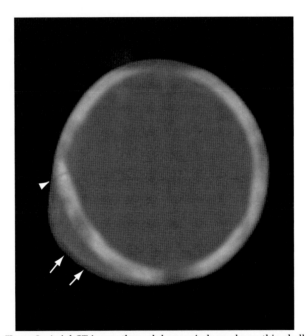

Figure 3. Axial CT image through bone windows shows thin shell of calcification (*arrows*) and fracture line (*arrowhead*).

Case 314

DEMOGRAPHICS/CLINICAL HISTORY

The patient is an 18-year-old male with facial swelling and nasal discharge.

FINDINGS

Near-complete opacification of the left maxillary sinus is seen on an axial contrast-enhanced computed tomography (CT) scan of the sinuses (Fig. 1). An air-fluid level is seen within the left frontal sinus on a more cranial CT image (Fig. 2). Inflammatory changes are seen in the subcutaneous tissues anterior to the frontal bone. A CT image further cranially (Fig. 3) shows a small midline periosteal fluid collection anterior to the frontal bone, which contains a few scattered foci of air.

DISCUSSION

Definition/Background

Osteomyelitis of the frontal bone (also known as Pott's puffy tumor) is a complication of sinusitis, along with intracranial infection and abscess formation.

Characteristic Clinical Features

When osteomyelitis of the frontal bone occurs as a direct complication of sinusitis, periosteal collections and extension into the subcutaneous tissues can cause redness, swelling, and tenderness over the frontal region. Patients typically have fever.

Characteristic Radiologic Findings

Extensive sinusitis is typically present and is usually visualized on CT or magnetic resonance imaging (MRI). Although osseous destruction of the frontal bone is an obvious sign of osteomyelitis, earlier signs include periosteal collections and extension of the sinus infection intracranially or into the subcutaneous soft tissues. If MRI is used, abnormal signal intensities in the frontal region and restricted diffusion within infected collections can be seen.

Diagnosis

Osteomyelitis of the frontal bone

Suggested Readings

Betz CS, Issing W, Matschke J, et al: Complications of acute frontal sinusitis: A retrospective study. Eur Arch Otorhinolaryngol 265:63-72, 2008.

Prasad KC, Prasad SC, Mouli N, Agarwal S: Osteomyelitis in the head and neck. Acta Otolaryngol 127:194-205, 2007.

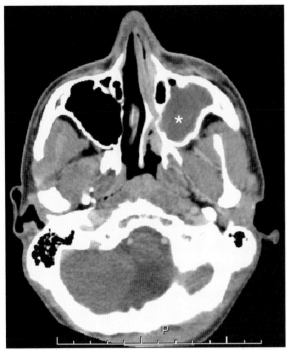

Figure 1. Axial contrast-enhanced CT scan of sinuses shows near-complete opacification of left maxillary sinus (*asterisk*).

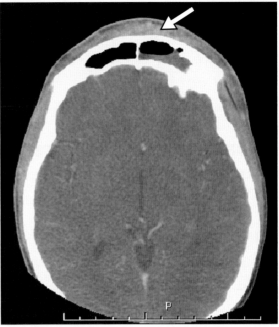

Figure 2. More cranial CT image shows air-fluid level within left frontal sinus. Inflammatory changes are seen in subcutaneous tissues anterior to frontal bone (*arrow*).

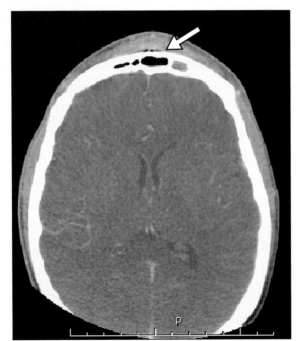

Figure 3. CT image further cranially shows small midline periosteal fluid collection anterior to frontal bone (*arrow*), which contains a few scattered foci of air.

Case 315

DEMOGRAPHICS/CLINICAL HISTORY

The patient is an 11-year-old child with lethargy, aphasia, and weakness.

FINDINGS

Axial computed tomography (CT) (Fig. 1) shows opacification of the left ethmoid air cells. A subdural-epidural low density collection can be seen adjacent to the falx on axial CT (Fig. 2). T2-weighted magnetic resonance imaging (MRI) (Fig. 3) shows complete opacification of the left maxillary sinus. Postcontrast coronal T1-weighted MRI (Fig. 4) shows a rim-enhancing collection along the falx, representing an abscess.

DISCUSSION

Definition/Background

Imaging of patients with sinusitis is done to determine whether there are complications, such as meningitis or abscess formation.

Characteristic Clinical Features

Sinusitis is often characterized by nasal drainage and sinus tenderness. Patients often have fever and an elevated white blood cell count.

Characteristic Radiologic Findings

CT and MRI show sinus opacification, air-fluid levels, and a bubbly appearance of the fluid within the affected sinuses. Intracranial extension of the infection can be seen as enhancement of the dura, meninges, subdural empyemas, epidural abscesses, venous thrombosis, and intracranial abscesses. Extracranial complications include cellulitis (particularly periorbital) and abscess formation.

Differential Diagnosis

- Juvenile nasopharyngeal angiofibroma (pediatric sinuses)
- Rhabdomyosarcoma (pediatric)
- Nasal polyps

Discussion

Juvenile nasopharyngeal angiofibroma, rhabdomyosarcoma, and nasal polyps appear as soft tissue masses, with enhancement, mass effect, and noninfectious history.

Diagnosis

Sinusitis with abscess formation

Suggested Readings

Eustis HS, Mafee MF, Walton C, Mondonca J: MR imaging and CT of orbital infections and complications in acute rhinosinusitis. Radiol Clin North Am 36:1165-1183, 1998.

Reid JR: Complications of pediatric paranasal sinusitis. Pediatr Radiol 34:933-942, 2004.

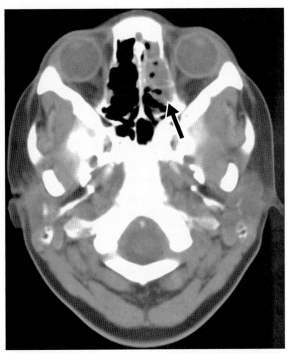

Figure 1. Axial CT image shows opacification of left ethmoid air cells (*arrow*).

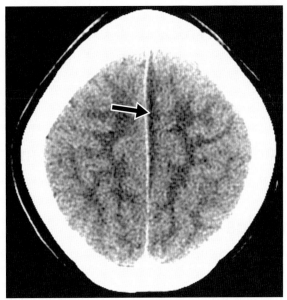

Figure 2. Axial CT image shows extra-axial low density collection adjacent to falx (*arrow*).

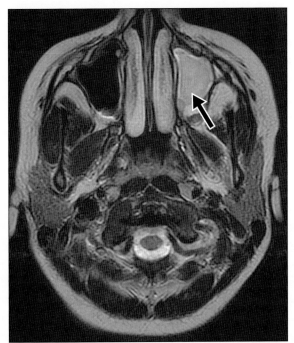

Figure 3. T2-weighted MR image shows complete opacification of left maxillary sinus (*arrow*).

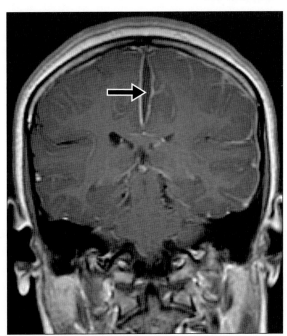

Figure 4. Postcontrast coronal T1-weighted MR image shows rim-enhancing collection along falx (*arrow*), representing abscess.

Case 316

DEMOGRAPHICS/CLINICAL HISTORY

The patient is a 12-week-old infant with a sacral dimple.

FINDINGS

Sagittal T1-weighted magnetic resonance imaging (MRI) of the spine (Fig. 1) shows a low-lying conus and tethered cord terminating in a large T1 hyperintense mass, representing a lipoma. Sagittal T2-weighted MRI (Fig. 2) shows a syrinx, low-lying conus, and dermal sinus. The large lipoma is well seen on axial T1-weighted MRI (Fig. 3), and the syrinx is seen within the distal cord on axial T2-weighted MRI (Fig. 4).

DISCUSSION

Definition/Background

Intradural lipomas are typically located in the terminal aspect of the cord and often cause tethering of the cord.

Characteristic Clinical Features

Many patients with intradural lipomas have a sacral dimple, birthmark, or overlying skin abnormality.

Characteristic Radiologic Findings

An echogenic mass can be seen on prenatal or neonatal spine ultrasound, associated with a low-lying conus. MRI shows the low-lying conus better and a T1 hyperintense mass at the caudal end of the cord, typically tethering the cord to the dorsal thecal sac.

Less Common Radiologic Manifestations

Intradural lipomas can communicate with the subcutaneous fat dorsal to the spine.

Differential Diagnosis

- Lipomyelomeningocele

Discussion

Lipomyelomeningocele is a closed spinal dysraphism and has a cystic mass associated with herniated neural elements and the fatty mass.

Diagnosis

Intradural lipoma

Suggested Readings

Grimme JD, Castillo M: Congenital anomalies of the spine. Neuroimaging Clin N Am 17:1, 2007.

Rossi A, Gandolfo C, Morana G, et al: Current classification and imaging of congenital spinal abnormalities. Semin Roentgenol 41:250, 2006.

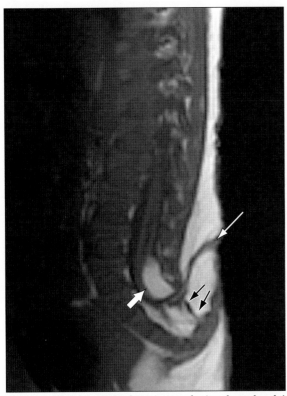

Figure 1. Sagittal T1-weighted MR image of spine shows low-lying conus and tethered cord terminating in large T1 hyperintense mass, representing a lipoma (*large arrow*). Low signal intensity extending from filum to dorsal cutaneous surface suggests dermal sinus tract (*small white arrow*). Sacral osseous abnormalities are also seen (*small black arrows*).

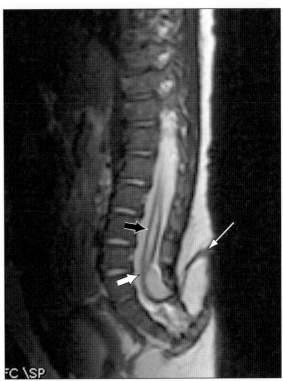

Figure 2. Sagittal T2-weighted MR image shows syrinx (*black arrow*) and low-lying conus (*large white arrow*) and dermal sinus tract (*small white arrow*).

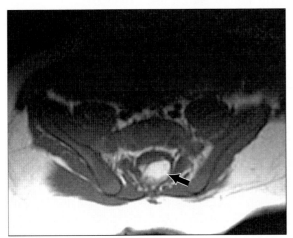

Figure 3. Axial T1-weighted MR image shows large lipoma (*arrow*).

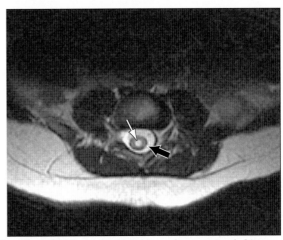

Figure 4. Axial T2-weighted MR image shows syrinx (*white arrow*) within distal cord (*black arrow*).

Case 317

DEMOGRAPHICS/CLINICAL HISTORY

A patient with abnormal findings on prenatal ultrasound, undergoing magnetic resonance imaging (MRI).

FINDINGS

Prenatal ultrasound (Fig. 1) shows a cystic mass at the base of the spine, superficial to the lumbosacral spine. A sagittal T1-weighted MR image of the spine (Fig. 2) shows the postnatal lumbosacral spine to be dysraphic with neural elements, the cystic mass, and no evidence of intradural fat. A sagittal T2-weighted MR image of the spine (Fig. 3) shows the low-lying hydromyelic cord, in continuity with a large cystic collection and neural elements. A sagittal T1-weighted MR image of the brain shows normal position of the cerebellar tonsils, and no significant abnormality.

DISCUSSION

Definition/Background

Terminal myelocystoceles occur at the lumbosacral region and are skin-covered cystic masses secondary to posterior spinal defects, herniated neural elements, and extension of the hydromyelic cord into a large terminal cyst.

Characteristic Clinical Features

Terminal myelocystoceles can be found prenatally or after birth with the presence of a skin-covered mass around the lumbosacral region. These lesions are often associated with cloacal exstrophy.

Characteristic Radiologic Findings

Imaging shows low-lying cord (typically L5-S1), posterior spinal fusion abnormalities, meningocele, involvement of the neural elements within the meningocele, and hydromyelia of the distal cord into a large cystic collection.

Less Common Radiologic Manifestations

Myelocystoceles can also occur in nonterminal (cervical and thoracic) locations. Other central nervous system abnormalities, such as Chiari malformations, can be seen.

Differential Diagnosis

- Meningocele
- Myelomeningocele
- Lipomyelomeningocele

Discussion

There are other covered spinal dysraphic defects with cystic masses containing cerebrospinal fluid with or without neural elements; however, a terminal myelocystocele also contains an ependymal and dysplastic glial-lined cystic collection (thought to be derived from severe cystic dilation of the terminal ventricle).

Diagnosis

Terminal myelocystocele

Suggested Readings

Byrd SE, Harvey C, Darling CF: MR of terminal myelocystoceles. Eur J Radiol 20:215, 1995.
Muthukumar N: Terminal and nonterminal myelocystoceles. J Neurosurg 107(2 Suppl):87, 2007.

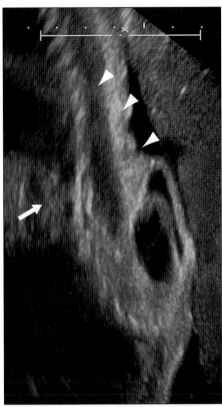

Figure 1. Prenatal ultrasound shows cystic mass (*arrow*) at base of spine, superficial to lumbosacral spine (*arrowheads*).

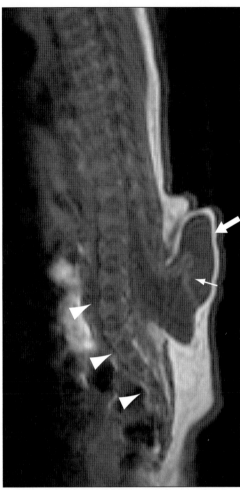

Figure 2. Sagittal T1-weighted MR image of spine shows postnatal lumbosacral spine (*arrowheads*) to be dysraphic with neural elements (*thin arrow*), cystic mass (*thick arrow*), and no evidence of intradural fat.

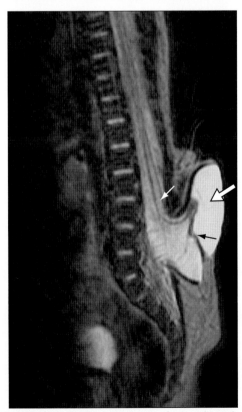

Figure 3. Sagittal T2-weighted MR image of spine shows low-lying hydromyelic cord (*thin white arrow*), in continuity with large cystic collection (*thick white arrow*) and neural elements (*black arrow*).

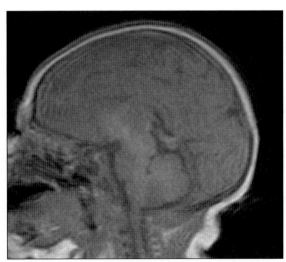

Figure 4. Sagittal T1-weighted MR image of brain shows normal position of cerebellar tonsils and no significant abnormality.

Case 318

DEMOGRAPHICS/CLINICAL HISTORY

The patient is a 1-year-old infant with a history of a frontal ridge on physical examination.

FINDINGS

An axial computed tomography (CT) scan (Fig. 1) shows a triangular configuration of the frontal bone. Coronal reconstruction (Fig. 2) shows the prominent ridge. Three-dimensional reconstruction (Fig. 3) allows better visualization of the triangular appearance of the frontal bone.

DISCUSSION

Definition/Background
Trigonocephaly is due to premature fusion of the metopic suture, which normally closes between 6 and 8 months, and sometimes by 3 months.

Characteristic Clinical Features
A frontal ridge and triangular-shaped forehead are often the presenting clinical features. In more prominent cases, hypotelorism can be seen.

Characteristic Radiologic Findings
Radiographic findings include nonvisualization or premature closure of the metopic suture and triangular configuration of the frontal bone. A "metopic notch" along the endocranial vault has been described in cases of metopic synostosis.

Diagnosis
Trigonocephaly

Suggested Readings

Schwartz RH: Congenital metopic craniosynostosis with secondary trigonocephaly: A case report. Clin Pediatr (Phila) 45:365, 2006.

Weinzweig J, Kirschner RE, Farley A, et al: Metopic synostosis: Defining the temporal sequence of normal suture fusion and differentiating it from synostosis on the basis of computed tomography images. Plast Reconstr Surg 112:1211, 2003.

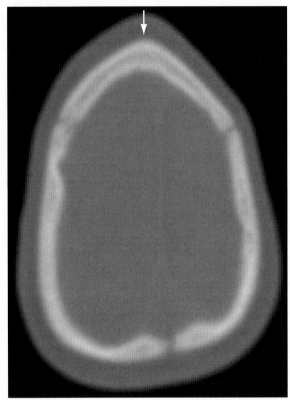

Figure 1. Axial CT scan shows triangular configuration of frontal bone (*arrow*).

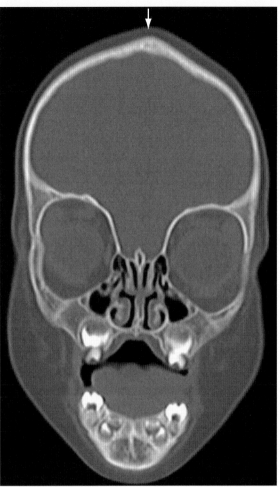

Figure 2. Coronal reconstruction shows prominent ridge (*arrow*).

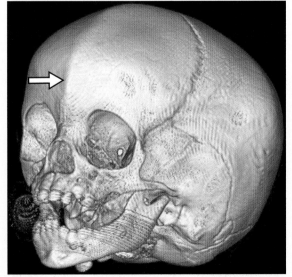

Figure 3. Three-dimensional reconstruction allows better visualization of triangular appearance of frontal bone (*arrow*).

Case 319

DEMOGRAPHICS/CLINICAL HISTORY

The patient is a 7-year-old Asian boy with occasional right-sided weakness.

FINDINGS

Axial postcontrast T1-weighted magnetic resonance imaging (MRI) (Fig. 1) shows narrowing of the middle cerebral arteries and multiple tiny collateral vessels ("moyamoya vessels"). Axial fluid attenuated inversion recovery (FLAIR) MRI (Fig. 2) shows a round hypointense area within the frontal white matter with minimal surrounding hyperintensity, likely representing a focal area of chronic ischemic injury and surrounding gliosis. Increased tiny parenchymal perforators are seen. In an older patient, axial FLAIR MRI (Fig. 3) shows high signal along leptomeningeal vessels ("ivy sign") and areas of gliosis secondary to chronic ischemia. Magnetic resonance angiography (MRA) (Fig. 4) in the same patient as in Fig. 3 shows the absence of the middle cerebral arteries, with multiple tiny collateral vessels.

DISCUSSION

Definition/Background

Moyamoya disease is an idiopathic vasoocclusive disease that causes progressive stenosis of the cerebral arteries (typically middle cerebral arteries), formation of collateral vessel formation, and strokes. Moyamoya syndrome is the constellation of findings seen in moyamoya disease; however, an underlying vasculopathic etiology is known, such as in sickle cell disease, Down syndrome, and neurofibromatosis (particularly postradiation neurofibromatosis).

Characteristic Clinical Features

Patients can present with strokes or transient ischemic symptoms.

Characteristic Radiologic Findings

Evidence of stenosis of the distal internal carotid arteries (and particularly the middle cerebral arteries), increased tiny parenchymal perforating vessels, leptomeningeal collaterals from the posterior cerebral arteries, and transdural collaterals from the external carotid arteries can be seen. Leptomeningeal enhancement and FLAIR high signal ("ivy sign") can also be seen. The "puff of smoke" sign seen on angiography is secondary to multiple tiny collateral vessels filling.

Less Common Radiologic Manifestations

Hemorrhage can rarely be seen in patients with moyamoya disease.

Differential Diagnosis

- Stroke from other causes (e.g., thromboembolic, MELAS, acute ischemia)

Discussion

Moyamoya disease or moyamoya syndrome has evidence of chronic ischemia with collateral formation and multiple tiny perforating vessels and stenosis of the distal internal carotid arteries, whereas the other entities typically do not have these findings.

Diagnosis

Moyamoya syndrome

Suggested Readings

Pereira PL, Farnsworth CT, Duda SH, et al: Pediatric moyamoya syndrome: Follow-up study with MR angiography. AJR Am J Roentgenol 167:526-528, 1996.

Yoon HK, Shin HJ, Chang YW: "Ivy sign" in childhood moyamoya disease: Depiction on FLAIR and contrast-enhanced T1-weighted MR images. Radiology 223:384-389, 2002.

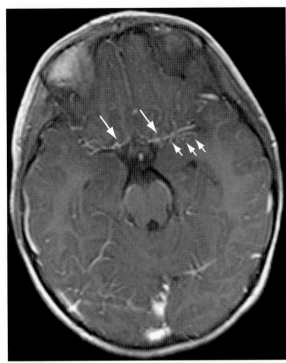

Figure 1. Axial postcontrast T1-weighted MRI shows narrowing of middle cerebral arteries (*large arrows*) and multiple tiny collateral vessels ("moyamoya vessels") (*small arrows*).

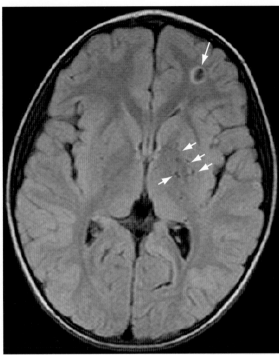

Figure 2. Axial FLAIR MRI shows round hypointense area within frontal white matter with minimal surrounding hyperintensity, likely representing a focal area of chronic ischemic injury and surrounding gliosis (*large arrow*). Increased tiny parenchymal perforators are seen (*small arrows*).

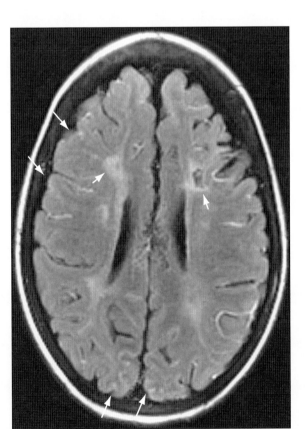

Figure 3. Axial FLAIR MRI in an older patient shows high signal along leptomeningeal vessels ("ivy sign") (*large arrows*) and areas of gliosis secondary to chronic ischemia (*small arrows*).

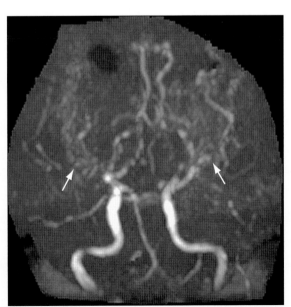

Figure 4. MRA in the same patient as in Fig. 3 shows the absence of the middle cerebral arteries, with multiple tiny collateral vessels (*arrows*).

Case 320

DEMOGRAPHICS/CLINICAL HISTORY

The patient is a 15-year-old girl status post lung transplant.

FINDINGS

Anteroposterior (Fig. 1) and lateral (Fig. 2) radiographs of the chest show a right-sided peripherally inserted central catheter (PICC) terminating in the superior vena cava (SVC). The patient is status post bilateral lung transplantation with two vertically oriented sternotomy wires and scarring and anastomotic chain suture material in the lingula from prior biopsy.

DISCUSSION

Definition/Background

A PICC is a catheter used to administer medications such as antibiotics, chemotherapy, or total parenteral nutrition. Most PICCs are placed in the upper extremity, although they may also be placed in the leg or scalp.

Characteristic Clinical Features

Patients receiving PICCs usually have need for long-term intravenous access, such as patients with osteomyelitis or perforated appendicitis or patients who are receiving chemotherapy or parenteral nutrition.

Characteristic Radiologic Findings

A PICC enters the arm via either the basilic or the brachial vein and can be identified on chest x-ray as it enters the axillary and subclavian vein on the side of placement. Ideal placement position for the tip of the catheter is the SVC to avoid complications such as infection, thrombosis, and catheter occlusion (which occur in smaller vessels) and arrhythmia and atrial rupture (which may occur when the tip is in the right atrium).

Diagnosis

Peripherally inserted central catheters (PICCs)

Suggested Readings

Connolly B, Amaral J, Walsh S, et al: Influence of arm movement on central tip location of peripherally inserted central catheters (PICCs). Pediatr Radiol 36:845-850, 2006.

Fricke BL, Racadio JM, Duckworth T, et al: Placement of peripherally inserted central catheters without fluoroscopy in children: Initial catheter tip position. Radiology 234:887-892, 2005.

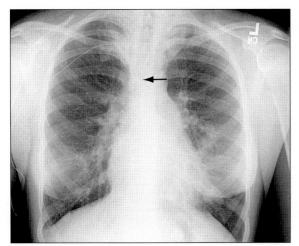

Figure 1. Anteroposterior radiograph of the chest shows right arm PICC terminating in SVC (*arrow*). Patient is status post bilateral lung transplantation with two vertically oriented sternotomy wires and scarring and anastomotic chain suture material in lingula from prior biopsy.

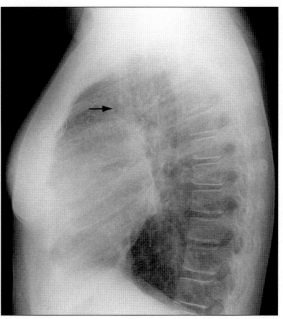

Figure 2. Lateral radiograph of the chest shows right-sided PICC terminating in SVC (*arrow*).

Index of Cases

Index

Page numbers followed by f indicate figures.